For the Health of the Enslaved

For the Health of the Enslaved

Slaves, Medicine and Power in the Danish West Indies, 1803–1848

Niklas Thode Jensen

MUSEUM TUSCULANUM PRESS
UNIVERSITY OF COPENHAGEN
2012

For the Health of the Enslaved:
Slaves, Medicine and Power in the Danish West Indies, 1803–1848

Consultants: Birgitte Holten and Michael Sterll
Copy editor: Jordy Findanis
Layout, composition and cover design: Erling Lynder
Set in Arno and printed by Tarm Bogtryk
ISBN 978 87 635 3171 9

Cover illustration: Estate Prosperity, St Croix 1838, by Frederick von Scholten
The Danish Maritime Museum.

This book is published with financial support from
Cand. Pharm. Povl M. Assens Fond
Carlsen-Langes Legatstiftelse
Danish Council for the Humanities
E. Lerager Larsens Fond
Farumgaard-Fonden
Den Hielmstierne-Rosencroneske Stiftelse
Konsul George Jorck og hustru Emma Jorck's Fond
Lademanns Fond
Landsdommer V. Gieses Legat
Lillian og Dan Finks Fond

Museum Tusculanum Press
126 Njalsgade
DK-2300 Copenhagen S
Denmark
www.mtp.dk

Contents

Chapter 4: Three Case Studies of the Health Policy of the Danish Colonial Administration 151

Preface

This book is the result of a long-standing interest in historical studies into disease and health in the colonial world. The inspiration originates from historians like David Arnold, Mark Harrison, Sharla M. Fett and others, who have shown that European medicine was used as a powerful tool for the colonisation and control of other people and countries.[1] However, the medical colonisation and control did not take place without resistance from the colonised and so opposing perceptions and traditions of disease and health emerges from the colonial situation. In this way, clashes of medical cultures can expose fundamental structures and processes in colonial societies, which can otherwise be difficult to distinguish. In this book, I have attempted to apply the perspective of colonial medical history to the Danish West Indian slave society in the period 1803–48. As will be shown, this was a society where health had a prominent position and where the tensions between the colonial masters and the colonised were extreme.

The book is an edited and translated version of my Ph.D. thesis *For Slavernes Sundhed. Sygdom, sundhed og koloniadministrationens sundhedspolitik blandt plantageslaverne på St Croix, Dansk Vestindien, 1803–1848,* submitted at the Department of History at the Saxo Institute, University of Copenhagen, Denmark, in 2006. A scholarship for the degree was graciously awarded by the Danish Council for the Humanities (FKK), and I received funds for books and other materials from the trust of Professor Ludvig Wimmer and his wife. The preliminary work on editing and translating the thesis for publication as a book was carried out as part of a postdoctoral fellowship sponsored by the Carlsberg Foundation. The FKK also sponsored the linguistic revision of the manuscript, while the publishing of the book was funded by several Danish foundations: Carlsen-Langes Legatstiftelse, Den Hielmstierne-Rosencroneske Stiftelse,

1 David Arnold, *Colonizing the Body: State Medicine and Epidemic Disease in Nineteenth-Century India* (London: University of California Press, 1993); Mark Harrison, 'The Tender Frame of Man: Disease, Climate, and Racial Difference in India and the West Indies, 1760–1860', *Bulletin of the History of Medicine* 70, no. 1 (1996); Mark Harrison, *Climates and Constitutions: Health, Race, Environment and British Imperialism in India, 1600–1850* (Oxford: Oxford University Press, 1999); Sharla M. Fett, *Working Cures: Healing, Health and Power on Southern Slave Plantations* (Chapel Hill: University of North Carolina Press, 2002).

E. Lerager Larsens Fond, Farumgaard-Fonden, Konsul George Jorck og hustru Emma Jorck's Fond, Lademanns Fond, Landsdommer V. Gieses Legat, Lillian og Dan Finks Fond and Cand. Pharm. Povl M. Assens Fond. I thank all sponsors for their generosity without which it would not have been possible to publish this book.

During my three years as a Ph.D. student at the Saxo Institute (2003 to 2006), I received a lot of help from a long list of staff and fellow students. I would like to thank them all for assisting with everything from practical to theoretical questions. Special thanks go to my supervisor, Associate Professor Ole Justesen, because he always found the time I needed for discussions at any time of day, and because he allowed me to fill his vacations with reading my texts. I would also like to thank Associate Professor Ole Hyldtoft for directing me towards important archival material, fellow Ph.D. student Maibritt Bager for expert advice on maritime biology, and Assistant Professor Michael Langkjær for linguistic advice on English translation. Finally, I owe a special thanks to the ever-changing group of Ph.D. students in the Department of History at the Saxo Institute for good teamwork, great intellectual agility, and a very social disposition.

Furthermore, a number of individuals and institutions deserve credit for their assistance. First, my thanks go to the staff at the Danish National Archive, whose knowledge and alacrity has been a great help during my work with the archival material. Particular thanks go to archivist Erik Gøbel and senior consultant Poul Olsen for expert advice on Danish West Indian matters. In addition, MA students Rikke Vindberg and Signe Trolle Gronemann graciously shared their knowledge of the Danish West Indian archives with me.

Outside Denmark, I received a lot of assistance during my research stay in Washington D.C. and in the US Virgin Islands. I would especially like to mention archivist Vernon Poul Rood and the staff at the National Archive and Records Administration, College Park, Maryland, USA, and staff in the libraries in the US Virgin Islands, the Enid Baa Library (St Thomas), the Elaine Sprauve Library (St John) and the Campus Library of the University of the Virgin Islands on St Thomas. At this point, I would also like to extend a special thanks to Dr Elisabeth Rezende who was at the time librarian at the St Croix Landmarks Society Archive and Library.

A number of Caribbean researchers are also entitled to great thanks due to their help and advice. George F. Tyson (St Croix) and his St Croix African Roots Project, whose help and kindness have been invaluable, because it made materials available that would otherwise have been inaccessible to me. Professor Emeritus Arnold Highfield (St Croix) deserves thanks for advice and for reading my manuscript. I am also grateful to Professor Emeritus Jerome Handler (Virginia Foundation for the Humanities) and Archive Director Dominique Taffin (Archives départementales de la Martinique) for letting me read parts of their unpublished manuscripts.

In addition, I owe a great thanks to my fellow Ph.D. students in the field of the Danish West Indies, Louise Sebro (University of Lund, Sweden) and Gunvor Simonsen (European University Institute, Florence, Italy) for fruitful discussions, good advice and access to valuable source material.

I would also like to express my thanks to fellow Ph.D. student and nurse Mette Rønsager (University of Copenhagen) who read and commented on everything in the thesis, and also listened to my frustrations, disappointments and victories in the academic process. Also many thanks to Curator Rikke Ilsted Kristiansen (Danish National Museum) who proof read my manuscript and imposed a meticulous discipline on the text.

I would also like to thank Professor Hans Jørn Kolmos, M.D., University of Southern Denmark, for reading and commenting on the manuscript as an expert on modern biomedicine, and Dr Juanita De Barros, Department of History at McMaster University, Canada, for reading and commenting on the manuscript as an expert on medicine in the early nineteenth-century Caribbean. My sincere thanks goes to the staff at Museum Tusculanum Press, and to the consultants Birgitte Holten and Michael Sterll and editors Trevor Curnow and Jordy Findanis, who did all they could to remove errors and turn heavy academic prose into a readable book.

Finally, I would like to thank family and friends for putting up with my mental and/or physical absence for weeks and months and for having tried to make my work easier when possible.

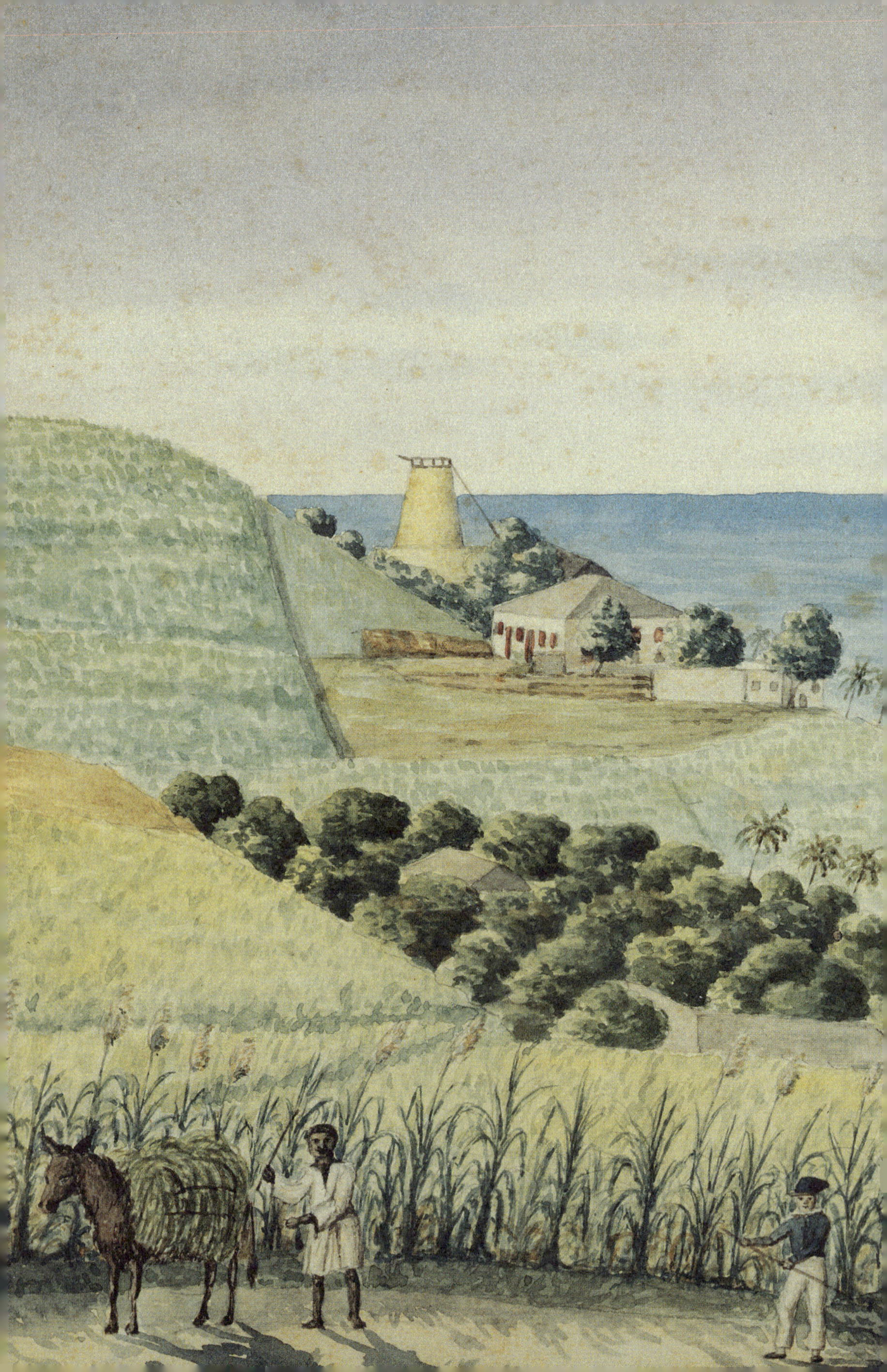

Chapter 1

Introduction

Subject and Research Questions

In the period 1803–48, safeguarding the health of enslaved workers became a central concern for the Danish West Indian plantation owners and colonial administrators. In 1803 the Danish government banned the importation of enslaved workers from Africa, but since the morbidity and mortality among the hardworking enslaved workers was high, they were not able to maintain their numbers through reproduction. This meant that the enslaved population in the Danish West Indies decreased steadily until the end of slavery in the Danish possessions in 1848. This excess mortality, with the death rate exceeding the birth rate, was a fateful problem for both the planters and the colony of the Danish West Indies as a whole because the enslaved workers were indispensable in the lucrative sugar production. Most other pre-emancipation Caribbean colonies suffered from the same problem. Consequently historical research into Caribbean slavery has investigated the reasons for the excess mortality in the enslaved populations, and how planters and colonial administrators tried to stop the demographic decline by improving the health of the enslaved. However, historical research into the Danish West Indies has not explored the health conditions of enslaved workers or the health related initiatives to promote the health of the enslaved. Accordingly, it is the aim of this book to investigate these questions for the period 1803–48.

The structure of the book follows two sets of research questions. First, a set of initial, contextual questions on how the health service was structured around the enslaved workers on the island of St Croix, which diseases the enslaved workers suffered from and what factors caused them. Second, a set of central questions focusing on what health policies the colonial administration initiated to promote the health of enslaved workers and prevent the excess mortality, and what kind of power relationships existed between the administration, the planters, and the enslaved workers in the field of health. Furthermore, embedded in both of these 'horizontal' levels of the book there is a 'vertical' comparative Caribbean perspective. It compares the health among the enslaved workers on the plantations of St Croix and the health policies of the Danish West Indian administration with the corresponding conditions and policies in the British and French West Indies.

Definitions

Following the arguments above, the chronological limits of the book are respectively the Danish ban on the import of enslaved workers from Africa in 1803 and the emancipation of the enslaved in the Danish colonies in 1848. As a geographical focus, I have chosen the island of St Croix, because this was the place in the Danish West Indies with the most plantations and the most extensive sugar production, and consequently the place with the highest number of enslaved workers. Because the sugar plantations contained the largest, the economically most important and the best documented group of enslaved workers in the Danish West Indies, I have limited the investigation to this group only. Enslaved workers on plantations producing other crops (rather unusual at the time) or living in the towns, as well as the free coloured Afro-Caribbeans, all lived under different circumstances.

The comparative Caribbean perspective has been limited to the enslaved workers on plantations in the British West Indies (1807–34) and French West Indies (1803–48).[2] The reason for this geographical focus is the limited linguistic abilities of the present author. The chronological frame for the British West Indies is set by the British ban on the slave trade in 1807 and emancipation of the enslaved in 1834. The French West Indian chronology is slightly different because slavery was banned as early as 1794, yet reinstated in 1802, the slave trade was banned in 1818 and emancipation proclaimed in 1848.

The research questions above contain a number of central concepts that require initial clarification. In the Caribbean context, the term 'slave' means a person over whom another person has full legal private ownership (chattel slavery). This means that legally the enslaved person was owned in the same way as a domestic animal or other movable property (chattels). In the period in question, the enslaved workers on St Croix were either of African or mixed

2 In this period, the British West Indies consisted of a number of colonies: Barbados, St Kitts, Nevis, Antigua, Montserrat, Virgin Islands (Tortola, Anegada, Virgin Gorda etc.), Jamaica, Dominica, St Lucia, St Vincent, Grenada, Tobago, Trinidad, British Guiana, British Honduras, Cayman Islands, Bahamas, Anguilla and Barbuda, whereas the French West Indies only consisted of the islands of Guadeloupe and Martinique (see Fig. 2.1).

African-European descent. Henceforward, free citizens on St Croix (Cruzians) of African descent will be referred to as 'Afro-Caribbeans', while free citizens of European descent will be termed 'Euro-Caribbeans'. The term 'the administration' refers to the local Danish colonial administrative system including the colonial government (headed by the Governor General), the courts and the other government bodies such as the Council of Citizens.[3] The term 'planter' is used as a collective designation for 'plantation owner' and 'plantation manager', i.e. the Euro-Caribbean individual who was in charge and had daily interaction with the enslaved workers on the plantation. The term 'health policies' refers to the various kinds of prophylactic measures initiated by the Danish colonial administration on St Croix. Finally, the central concept of 'the health of the enslaved' will be dealt with in detail as the discussion unfolds.

Methods and Structures

This book is fundamentally an empirical study. The investigation of the research questions is not governed by one overriding theoretical perspective. Instead, I apply different methods and theories as tools to handle different kinds of source material at different levels of the investigation. This approach is well suited to, and to some extent contingent on, the fact that the book deals with an interdisciplinary field. Historical studies of disease and health combine the methods and theories of history and medicine, as well as science, which means that methods from these disciplines can be employed beneficially to investigate issues in the historical materials. In this way, the choice of methods in this book has been made according to the kind of source material in question. The intention was to make different kinds of source material and approaches act as correctives to each other.[4] This may become clearer after the following presentation of the stepwise structure in answering the research questions and of the methodological and theoretical approaches related to each step.

The overall approach of the book can be characterised as structural. This means that the focus is not on single actors but on the interactions of groups (the administration, the planters, and the enslaved workers) and of the physi-

3 The Council of Citizens (*Borgerrådet*) consisted of a group of the most influential men and largest taxpayers (mainly planters) on the island of St Croix. The council operated as an advisory body to the Governor General, particularly in financial matters.

4 Joseph C. Dorsey, *Slave Traffic in the Age of Abolition: Puerto Rico, West Africa, and the Non-Hispanic Caribbean, 1815–1859* (Gainesville: University Press of Florida, 2003), 10–11.

cal environment with the health of the enslaved, and on the results of such interactions. On the first level of the book, where the focus is on the first two research questions, I use both a quantitative demographic approach to establish the framework for the demography, morbidity, and mortality of the enslaved population, and a qualitative approach to fill in this frame with descriptions of diseases, treatments, and systems. Both the quantitative and the qualitative approach are influenced by and take their departure from the existing international literature on the health of enslaved workers in the Caribbean. To a large extent, this literature has been based on demographic studies, the most influential being those of Barry W. Higman. In comparison, the qualitative approach as represented by, for instance, Richard Sheridan has a weaker presence in the literature.[5]

On the second level of the book, I go into greater detail and answer the two central research questions through three case studies of selected areas of the administration's health policy regarding enslaved workers. The case studies have been chosen to fulfil two purposes. First, to elucidate some of the elements in the complex of synergic factors surrounding the sugar plantations that caused the excess mortality among the enslaved. As will appear from Chapter 2, the workload of the enslaved has previously been the focus of attention. However, the Danish West Indian materials suggest that other factors were also important and deserve a closer investigation. Second, the aim is to elucidate different levels of the administration's health policy towards the enslaved workers. The hypothesis is that a continual struggle or negotiation for power over the health of the enslaved took place between the administration, the planters, and the enslaved workers. The first case study concerns the nutrition of the enslaved workers and covers a central area of the health of the enslaved strongly related to the surrounding environment. Inspiration for this has been drawn from the investigations of Kenneth Kiple into the nutritional state of enslaved workers in other Caribbean colonies. However, the focus on the importance of the resources in the surrounding environment follows a more recent trend in research into Caribbean slavery (see Chapter 4). The second case study deals with smallpox vaccination among the enslaved workers and so with a far narrower field. However, vaccination was the only effective prophylactic method known at the time. The third case study concerns the system of midwives and

5 Barry W. Higman, *Slave Populations of the British Caribbean, 1807–1834* (Baltimore: Johns Hopkins University Press, 1984); Richard Sheridan, *Doctors and Slaves: A Medical and Demographic History of Slavery in the British West Indies, 1680–1834* (Cambridge: Cambridge University Press, 1985).

the birth practices of the enslaved. The case therefore connects to the reproductive health of the enslaved, which was of central importance in safeguarding the size of the enslaved population because of the soaring child mortality. In all three case studies, the qualitative approach dominates, yet particularly the first case study also utilises quantitative approaches (estimates, calculations etc.).

The third step is the conclusion of the book. Here, the approach is expanded again using the recurrent comparative Caribbean perspective, which frames the results from the Danish West Indies.

Hypotheses and Theories

Power and Medicine in Colonial Perspective

As mentioned, the two central research questions of the book focus on the health policy of the Danish administration regarding enslaved workers. This is due to a number of circumstances. Previous research has shown that the health service was a field to which the Danish West Indian administration paid special attention.[6] This approach points back to the absolute Danish monarchy and state, which had been deeply involved in establishing a centralised health policy in Denmark from the middle of the eighteenth century.[7] Because safeguarding the health of the enslaved workers was made urgent by the negative demographic growth, it is interesting to look at the kind of health policies the Danish colonial administration employed – especially when viewed in a comparative Caribbean perspective.

Another interesting problem of the colonial administration's health policy relating to enslaved workers is the fact that the vast majority of slaves were private property and so not directly subject to the authority of the administration in the same way as the free citizens of the islands. This meant that the administration did not have the authority to implement a health policy, unless it assumed powers that limited the planters' rights of disposal over their slaves. On this basis, my hypothesis for the second central research question is that the administration succeeded in assuming new powers relating to the health of the enslaved, but that this happened in a continual process of negotiation or

6 Niklas Thode Jensen, *En verden til forskel? Undersøgelser af sundhedsvæsenet og lægerne i Dansk Vestindien, 1755–1830* (Unpublished MA thesis, University of Copenhagen, Department of History, 2002).

7 See for instance Gerda Bonderup, '"Omsorg for at afværge smitsomme sygdomme': Sundhedspolitiet ca. 1750–1900",' *Årsskrift, Politihistorisk Selskab København* (1992), 5–38; Anne Løkke, *Døden i Barndommen. Spædbørnsdødelighed og moderniseringsprocesser i Danmark 1800 til 1920* (Copenhagen: Gyldendal, 1998), 70–71 et passim.

struggle between the planters and the administration. At the same time, similar negotiations or struggles took place in other areas related to the enslaved, for instance concerning punishment.[8] However, the struggle for power over the health of the enslaved was not only a matter between the administration and the planters. The enslaved workers themselves sought actively to gain influence over their own lives through negotiation and conflict. Inspired by historian Sharla M. Fett's research into the connections of health and power among whites and enslaved workers in the southern United States before the Civil War, it is my hypothesis that the enslaved workers in the Danish West Indies participated actively in negotiations and/or conflicts about matters relating to their own health.[9] To the same extent as in other areas of enslaved life, if not more so, health was a field where the fundamental contest for power between masters and enslaved was played out.

My inspiration for viewing health as an instrument in the colonial administration's exercise of power over the colonial population originates from the book *Colonizing the Body: State Medicine and Epidemic Disease in Nineteenth-Century India* (1993) by David Arnold. Here, Arnold views the indigenous, colonised body as 'a site for the construction of its [colonialism's] own authority, legitimacy and control', and he argues that the body was 'a site for contestation and not simply a colonial appropriation.'[10] In other words, the colonial state (in Arnold's case the British administration in India) tried to use European medicine as a tool to extend its authority and control to include the physical wellbeing of the colonised subjects (or at least their physical function), but this endeavour met with resistance from the colonised. The body, and more precisely its physical health, became a field of the struggle for power between the colonised and the colonisers. However, Arnold does call attention to the fact that the colonial state's use of medicine to exercise power was by no means unique to the colonial situation, but followed patterns also found in Europe. So, he emphasises that this perspective is inspired by Michel Foucault's ideas of medicine as an instrument in the modern European state's exercise of power.[11]

The reason why I, unlike Arnold, have not chosen to focus on the attempts

8 Poul Erik Olsen, 'Fra ejendomsret til menneskeret', in *Fra slaveri til frihed: Det dansk-vestindiske slavesamfund 1672–1848*, ed. Per Nielsen (Copenhagen: Nationalmuseet, 2001), 47; Poul Erik Olsen, 'Danske Lov på de vestindiske øer', in *Danske og Norske Lov i 300 år*, ed. Ditlev Tamm (Copenhagen: Jurist- og Økonomforbundets Forlag, 1983), 312–14.

9 Fett, *Working Cures*.

10 Arnold, *Colonizing the Body*, 8, 10.

11 See for instance Michel Foucault, *The Birth of the Clinic* (London: Tavistock Publications, 1979).

of European medicine to control the 'bodies' of the enslaved but only on their 'health', is because a 'colonisation' of the body also implies other forms of disciplining than the medical. For instance, corporal punishment featured prominently in disciplining enslaved workers in the Danish West Indies. As I am not dealing with the punishment of the enslaved but only with the initiatives carried out to keep them healthy, I have chosen to describe my focus as 'the health of the enslaved'.

Perspectives of Medical Anthropology: 'Health' and 'Disease'

The conceptual pair of 'health' and 'disease' is central to the following investigations. Accordingly, it is necessary to give a more detailed explanation of the terms, and to this end, I have utilised theories from medical anthropology. In this theoretical frame, to be 'healthy' does not only imply absence of disease. It is not a physically determined definition independent of time and place but a concept linked to perceptions of good and evil, and so defined culturally, socially, politically, personally etc. One expression of this relation has been that 'health only exists as positively charged notions about life, about characteristics and conditions, which we perceive as valuable.'[12] One example of a definition of health that has been prominent in the Western world in recent times is WHO's definition from 1948, stating that: 'Health is a state of complete physical, mental and social well-being and not merely the absence of disease or infirmity.'[13] Based on the contextual character of the concept of health it is no wonder that several different perceptions of health existed on St Croix in the period 1803–48.

In general, three different perceptions of health and disease will appear in this book. First, the two diverging perceptions found in the source materials, namely the perceptions of the Euro-Caribbean doctors and of the enslaved workers respectively. Because of the origin of the source materials in the Danish West Indian administration and among the Euro-Caribbean doctors, the former perception will be dominant in what follows. However, the perceptions of the enslaved will also be presented and discussed separately (Chapter 2). Still, not even the perception of health and disease among the doctors and the Euro-Caribbean public is immediately comprehensible for contemporary readers. In particular, the medical terminology is different from current biomedical terminology. Consequently, it has been necessary to include a third definition of

12 Hans Stifoss-Hansen and Kjell Kallenberg, *Livssyn, sundhed og sygdom: Teoretiske og kliniske perspektiver* (Copenhagen: Hans Reitzels Forlag, 1999), 53.
13 Stifoss-Hansen and Kallenberg, *Livssyn*, 54.

health and disease in the investigations, namely the modern biomedical definition. This makes it possible to interpret the definitions of health and disease of the period 1803–48 within a modern biomedical conceptual frame.

The Structure of Health Perception: 'Illness', 'Disease' and 'Sickness'

Since the definition of health and disease is generally contextual and so potentially always changeable, it becomes important to distinguish the fundamental structures that guide the definition. Medical anthropology utilises several different models of how disease can be defined. One of the most commonly used is the tripartite model of 'Illness', Disease' and 'Sickness'. It focuses on who defines the disease: the patient, the doctor or the society. The 'Illness' perspective characterises the patient's perspective, that is, the subjective perception of the patient and his nearest relations. The illness interpretation of the causes and meanings of the symptoms determines the patient's reaction to the disease and his relation to the surroundings, and which treatment strategy he chooses. The illness interpretation depends on the patient's personality, cultural background, and experience, as well as on the specific cultural, social, and economical context in which the symptoms arise. So, what to modern biomedicine would appear to be one disease or symptom could be interpreted as very different 'illnesses' in different cultures and periods, and lead to very different treatment strategies. In many past and present non-industrialised societies, health is a sign of a balanced relationship between humans, between humans and nature, and between humans and the supernatural world. Upsetting the balance between any of these groups will cause physical and/or emotional symptoms, which point to the 'disease'.[14]

The second perspective in the model, the 'Disease' concept, is the doctor's professional interpretation of the disease. For doctors trained in modern biomedicine this special perspective is based on a number of premises, namely scientific rationality, objective measurement, physical/chemical data, dualism between body and mind, diseases understood as units (i.e. each with its own specific cause, signs and symptoms), and reductionism. The focus of this perspective is on the individual patient instead of on the family or the community. On this basis, disease phenomena only become 'real' – become facts – when they have been observed objectively, measured and the logical causal con-

14 Cecil G. Helman, *Culture, Health and Illness* (London: Hodder Arnold, 2000), 83–84.

nection behind them has been found.[15] Regardless of these modern scientific criteria, I would argue that the perception of disease among the doctors on St Croix in the first half of the nineteenth century was also based on the 'Disease' concept. Of course, their knowledge of physical and chemical matters was significantly smaller than that of modern doctors, yet the characteristics of their approach to disease were also a dualism between body and mind, the focus on the individual patient instead of the family and the demand for scientific rationality. They did not necessarily share the patient's subjective understanding of what ailed him, and for them disease could not be attributed to witchcraft, but had to be a natural phenomenon treatable by physical remedies.

The third perspective in the model is the concept of 'Sickness'. This is the broad, popular perception of disease. In the sickness perspective, the popular perception is related to the broader social, economic, political context. For instance, in relation to environmental conditions that could expose one part of the population to an increased risk of developing a certain disease.[16]

The Structure of Therapy: The 'Popular', the 'Folk' and the 'Professional' Sectors

Based on the different perceptions of disease and health among patient, doctor, and society respectively, it is useful to investigate the ways these perceptions are reflected in the structures of medical therapy. Arthur Kleinman has suggested a model to explain how the treatment of diseases is structured in complex societies. He argues that three overlapping sectors can be identified, the 'Popular', the 'Folk' and the 'Professional' sectors.

The 'Popular' sector is the non-professional, non-specialised part of society, where the disease is first discovered and defined, and where therapy is initiated (see Fig. 1.1). The therapy is carried out by the patient himself, by family, friends, neighbours, by religious or other societies, or by a person with personal experience of the disease. Therapy is informal and carried out without charge within the patient's own social networks. The most important of these networks is the family where the vast majority of primary therapy is carried out in all societies.[17]

The 'Folk' sector consists of individuals who are specialised in therapies, which are either religious or secular or a mixture of the two. These healers are not a part of the government-sanctioned medical system, and range from tech-

15 Helman, *Culture*, 79–81.
16 Peter Elsass, *Sundhedspsykologi* (Copenhagen: Gyldendal, 1992), 82–83.
17 Helman, *Culture*, 51–52.

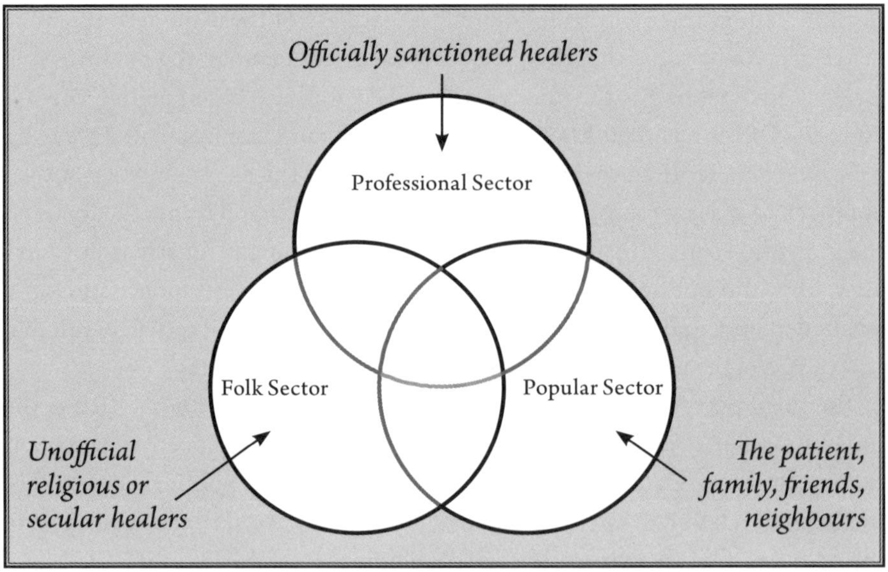

Fig. 1.1: Simplified version of Arthur Kleinman's model for the sectors in the system of healers in developed societies. See Arthur Kleinman, *Patients and Healers in the Context of Culture: An Exploration of the Borderland between Anthropology, Medicine and Psychiatry* (London: University of California Press, 1980), 50.

nical specialists as tooth extractors to spiritual healers as shamans and clairvoyants.[18] In cultures other than the modern Western one, most of these healers share the same fundamental cultural values and worldviews as the societies they live in, and so also the same perceptions of the cause and treatment of disease.[19] Often, their approach is holistic in as much as they treat all aspects of the patient's life (cf. the illness perspective above), the relation to other humans, nature and the spirit world as well as physical and emotional symptoms. Their therapy usually involves the entire family and not just the individual patient. The folk healer may have acquired his skills from his own family as an inherited ability, as a revelation or from working as an apprentice with another healer. Generally, folk healers are not organised into larger bodies, although they may form smaller networks.[20]

18 Helman, *Culture*, 53.
19 Elsass, *Sundhedspsykologi*, 76.
20 Helman, *Culture*, 53–55.

The 'Professional' sector consists of the organised and officially authorised health professions. In the case of Western biomedicine, this sector includes not only doctors but also nurses, midwives etc. The professional sector is supported by legislation that furnishes the members of the sector with powers, rights and obligations that other members of the society do not have.[21]

According to Kleinman, patients are in principle able to move freely between the three sectors during therapy. However, the legal complex sanctioning the 'Professional' sector has an inhibitory effect on the 'Popular' and 'Folk' sectors. Often a patient avails himself of treatments from all three sectors at the same time, especially when the treatment in one sector does not alleviate the physical symptoms or emotional problems.[22]

In relation to the investigations of this book, Kleinman's model gives a general theoretical framework for all the various therapists who took care of the health of the enslaved workers. This is useful because the source material utilised is primarily Euro-Caribbean in origin and accordingly focuses almost entirely on only one third of the therapeutic landscape, namely the 'Professional' sector. Because of this, the model can compensate for some of the bias in the sources. Furthermore, the model can position the healing carried out by the enslaved workers themselves (see Chapter 2) in relation to Euro-Caribbean medicine and in this way help to fill out the picture of the medical world on St Croix.

The Source Material

As is evident from the bibliography and list of sources, I have used both printed and especially manuscript archival material from the period in question. In general, a Euro-Caribbean (or European) perspective dominates these sources. The perspectives of the public authorities and the doctors are particularly prominent, whereas the perspective of the planters is less so. The representation of the perspective of the enslaved and the Afro-Caribbeans as such is very weak and only becomes visible through Euro-Caribbean interpretations of enslaved workers' views and reactions. This bias in the source material is, on the one hand, a universal problem in research into the history of Caribbean slavery caused by the simple fact that the enslaved workers were rarely able to write. On the other hand, the bias is also caused by the fact that the sources utilised for this investi-

21 Elsass, *Sundhedspsykologi*, 77.
22 Helman, *Culture*, 53.

gation have primarily been chosen with the aim of elucidating the health policy of the colonial administration towards the enslaved.

The source materials utilised, both printed and manuscript, divide into two main groups. The first group is material used primarily in only one of the investigations of the book. This applies to the doctors' annual medical reports, the records from plantation hospitals, plantation records, and church records (see Chapter 3). The characteristics of each of these source groups are dealt with in each chapter. The other group of materials is used throughout the book and so needs to be specified here. This group of records also consists of two parts. One part is the correspondence and legislation of various public authorities. Generally, they express the views and intentions of the administration and to some degree of the planters concerning the health of the enslaved workers. The second part of the group, however, is much more diverse. It consists of publications by a number of authors who visited St Croix sometime between the 1820s and 1840s and described different aspects of the health conditions surrounding the enslaved workers there. The most detailed and important of them were written in the later years of the 1820s by a certain Lieutenant Brady of the British navy.[23] Later, during the 1830s and 1840s a number of travel accounts were published by a number of individuals who for various reasons had visited St Croix for some months. In chronological order the authors were the North American abolitionist Sylvester Hovey (winters of 1835/6 and 1836/7),[24] the North American convalescents Joseph Tuckerman (winter of 1836/7)[25] and James Smith (winter of 1839/40),[26] the leader of the French anti-slavery movement Victor Schoelcher (first years of the 1840s),[27] and the North American publisher Thurlow Weed (winter 1844/45).[28]

23 Arnold R. Highfield, ed., *Observations on the State of Negro Slavery in the Island of Santa Cruz, the Principal of the Danish West India Colonies, with Miscellaneous Remarks upon Subjects Relating to the West India Question and a Notice of Santa Cruz* (St Croix: Antilles Press, 1996. Originally published by Simpkin and Marshall and Longman Reid and Co., London 1829), vi–ix, xxi–xxxi.

24 Sylvester Hovey, *Letters from the West Indies: Relating Especially to the Danish Island of St Croix and to the British Islands of Antigua, Barbados and Jamaica* (New York: Gould and Newman, 1838).

25 Joseph Tuckerman, *Letter Respecting Santa Cruz as a Winter Residence for Invalids* (Boston, 1837).

26 James Smith, *Winter of 1840 in St Croix with an Excursion to Tortola and St Thomas* (New York, 1840).

27 Original title: Victor Schoelcher, *Colonies Étrangères et Haiti* II (Paris, 1843). I have used excerpts from George F. Tyson and Arnold R. Highfield, eds., *The Kamina Folk: Slavery and Slave Life in the Danish West Indies* (US Virgin Islands: Virgin Islands Humanities Council, 1994), 207–10.

28 Original title: Thurlow Weed, *Letters From Europe and the West Indies, 1843–1852* (Albany, 1866). I have used excerpts from Tyson and Highfield, *The Kamina Folk*, 211–17.

Historiography

As mentioned earlier, this book covers a field where different scholarly disciplines and historical research areas meet. In general, the field consists of two areas: research into Caribbean slavery and research into the connection between medicine and colonialism. Obviously, this makes it complicated to locate the field historiographically, yet at the same time, it also makes it all the more necessary to attempt to situate it. In the following, I shall attempt to give a brief sketch of the historiographical development and connections which this field is a part of, and a sketch of the location of the book within the field.

Historical Research concerning Caribbean and Danish West Indian Slavery, ca. 1950–2006

The historiography of Caribbean slavery is a problematic entity. First, the area is geographically, linguistically, politically, culturally and racially complex, which makes it difficult to speak of one historiographical development. However, slavery is one of only a number of institutions that unite the area even though Caribbean slavery has many different modes of expression depending on economy, system of government, crops etc. Nonetheless, the common reference point in slavery and European colonialism makes it possible to operate with a common historiography for historical research into Caribbean slavery.[29] That said, very few publications attempt to draw together and compare historical research into the different areas in the Caribbean and so the historiography is still fragmentary.[30] Regardless, in the following, I shall discuss Caribbean historiography as if it were unambiguous, knowing quite well that the literature I use focuses on the historiography of the Anglophone areas.

Second, a special problem appears when we move from the general Caribbean level down to the historiography of the Danish West Indian Islands/US Virgin Islands. The islands are a part of both the Caribbean and the USA and they have received influences from historical research in both places, yet at the same time they are also a part of Danish history and so of the historiography of Danish colonial history, which is quite different from Caribbean or North

29 Francisco A. Scarano, 'Slavery and Emancipation in Caribbean History', in *General History of the Caribbean: Methodology and Historiography of the Caribbean* VI, ed. Barry W. Higman (London: UNESCO publishing, 1999), 233–35.

30 Barry W. Higman, 'Introduction', in *General History of the Caribbean: Methodology and Historiography of the Caribbean* VI, ed. Barry W. Higman (London: UNESCO publishing, 1999), 16.

American historiography. Therefore, the following discussion of the historiography of the Danish West Indies will include both perspectives.

Caribbean Research concerning the History of Slavery, ca. 1950–2006

Since the 1950s, research into the history of slavery has become a part of a national project in several parts of the Caribbean inspired by the process of decolonisation and the anti-colonial and national popular independence movements of the time. In the 1960s, the influence of slavery research, especially in the USA, meant that the volume of research on social aspects, *history from below*, and economical aspects of slavery in the Caribbean increased greatly. Previously, research had mainly focused on the legislation and institutions, of which the enslaved were the victims. Yet now, the interest centred on structures and the enslaved workers' ability to resist and fight slavery, their agency. This *resistance motif* seems to have originated with both the struggle for national independence and the struggle for racial equality, which in those years radiated from the civil rights movement in the USA. To gain insight into the world the slaves made, despite the lack of any source materials they produced themselves, the historians of social history used both quantitative methods from the social sciences, for instance demography and historical anthropology, to write a history seen from 'below'.[31] Researchers attempted to explain slavery as a system, viewed either from a sociological position in the theory of social classes or from an anthropological perspective as a special culture.[32]

The end of the 1960s and the beginning of the 1970s saw a growing dissatisfaction with the dominant dualistic approach in slavery research, which contrasted the Euro-Caribbean part of colonial society with the Afro-Caribbeans, and was only able to portray slavery as the struggle against Euro-Caribbean oppression. Rather than this diametrical contraposition, the historian Edward Braithwaite used concepts like 'interculturation' and 'creolisation' for the development of the slavery-based colonial societies that fused the different original racial,

31 Joseph C. Miller, 'Historical Approaches to Slavery: Bibliography of Slavery', in Paul Finkelmann and Joseph C. Miller, *Macmillan Encyclopedia of World Slavery* I (New York: Macmillan Reference, 1998), 394–95.

32 The most influential books with this approach are Elsa Goveia, *Slave Society in the British Leeward Islands at the End of the Eighteenth Century* (New Haven and London: Yale University Press, 1965); Philip Curtin, *Two Jamaicas: The Role of Ideas in a Tropical Colony, 1830–1865* (Cambridge: Harvard University Press, 1955); Douglas Hall, *Free Jamaica, 1838–1865* (New Haven and London: Yale University Press, 1959); Orlando Patterson, *The Sociology of Slavery* (London: MacGibbon and Kee, 1967); and Richard Sheridan, *Sugar and Slavery: An Economic History of the British West Indies, 1623–1775* (Barbados: Caribbean University Press, 1974).

linguistic and cultural elements into new unique societies.[33] Some years later, anthropologists Sidney W. Mintz and Richard Price developed these concepts further in their book *An Anthropological Approach to the Afro-American Past: A Caribbean Perspective* (1976). Consequently, creolisation is today a standard concept in Caribbean slavery research.[34] Returning to the resistance motif, it was further nuanced in the 1990s with the addition of an element of accommodation. Now, the resistance of the enslaved workers was not perceived solely as a direct struggle against slavery and Euro-Caribbean suppression, but it was pointed out that the enslaved were also able to change the scope of the system from within through a 'negotiation' of power, and in this way create a better life for themselves.[35] In my opinion, this view of the relationship between Euro-Caribbeans and enslaved workers is also warranted in the case of the power over the health of the enslaved.

Among the approaches applied in slavery research since the 1970s, I would like to emphasise the relevance of demography to the investigations of this book. Historical investigations into the demography of Caribbean slavery were central to slavery research from the 1970s to the 1990s and they have often discussed issues relating to the health conditions of the enslaved, diseases, mortality, and fertility. In particular, studies of British and Dutch colonies in the Caribbean have offered an insight into the connections between diet, work, and environmental factors in relation to the demography of the enslaved workers. One major discovery of this work has been that the enslaved workers of the USA were able to maintain their population levels through reproduction from the early eighteenth century, whereas most enslaved populations in the Caribbean were never able to.[36] In the investigations of this book, the demographic and statistical approach to the morbidity and mortality of the enslaved workers is represented particularly by the most thorough study so far of an enslaved population, namely Barry W. Higman's *Slave Populations of the British Caribbean, 1807–1834*. However, since the 1980s the so-called 'cliometric'[37] approach to history of the demographic and quantitative studies has been attacked by researchers using a

33 Edward Braithwaite, *The Development of Creole Society in Jamaica 1770–1820* (Oxford: Clarendon, 1971).

34 Scarano, 'Slavery and Emancipation', 263.

35 Stephan Palmié, ed., *Slave Cultures and the Cultures of Slavery* (Knoxville: The University of Tennessee Press, 1995), xvii–xviii, xx–xxi.

36 Miller, 'Historical Approaches to Slavery', 394.

37 Cliometry: historical investigations based on quantitative data and calculations, mostly economic and demographic history.

qualitative approach because they find that cliometrics make the human tragedy and destruction of slavery impersonal.[38] In recent years, the attitude among leading scholars to this problem has been that quantitative and qualitative approaches cannot do without each other.[39] They need each other to interpret each other's results, and from this point of view the investigations of this book attempt to integrate quantitative and qualitative methods and sources.

From the 1970s until the mid-1990s, slavery research followed the empirical and methodological lines of development in the international historical research and moved from the general investigation of entire enslaved societies towards detailed investigations of single subjects in shorter periods. The subjects investigated have been, for instance, the slave trade and the Atlantic perspective, demography, family life, rebellion, marronage, women/gender, leisure and entertainments.[40] One might view the traditional qualitative investigations of aspects of health and disease surrounding the life of the enslaved workers as a part of this trend. Two central books in this genre are Richard Sheridan's *Doctors and Slaves: A Medical and Demographic History of Slavery in the British West Indies, 1680–1834* and the precursor of that book Todd L. Savitt's *Medicine and Slavery: The Diseases and Health Care of Blacks in Antebellum Virginia*.

The apparent fragmentation of slavery research into single subjects and periods is probably due to a growing recognition that the local historical circumstances – be they ecological, demographic, economic, social, or political – have had a tremendous impact on the way in which the conflict and/or negotiation of power has taken place between various actors in various slavery-based societies. For instance, research concerning the British Caribbean has shown the importance of ecology, climate, topography, epidemiology, and demography on the development of the slave societies.[41] Many different types of interdisciplinary methodology have been employed in the investigation of these local circumstances of slavery, for instance archaeology and physical anthropology.[42] Based on these and other results, the investigations of this book emphasise the local meteorological, geographical and ecological circumstances and thus the interdisciplinary use of data from natural science and medical science concern-

38 Robert W. Fogel and Stanley L. Engerman's controversial book *Time on the Cross: The Economics of American Negro Slavery* (Toronto: Little, Brown and Company, 1974) has been made the scare example of the cliometric method.

39 Dorsey, *Slave Traffic*, 10–11.

40 Scarano, 'Slavery and Emancipation', 264–65.

41 Palmié, *Slave Cultures*, xx–xxi.

42 Miller, 'Historical Approaches to Slavery', 409.

ing the physical basis of the slave society. Further to this, I would like to add a third central book in the genre of 'the health of the enslaved', namely Kenneth F. Kiple's *The Caribbean Slave: A Biological History*. Here, Kiple investigates the nutritional state of the Caribbean enslaved workers, which was the inspiration for the investigation of the nutritional state of the enslaved workers on St Croix (see Chapter 4).

Historical Research concerning the Danish West Indies, ca. 1950–2006

The historical research concerning the Danish West Indies, the present US Virgin Islands, including research into slavery in these islands, differs from research into slavery in other areas of the Caribbean by being structurally separated into two parts, a Danish-language part and an English-language part. This division has been and still seems to be an impediment to both the investigation and the communication of the history of the islands. The problem is greater for Anglophone researchers, who are often unable to read Danish and thus unable to access the majority of the source material which is in Danish and housed in Danish archives.[43] Danish researchers are usually better off as they normally read and use sources in English, yet many of them have not published their findings in English. In addition, until the 1980s Danish researchers showed an inclination towards a somewhat nationalistic approach to Danish colonial history and to Danish West Indian history in particular.[44] Consequently, two only partially overlapping circuits of research have emerged concerning the history of the islands, which means that the population of the islands is cut off from a part of their past, while the population in Denmark maintains an often simplified and national romantic idea of the Danish West Indian past. However, since the 1990s a number of English translations of central Danish-language sources, plus detailed English-language bibliographies and catalogues of Danish West Indian archival material in Denmark, have contributed significantly to making the history more accessible to the population of the islands.[45] Only time will

43 See for instance Barry W. Higman, 'Danish West Indian Slavery in Comparative Perspective: An Appreciation of Neville Hall's Contribution to the Historiography', in *Bondmen and Freedmen in the Danish West Indies: Scholarly Perspectives*, ed. George F. Tyson (US Virgin Islands: Virgin Islands Humanities Council, 1996), 1.

44 See for instance Karen Fog Olwig, 'Narrating deglobalization: Danish Perceptions of a Lost Empire', in *Global Networks* 3, no. 3 (2003).

45 For instance Reimert Haagensen, *Description of the Island of St Croix in America in the West Indies* (US Virgin Islands: Virgin Islands Humanities Council, 1995); Johan Christian Schmidt, *Various Remarks Collected on and about the Island of St Croix in America* (US Virgin Islands: The Virgin Islands Humanities Council, 1998 [First published in Copenhagen, 1788]); Arnold R. Highfield and George

tell if this will also bring Danes up to date with their knowledge of the common West Indian past.

The development of Danish research into Danish West Indian history for the period up to 1848 has followed the main currents in international historical research – albeit occasionally with some delay. The broadest and most comprehensive Danish-language account of Danish West Indian history is still *Vore gamle tropekolonier* (Our Old Tropical Colonies) edited by historian Johannes Brøndsted and published in 1952/3.[46] In line with history writing at the time, this series of books describes the Danish West Indies from the viewpoint of the Danish colonial power. So, the focus is on administrative issues, institutions, legislation, trade, and economy. The conditions of the enslaved workers and the free Afro-Caribbeans are dealt with in separate sections without much reference to the rest of the account. As a result, the enslaved and free Afro-Caribbeans appear to be passive victims of European oppression without having any agency of their own.[47] In the 1960s and 1970s, historical research kept focusing on economic and commercial history, and the theoretical approach was almost exclusively the empirical inductive method of the so-called 'Copenhagen School' which attached great importance to the analysis and criticism of the sources.[48] For instance, historian Svend E. Green-Pedersen made important contributions with his research in the 1970s concerning aspects of the islands' economy, the demography of the enslaved workers, the slave trade, and the abolition of the trade.[49] As previously mentioned, these approaches were in line with the then dominant methods of the social sciences and statistics. With Green-Pedersen, the enslaved workers became the focus of historical research, though they still assumed a passive role. However, at the same time other initiatives went in the direction of cultural history, although still in a traditional national form. For instance in 1960, the Royal Danish Academy of Art undertook a number of investigations into the architectural history of townhouses built on the islands during Danish times. One of the participants was Inge Mejer Antonsen, who in the following years published several articles on paintings,

F. Tyson, *Slavery in the Danish West Indies: A Bibliography* (US Virgin Islands: The Virgin Islands Humanities Council, 1994); Erik Gøbel, *A Guide to Sources for the History of the Danish West Indies (US Virgin Islands), 1671–1917* (Odense: University Press of Southern Denmark, 2002).

46 Peter Hoxcer Jensen et al., eds., *Dansk kolonihistorie. Indføring og studier* (Aarhus: Forlaget Historia, 1983), 10–12, 29–30.

47 Gunvor Simonsen, 'Nye og gamle perspektiver på dansk kolonihistorie', *1066 – Tidsskrift for Historie* 33, no. 2 (2003), 4–5.

48 Hoxcer Jensen et al., *Dansk kolonihistorie*, 29–30.

49 Higman, 'Danish West Indian Slavery', 9.

furniture, and interiors from the Euro-Caribbean upper class on the islands.[50] In 1980, the successor of *Vore gamle tropekolonier* was published as the three-volume book *Danmarks Historie – uden for Danmark* (The History of Denmark – Outside Denmark) edited by Svend Ellehøj and Kristof Glamann. However, in the volume *Kolonierne i Vestindien* (The Colonies in the West Indies) Ove Hornby continued the tradition of earlier Danish colonial history by focusing on the economy and administration with little interest shown in the enslaved workers. On this basis, we can generally conclude that until 1980 Danish historians predominantly engaged with the Danish West Indies from a European perspective.[51]

Since 1980 however, research has followed a somewhat different trajectory. An ever increasing and more important part of historical research concerning the Danish West Indies has come from American researchers based on the islands themselves. From the mid-1980s to the 1990s new and groundbreaking contributions have come from Karen Fog Olwig, who has investigated the Afro-Caribbean population on the island of St John.[52] One example of her work is the book *Cultural Adaptation and Resistance on St John: Three Centuries of Afro-Caribbean Life*. In her approach and presentation, Olwig was strongly inspired by historical research in the USA, and by extension in the Caribbean, for instance the book *The Birth of African-American Culture: An Anthropological Perspective* by Sidney W. Mintz and Richard Price (cf. above). From an anthropological-historical perspective, she has criticised traditional Danish historical research on the Danish West Indies following *Vore gamle tropekolonier* for not considering the possibility that the enslaved workers might have taken any action against their oppressors.[53] Parallel to Olwig's new approach, research with more traditional approaches carried out since the 1980s has also made important contributions concerning the enslaved workers. In the field of enslaved demography, Hans Christian Johansen has used quantitative methods to show that just as in most other Caribbean sugar-growing societies the enslaved population in the Danish West Indies was not able to maintain a stable population through

50 Peter Bredsdorff et al., 'Kunstakademiets studier af byer og bygningskunst på de Dansk-Vestindieske Øer', *Arkitekten* 62 (1960); Inge Mejer Antonsen, 'Møbler og boligkultur i Dansk Vestindien', *Dansk Kunsthåndværk* 40 (1967–68).

51 Hoxcer Jensen et al., *Dansk kolonihistorie*, 11–15.

52 Margaret D. Rouse-Jones, 'Historiography of the Leeward Islands and the Virgin islands', in *General History of the Caribbean: Methodology and Historiography of the Caribbean* VI, ed. B.W. Higman (London: UNESCO Publishing, 1999), 542.

53 Simonsen, 'Nye og gamle perspektiver', 7.

reproduction.[54] At the same time, the same demographic-quantitative approach was used in a number of historical MA theses from the University of Aarhus, for instance Jesper Bering Asmussen and Peter Hoxcer Jensen.[55] Poul E. Olsen and Erik Gøbel have, respectively, examined subjects like legislation concerning the enslaved, administration and customs, and shipping, slave trade and the triangular trade.[56] In the 1990s Per Nielsen joined them with contributions on trade, shipping, architectural history and free Afro-Caribbeans in the Danish West Indies.[57]

From around the turn of the millennium Danish historical research concerning the Danish West Indies has been growing. An important reason has been the Danish National Archive's thorough re-cataloguing, repacking, and refurbishing of the so-called West Indian Local Archives, which took place from 1999 to 2001.[58] An important result of this work was Erik Gøbel's *A Guide to Sources for the History of the Danish West Indies (US Virgin Islands), 1671–1917*, which is and for the foreseeable future will remain the natural point of departure for research into Danish West Indian history.[59] In the first years of the new millennium, the possibilities created by the re-cataloguing sparked off new research in MA theses by a number of history students.[60] Three of these students have since embarked on Ph.D. projects focusing on the enslaved population in the Danish West Indies.[61] This book is the result of one of those projects.

Until the end of the 1960s, Caribbean historical research into slavery in the Danish West Indies was predominantly carried out by a few local amateur his-

54 Higman, 'Danish West Indian Slavery', 9.

55 Jesper Bering Asmussen, *Slavedemografi: St Croix' Landdistrikter, 1803–1848* (unpublished MA thesis, University of Aarhus, 1983); Peter Hoxcer Jensen, *From Serfdom to Fireburn and Strike: The History of Black Labour in the Danish West Indies, 1848–1916* (St Croix: Antilles Press, 1998).

56 For instance Poul Erik Olsen, 'De dansk-vestindiske øer og junigrundloven', *Historie* 18, no. 1 (1989); Erik Gøbel, 'Danish Trade to the West Indies and Guinea, 1671–1754', *Scandinavian Economic History Review* 31 (1983).

57 See for instance: Nielsen, *Fra Slaveri til Frihed*.

58 Gøbel, *A Guide to Sources*, 60.

59 See also: www.virgin-islands-history.dk/ (accessed 30-05-2011).

60 The following list is not exhaustive: Gunvor Simonsen, *En fortræffelig Constitution – om konstruktion af social orden på de Dansk Vestindiske øer i sidste halvdel af 1700-tallet* (unpublished MA thesis, University of Roskilde, 2000); Louise Steensgaard, *På sporet af den 'Vestindiske Philosophie': en undersøgelse af kreoliseringen af eurocaribierne i Dansk Vestindien i det 18. Århundrede* (unpublished MA thesis, University of Copenhagen, 2002); Jensen, *En verden til forskel?* (unpublished MA thesis).

61 Besides the thesis forming the basis of this book, the other theses are: Gunvor Simonsen, *Slave Stories: Gender, Representation, and the Court in the Danish West Indies, 1780s–1820s* (European University Institute, Department of History and Civilisation, Florence, Italy, 2007); Louise Sebro, *Mellem afrikaner og kreol: Etnisk identitet og social navigation i Dansk Vestindien, 1730–1770* (University of Lund, Sweden).

torians.[62] According to Barry W. Higman, until the 1970s this research was characterised by a recurring theme relating to the subject of this book, namely to what extent the planters in the Danish West Indies had treated their slaves better than planters in other colonies did.[63] So, in the 1950s, Jens Larsen[64] and Lawrence Spingarn[65] advanced the opinion that the enslaved in the Danish West Indies were treated better than those in other colonies. The claim persisted well into the 1960s despite the above-mentioned upheaval in Caribbean historical research, which brought the focus closer to the life the enslaved workers lived on the islands. In 1969, Patricia Murphy[66] positioned the Danish slave regime on a par with the Spanish and Portuguese using the hypothesis of Frank Tannenbaum and Stanley Elkins that in the eighteenth century Spaniards and Portuguese were more lenient slave owners than all other European nations because of the influence of Catholicism and traditions from Roman law.[67] In 1970 Florence Lewisohn nuanced the assertion of the better treatment of Danish West Indian enslaved workers by claiming that the handling of them was good by the middle of the eighteenth century yet deteriorated markedly in the years between 1820 and 1840 along with the planters' economic situation.[68] In 1974, Isaac Dookhan mentioned the claim for the last time;[69] however, he carefully avoided taking a position on its accuracy.[70]

Today, the claim of better treatment of the enslaved workers in the Danish West Indies seems irrelevant to historical research for several reasons. Accordingly, I would like to clarify that the intention of this book is *not* to resurrect or answer this claim. As Higman has duly noted, the reason why the question has not been investigated since the 1970s is that it is too broad. To begin with, 'treatment' can refer to a number of things. For instance the amount of food handed out, the brutality of the punishments or the enslaved workers' access to

62 The exception is the classic book by Waldemar Westergaard, *The Danish West Indies under Company Rule* (New York, 1917). I have discarded Westergaard because this historiographic examination focuses on the years after 1950.

63 Higman, 'Danish West Indian Slavery', 3–6.

64 *Virgin Islands Story* (Philadelphia: Muhlenberg Press, 1950).

65 'Slavery in the Danish West Indies', *The American-Scandinavian Review* 45 (1957), 35–43.

66 *The Moravian Mission to the African Slaves of the Danish West Indies, 1732–1828* (St Thomas: Caribbean Research Institute of the College of the Virgin Islands, 1969).

67 Frank Tannenbaum, *Slave and Citizen: The Negro in the Americas* (New York: Vintage Books, 1946); Stanley Elkins, *Slavery: A problem in American Institutional and Intellectual life* (Chicago and London: University of Chicago Press, 1959).

68 *St Croix under Seven Flags* (Hollywood, Florida: The Dukane Press, 1970).

69 *A History of the Virgin Islands of the United States* (St Thomas: Caribbean Universities Press for the College of the Virgin Islands, 1974).

70 Higman, 'Danish West Indian Slavery', 3–6.

manumission. Furthermore, comparative studies always require that the entities compared are in fact comparable, for instance that the economic, agricultural or other circumstances in the colonies are comparable, which was often not the case in the comparative studies that the claim was based on. In addition, the arguments in the discussion were founded on phenomena as vague as the national characters of different colonial powers, which can hardly be the basis of any precise comparison – especially in relation to a society as multinational as the Danish West Indian.[71] Finally, it is evident that the entire discussion is apologetic in relation to slavery. Based on the research in existence today it seems uninteresting at best to discuss who had the honour of the least gruesome treatment of the enslaved workers. Accordingly, the aim of this book is something else. As mentioned earlier, the enslaved population in the Danish West Indies continued to decrease until emancipation in 1848 and even beyond that date. This means that the 'result' of this book is in a sense given from the beginning, namely that the health policies of the Danish colonial administration did not accomplish their aim of keeping enslaved workers healthy and fit for work. Consequently, the administration did not 'treat' the enslaved workers 'better' than other colonial authorities – or at least it did not generate a demographic result. However, what we do not know is what the health conditions of the enslaved workers were like in the Danish West Indies and what was done to improve them, if anything. So, the aim of this book is, in line with the research questions above, to investigate the health conditions of the enslaved workers, and the comparative Caribbean perspective makes it possible to see the administration's health policies in a wider historical context. Finally, it also becomes possible to see the health policies as a tool used by the administration in its attempt to gain control of the enslaved workers.

If we return to the historiographical development in Caribbean historical research concerning slavery in the Danish West Indies since the 1970s, we see a very different development from the previous period. In the 1970s and 1980s historical research was dominated by trained historians based in the Caribbean and even in the US Virgin Islands, for instance Isaac Dookhan and Neville Hall.[72] Hall in particular contributed greatly to research into slavery in areas that had not been touched upon previously. He addressed issues concerning the social control of the enslaved, the culture of the enslaved and their resist-

71 Higman, 'Danish West Indian Slavery', 7–8.

72 Rouse-Jones, 'Historiography of the Leeward Islands', 540.

ance to the Euro-Caribbean regime. Contrary to many of the above-mentioned authors, Hall was able to read Danish and so had access to the extensive Danish-language source material.[73] In the 1990s Arnold R. Highfield, George F. Tyson, and Svend E. Holsøe took over. The first two in particular have contributed a number of books and most importantly a series of English translations of key historical sources in Danish. Here again, it has been of central importance that Highfield and Holsøe understand Danish and so have had access to materials in Danish. After the turn of the millennium, the influence of Highfield and Tyson is undiminished in the sense that the former has translated Hans West's central account of the Danish West Indies dating from 1793,[74] whereas the latter has been the main force behind a large demographic survey of all Afro-Caribbean inhabitants on St Croix during Danish times (1733–1917) entitled the 'St Croix African Roots Project'.[75] There is no doubt that this project will be of great importance to any future research into the demography and social history of the enslaved society in the Danish West Indies.

In the above examination of the previous historiography, the subject of the health conditions among the enslaved in the Danish West Indies is not mentioned at all for the simple reason that it has never previously been the subject of an independent investigation.[76] However, as mentioned in the examination of Caribbean slavery research, the field has been thoroughly investigated for the British West Indies (and the USA and French West Indies). Regarding the Danish West Indies, research into other subjects has occasionally touched upon aspects of slave health, for instance demographic studies, and they incidentally mention issues of workload, rations, housing, clothing etc. Accordingly, this book is situated in an empty field in the historical research of the Danish West Indies.

Historical Research concerning Medicine and Colonialism, ca. 1950–2006

The second area of historical research included in this book is the connection between medicine and colonialism. The area is part of a larger research field

73 Higman, 'Danish West Indian Slavery', 8–12.

74 Original title: *Beskrivelse over St Croix med en kort Udsigt over St Thomas, St Jean, Tortola, Spanishtown og Crabeneiland* (Copenhagen, 1793).

75 See: http://stx.visharoots.org/scarp.html (accessed 30-05-2011).

76 The health service and the doctors in the Danish West Indies have been investigated in my MA thesis *En verden til forskel?* (unpublished). The relation between the health service and the enslaved workers was investigated for the first time in my Ph.D. thesis, *For Slavernes Sundhed*. Concerning the years after 1848 the same subjects have been investigated in a number of articles by Torben Geill (see Bibliography).

focusing on medicine and health, and in short, it deals with the position of medical science within the colonial project of dominating and controlling colonised populations.

Until the end of the 1960s, medical history was predominantly a positivist account of medical triumphs and of the great doctors who saved thousands of lives with their discoveries. Since then, medicine has become integrated with social history, so moving the focus to the context, to the society and the patients whose bodies and minds suffered both the diseases and medicine. This development has opened up the discipline to an extensive use of interdisciplinary approaches from literary studies through sociology, anthropology, and demography to approaches of natural science such as nutritional science. For instance, the work of medical anthropologists in developing countries has revealed the fundamental structures of very different medical systems.[77] Furthermore, in the same period, a new cultural history of medicine has developed in the qualitative part of the social history of medicine. Here the influence comes from the French 'Annales' school and particularly from Michel Foucault.[78]

One of the most important trajectories in the future development of medical history is comparative studies, and colonial medical history is one of the fields that almost inevitably leads to comparisons between different perceptions and systems of health. In traditional medical history, colonial medicine more than other kinds of medicine was regarded as the most admirable and humane expression of enlightened science. However, recent research has positioned medical history in the political, economic, and cultural context of colonisation and focused critically on how colonialism used medicine as a strong ideological and practical tool for social control and suppression. It has also been revealed that European medicine in the colonies was only one of several competing medical systems and not necessarily the most effective or acceptable for the colonised populations.[79]

The field of colonial medical history has been subdivided in many ways, but historian David Arnold has suggested a geographical division between Euro-

77 For instance the work of anthropologist Arthur Kleinman on the system of healers in Taiwan. See for instance: Arthur Kleinman, *Patients and Healers in the Context of Culture: An Exploration of the Borderland between Anthropology, Medicine and Psychiatry* (London: University of California Press, 1980).

78 Gert Brieger, 'The Historiography of Medicine', in *Companion Encyclopedia of the History of Medicine*, ed. W.F. Bynum and Roy Porter (London: Routledge, 1993), 24–42.

79 David Arnold, 'Medicine and Colonialism', in *Companion Encyclopedia of the History of Medicine*, ed. W.F. Bynum and Roy Porter (London: Routledge, 1993), 1393–94.

pean settler colonies (for instance USA, Australia, New Zealand) and tropical colonies (Caribbean, India, South East Asia, Africa). This division is justified because in contrast to the settler colonies the tropical colonies had a predominantly non-European population, which made European medicine more dependent on and oriented towards the needs and aims of the colonial state. In these colonies, of which the Danish West Indies was one, European medicine was often extended only to the enclaves where Europeans lived, for instance military camps and the European quarters of colonial towns. Where European medicine was extended to the native population, one of the main objectives was to make the workforce more productive and profitable. This motive is extremely clear in the West Indian colonies in the planters' employment of European doctors for their enslaved workers and in the interventions of the colonial authorities to maintain certain minimum standards concerning the treatment of the enslaved. This ensured a continuation of the profits from the production of the enslaved and deflected humanitarian criticism from Europe.[80]

Nevertheless, the relation between government medical science and the enslaved workers in the different Caribbean colonies has not been the object of research. The closest we get is the above-mentioned book by Richard Sheridan and here the focus is not on the role of colonial authorities or on medicine as a tool for discipline, even if the latter function is of course present implicitly. However, in the field of enslaved workers and medicine in the USA there has been a focus on the disciplinary functions of medicine. Here, Sharla M. Fett has taken up the work of Todd Savitt, but with a new focus on the conflict and/or negotiation concerning power over health between enslaved workers and slave owners.[81] But in the USA the opponents of the enslaved were the planters and not the state. Accordingly, the European medicine Fett describes being used on the enslaved workers was not part of a state health policy towards the enslaved, but only a result of the ideology of white planter society in general. The reason for the absence of a state-controlled colonial medicine in the USA may have been the British tradition of a relatively free market for medical services. In contrast, continental European and absolutist states like Denmark had a long tradition of state control of all medical services and so it is important to investigate the role of the colonial administration in relation to the health of the enslaved workers in the Danish West Indies.

80 Arnold, 'Medicine and Colonialism', 1394–1401.
81 Fett, *Working Cures.*

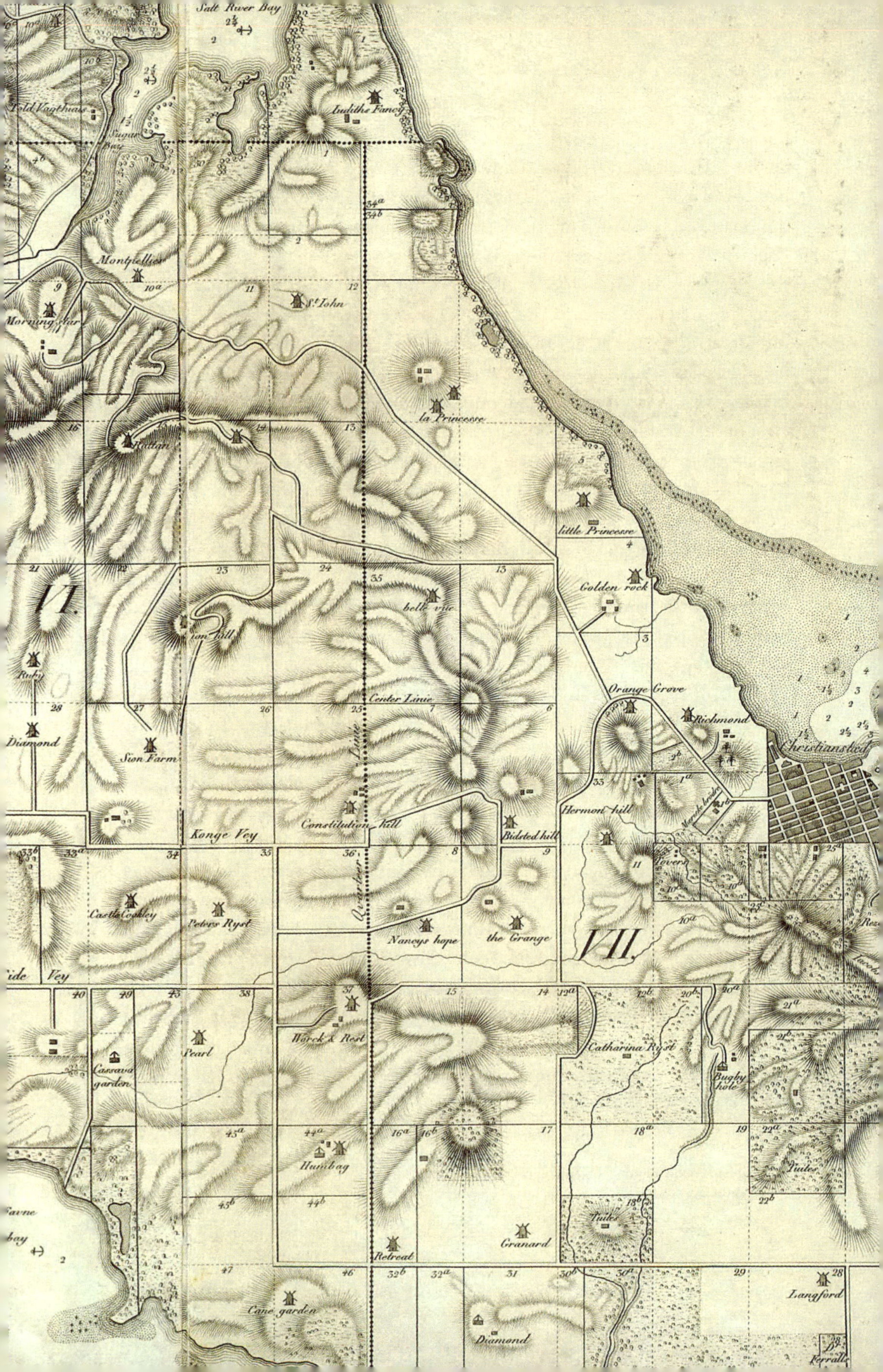

Salt River Bay
Judiths Fancy
Montpellier
St. John
Morning Star
la Princesse
little Princesse
Golden rock
VI.
VII.
Ruby
Diamond
Sion Farm
belle vue
Center Linie
Orange Grove
Richmond
Christiansted
Hermon hill
Constitution hill
Bidsted hill
Konge Vey
Castle Coakley
Peters Ryst
Nancys hope
the Grange
Work & Rest
Pearl
Cassava garden
Catharina Ryst
Bugby hole
Humbug
Retreat
Granard
Tuites
Langford
Cane garden
Diamond
Ferrall

Chapter 2

Context

The state of health among enslaved workers in the Danish West Indies depended to a large extent on the distinctive context of the islands. In order to facilitate the following analyses, this chapter sets out to establish these background factors. I will investigate the general history, geography and ecology of the Danish West Indies, outline the annual production cycle on the sugar plantations, examine the general demography of the West Indian enslaved populations, and present the general development of western medicine, of the health services on the island of St Croix and the medicine of the enslaved. In addition, information about the similar contexts in the British and French West Indies will facilitate the comparative Caribbean perspective.

Danish, British and French West Indian History, Geography and Ecology

The History of the Danish West Indies, 1672–1917

In 1672, the Royal Danish West Indian Company (*Det Kongelige Octroyerede Danske Vestindiske Compagnie*) occupied the island of St Thomas. The purpose was to follow the example of other Western European nations and establish a colony to produce lucrative West Indian goods like coffee, tobacco, indigo, cotton, and sugar. Accordingly, the island was quickly divided into plantations. The knowhow required for plantation production came with English, French, and especially Dutch immigrants whose presence made the Danish West Indian society international from the very beginning.[82]

The first years from colonisation to the War of the Spanish Succession (1701–14) were characterised by a lack of leadership and failing connections with Denmark. However, the wartime conditions meant an upturn in the neutral Danish trade on St Thomas. When peace returned, the positive trends were replaced

82 Ove Hornby, 'Kolonierne i Vestindien', in *Danmarks historie – uden for Danmark*, ed. Svend Ellehøj and Kristof Glamann (Copenhagen: Politiken, 1980), 31–38.

by a recession back to a more normal level, a pattern that was to repeat itself several times in the history of the Danish West Indies. In 1718, the Danish West Indian Company occupied the neighbouring island of St John, which was also laid out for plantations and settled by planters from St Thomas. The expansion continued until 1733 when the company bought the nearby island of St Croix from France. St Croix, or Santa Cruz, was also surveyed and laid out for plantations, but since neither venture capital nor inhabitants could be attracted from Denmark, British planters came to dominate this island.[83]

Plantation agriculture was quickly dominated by the production of sugar, but other crops like cotton and various foodstuffs were also grown. At the same time the workforce became completely dominated by enslaved workers imported from Africa. However, as they died faster than they could reproduce, it was necessary to keep importing fresh enslaved workers in order to maintain the sugar production.[84]

In 1755, the Danish Crown bought the three Danish West Indian islands from the company and initiated a profound change in the administrative system, including the health services. The following year saw the beginning of The Seven Years War (1756–63) which again created a boom in Danish West Indian trade. The reason for this was that Britain's enemies, France, Spain, and the Netherlands, sent their West Indian goods via front men in the Danish West Indian harbours to avoid the British trade embargo. From the Danish West Indies the cargoes were shipped under escort by Danish naval vessels via Copenhagen to the European markets. When the war ended, so did the lucrative trade and a peace depression followed. However, the pattern repeated itself with even greater profits during the American War of Independence (1775–83), the French Revolutionary Wars (1792–1801), and the Napoleonic Wars (1803–15). Yet, this profitable exploitation of Denmark's neutrality had its price. During the French Revolutionary Wars the relationship between Denmark and Britain grew increasingly tense, and a few days before the culmination in the Battle of Copenhagen on 2 April 1801, the Danish West Indies were occupied by Britain. The war ended in 1801 but not until the beginning of 1802 did Denmark regain the islands.[85]

By the beginning of the period 1803–48 two decisive events occurred. First and foremost, the Danish ban against importation of enslaved workers took

83 Hornby, 'Kolonierne i Vestindien', 47–61, 65–67, 75–87, 101–6.

84 Hornby, 'Kolonierne i Vestindien', 127, 184.

85 Hornby, 'Kolonierne i Vestindien', 110–16, 145–46, 151–54, 157–58, 204–11.

effect after a grace period of ten years. However, it was still legal to trade enslaved workers internally in the Danish West Indies. The prohibition was caused by humanist and abolitionist movements, yet also by political and economic considerations, since the British parliament had long been discussing a similar ban, which was eventually implemented in 1807. The prohibition of the slave trade made it necessary for the planters and the colonial administration on St Croix to try to preserve the health and lives of the enslaved workers. The other event was the outbreak of the Napoleonic Wars, which caused Britain to occupy the Danish West Indies in 1807 when Denmark allied itself with Napoleon. Only after the end of the war in 1815 did the islands return to Denmark.[86]

During the years 1815–20, the prosperity in the Danish West Indies reached its zenith. The price of sugar on the world markets was still as high as it had been during the wars, which benefited the Cruzian planters immensely.[87] However, many of the planters had massive debts, which they could only pay instalments on if the income from sugar remained high. Consequently, the drastic fall in sugar prices in the 1820s sent many planters into bankruptcy, and a number of plantations reverted to the Danish state as the planters' main creditor. The economic situation improved somewhat towards the end of the 1830s and in the 1840s, yet at the same time the soil started to show signs of exhaustion and decreasing yields. Furthermore, there was an increasing shortage of labour because of the constantly shrinking population of enslaved workers. Accordingly, by emancipation in 1848 the economic and production situation on St Croix was generally not good.[88]

In the years between 1848 and the sale of the islands to the United States in 1917 conditions did not improve. As early as the 1840s, the Danish state's net profit from owning the Danish West Indies had turned into a deficit.[89] With the emancipation of the enslaved workers, the shortage of labour became chronic despite attempts to import workers from other Caribbean islands and India. Sugar production decreased further, which made the deficit on the colonial finances permanent. The Danish government began to view the islands as an

86 Hornby, 'Kolonierne i Vestindien', 180–89, 255–61.

87 P.P. Sveistrup, *Bidrag til de tidligere dansk-vestindiske Øers økonomiske Historie: Med særligt Henblik på Sukkerproduktion og Sukkerhandel* (Copenhagen: Institut for Historie og Samfundsøkonomi, 1942), 79.

88 Jens Vibæk, 'Dansk Vestindien, 1755–1848: Vestindiens storhedstid', in *Vore gamle tropekolonier* II, ed. Johannes Brøndsted (Copenhagen: Forlaget Fremad, 1966), 312–29.

89 Vibæk, 'Dansk Vestindien, 1755–1848', 331.

economic burden and considered potential buyers. In 1917, Denmark sold the islands to the United States.[90]

Geography, Topography, Meteorology, and Ecology

The former Danish West Indian islands, St Croix, St Thomas, and St John, form part of the cluster of islands called the Virgin Islands and the greater archipelago of The Lesser Antilles. The islands are located east of Puerto Rico between the Atlantic and the Caribbean (see Fig. 2.1 and Fig. 2.2). St Croix is the largest of the three, approximately 213 square kilometres in area. Unlike the two smaller islands, St Croix is not rocky but contains three dominant kinds of landscape. The north-west is mountainous with the highest point being 380 metres above sea level (Mount Eagle). The eastern end is hilly but the elevation is lower than in the north-west. The rest of the island is generally covered by a large plain, which slopes from the mountains in the north to the ocean in the south (see Fig. 2.3).[91] Because of the absence of high mountains to catch, lift, and cool the humid trade winds from the Atlantic, the climate of St Croix is dry tropical.[92] The average monthly temperature ranges between 22 and 32 degrees Celsius.[93] The annual precipitation has been about the same for the last 144 years, and varies between 1400 mm in the north-western mountains and 600 mm on the eastern end and in the south-western area. However, there are great variations in the quantity of precipitation from year to year, especially in the mountains on the north side. The lowest precipitation is in March and the highest from September to November.[94] Generally, the rainy season is from May to November and the dry season from December to April.[95] Compared to other islands in the area the amount of rainfall on St Croix is low, since the annual average is 1,176 mm (measured in the period 1852–1911) whereas Puerto Rico receives about 1,460 mm and Martinique about 2,000 mm per year.[96] Because of the relatively low and variable amount

90 Hornby, 'Kolonierne i Vestindien', 278–79, 283–84, 289–93, 380–83.

91 Sveistrup, *Bidrag*, 1–3.

92 H. Gray Multer and Lee C. Gerhard, eds., *Guidebook to the Geology and Ecology of Some Marine and Terrestrial Environments, St Croix, US Virgin Islands*, Special publications no. 5 (US Virgin Islands: West Indies Laboratory, Fairleigh Dickinson University, 1974), 204.

93 John Cappelen and Jens Juncher Jensen, *Jordens Klima – Guide til vejr og klima i 156 lande* (Copenhagen: Danmarks Meteorologiske Institut, 2001), www.dmi.dk/dmi/tr01-17.pdf (accessed 30-05-2011).

94 Multer and Gerhard, *Guidebook*, 202–5.

95 Charles Frederick Millspaugh, *Flora of the Islands of St Croix* (Chicago: Field Columbian Museum, 1902), 442.

96 Sveistrup, *Bidrag*, 3.

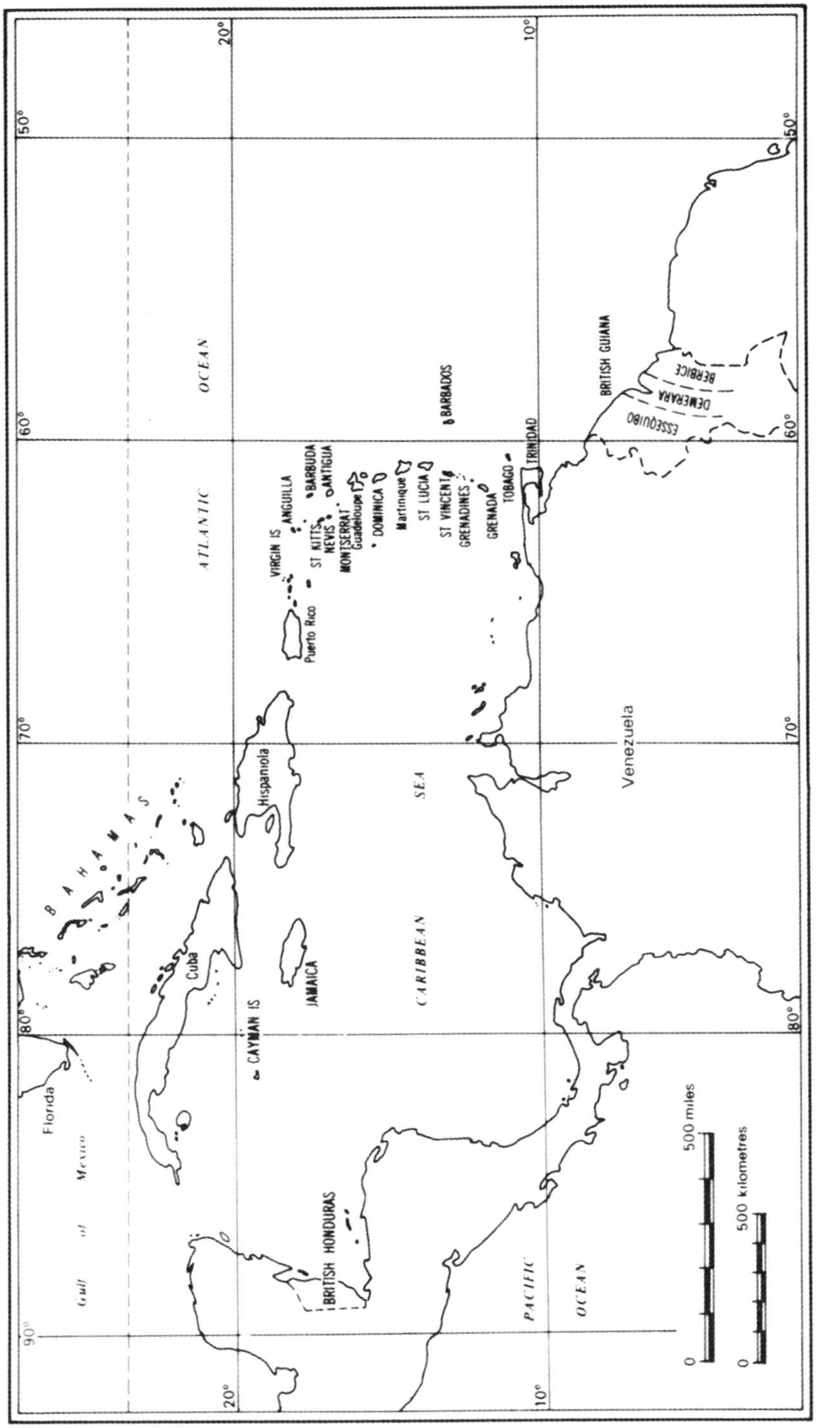

Fig. 2.1: The Caribbean Sea. Higman, *Slave Populations*, xxvi.

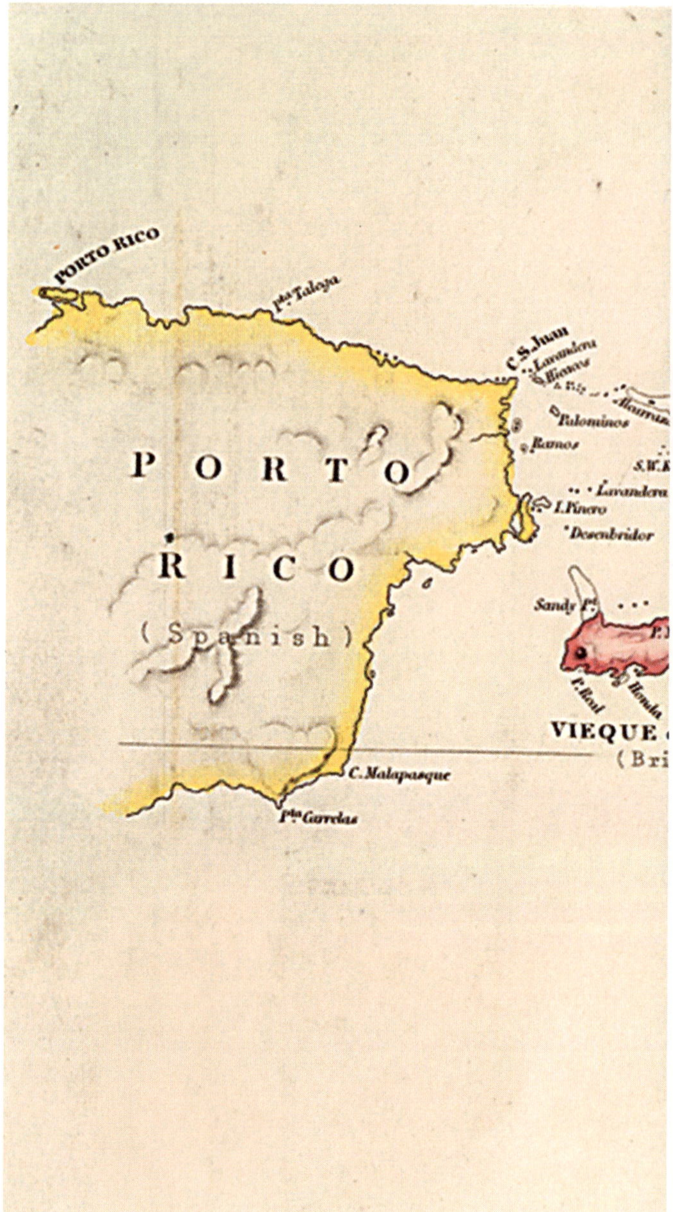

Fig. 2.2: The Danish West Indies with neighbouring islands. Section of *Map of The Leeward Islands*, John Arrowsmith (London, 1844). David Rumsey Historical Map Collection, www.davidrumsey.com (accessed 30-05-2011).

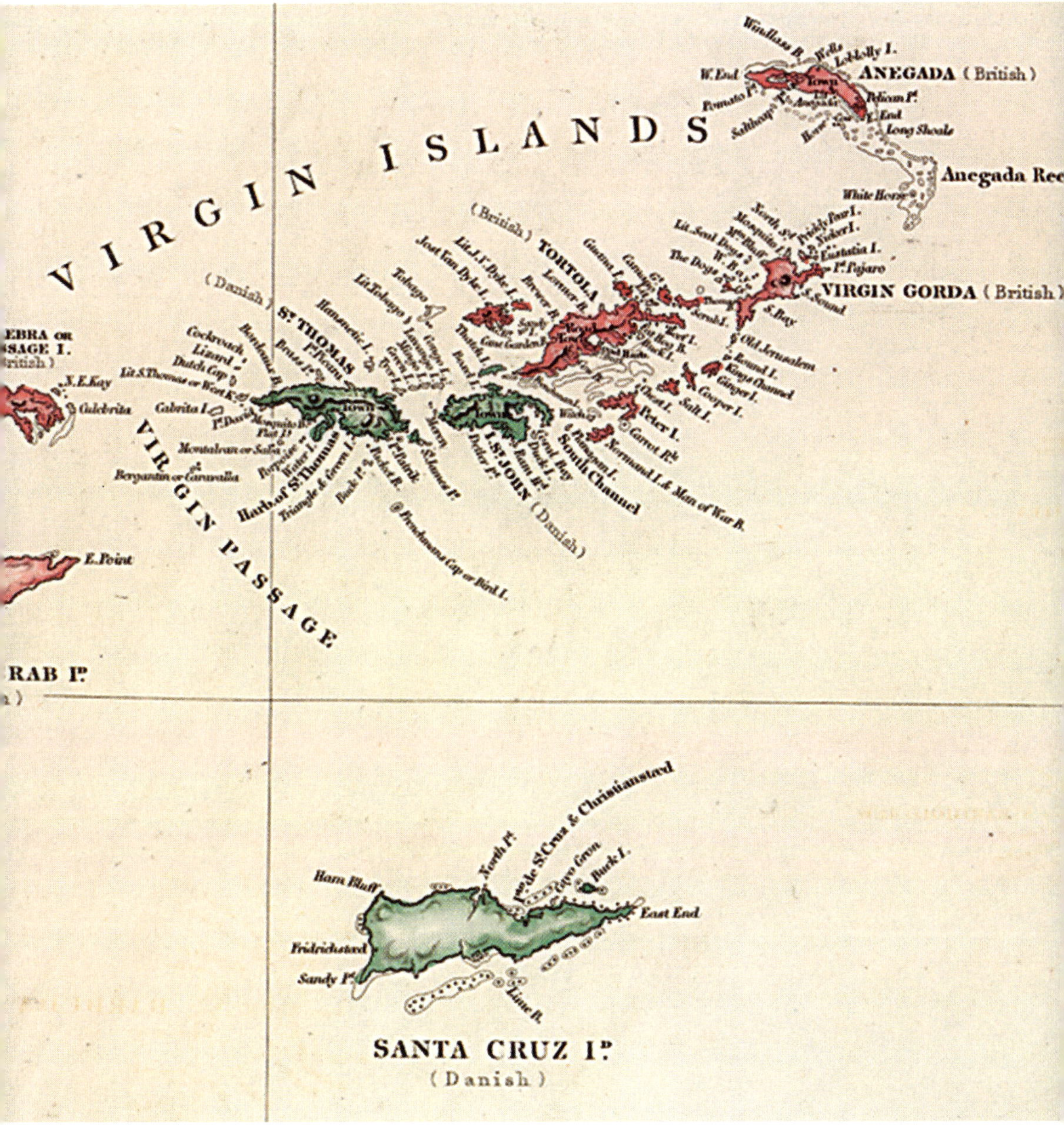
VIRGIN ISLANDS
ANEGADA (British)
Anegada Reef
TORTOLA
(British)
VIRGIN GORDA (British)
St. THOMAS
(Danish)
I. St. JOHN
(Danish)
VIRGIN PASSAGE
South Channel
Old Jerusalem
RAB I.
E. Point
Ham Bluff
North Pt.
East End
Fridrichstad
Sandy Pt.
Buck I.
SANTA CRUZ I.
(Danish)

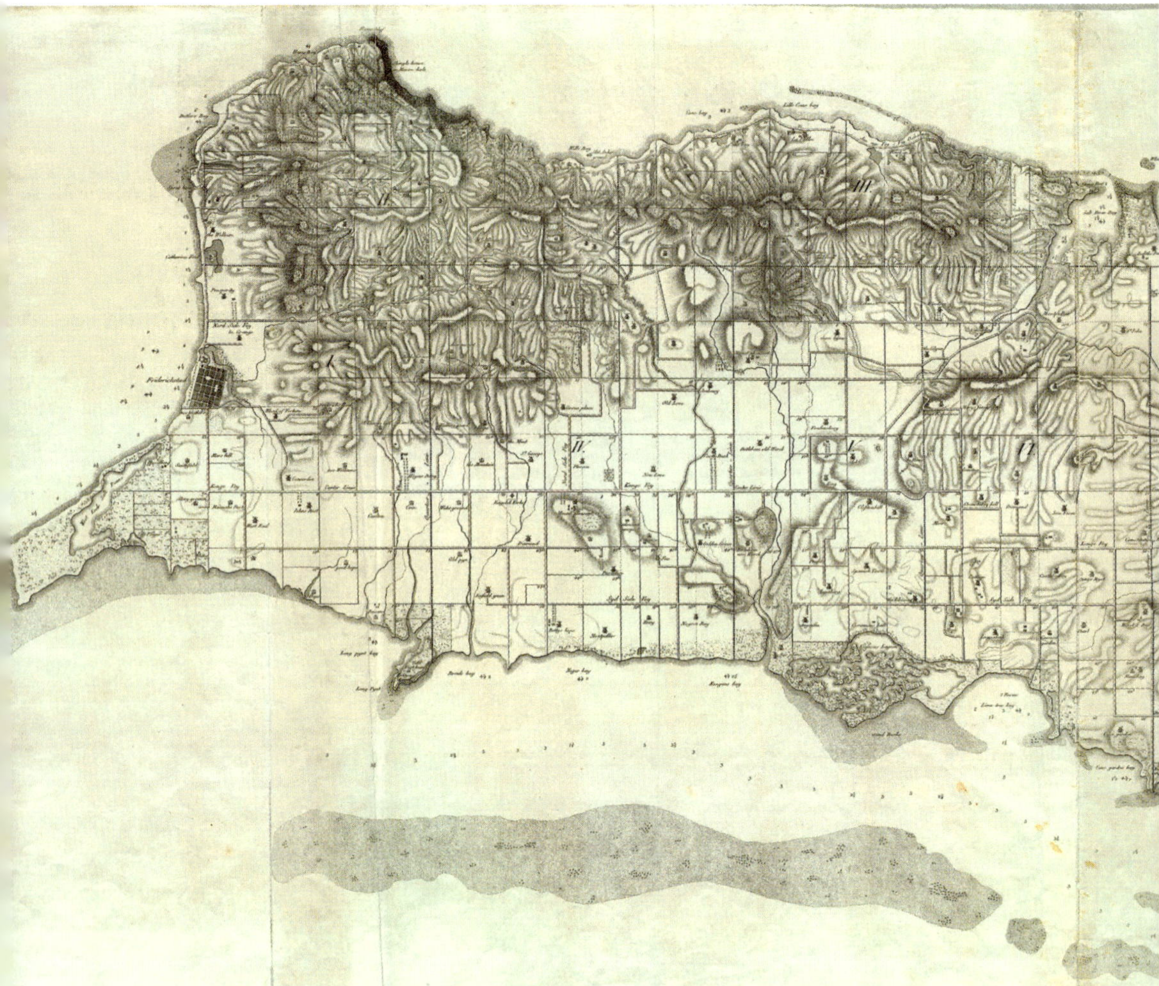
Frederiksted

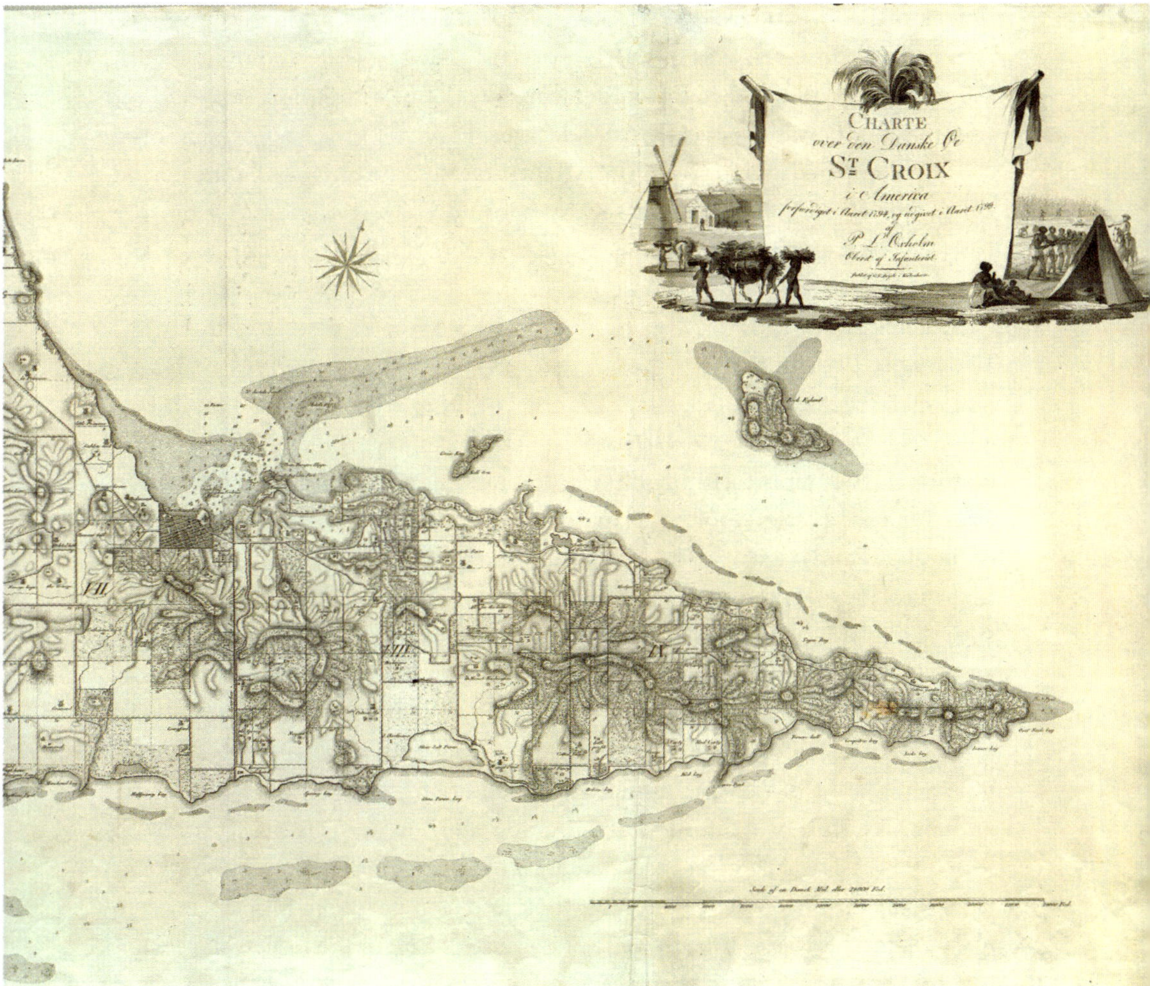

Fig. 2.3: St Croix, 1794. *Charte over den Danske Øe St. Croix i America: forfærdiget i Aaret 1794, og udgivet i Aaret* 1799 by P.L. Oxholm and G.N. Angelo (Copenhagen, 1799). The Royal Library, Collection of Maps and Pictures, Copenhagen.

of precipitation, drought is a recurring problem on St Croix. Furthermore, the rain on St Croix often falls in short, powerful showers, which combined with the constant wind and high temperature results in a high level of evaporation that further desiccates the island.[97] From around June to November the warm, humid trade winds from the Atlantic blow constantly, while the period December to May is characterised by cool north-westerly winds from the North American continent. From August to October, St Croix is occasionally visited by tropical storms and hurricanes.[98]

The Sugar Production

During the period 1803–48, the production of sugar in the various West Indian colonies was carried out in virtually the same way regardless of the national, historical, geographical, and other differences between the colonies. On St Croix, the production took place in the same way it had done since the middle of the eighteenth century. The cultivation started by the 'holing', which meant that the slaves worked the ground with hoes and prepared it for planting the sugar cane. The work was hard and organised as gang labour in which the enslaved worked side by side in a long row hacking their way backwards across the field. They were supervised by the 'driver', an enslaved worker appointed to be foreman or boss. For every four square feet[99] the enslaved dug a square hole with banks of earth around it and filled it with two sticks of sugar cane and a basket full of manure and soil. Soon after, new sugar plants grew up, which the enslaved then had to weed until the plants reached a certain size. If the sugar cane was newly planted, it took fourteen or fifteen months for it to mature, but if it was a 'rattoon' cane, i.e. a cane of a plant previously harvested, it would mature in about twelve months. When the cane went yellow and the leaves withered, it was time to harvest. The strongest enslaved workers worked at the front, cutting down the cane while the other enslaved gathered the cane, tied it into bundles and loaded it onto mules. The children drove the mules to the sugar mill, which was driven by either wind or horse power, and

97 Multer and Gerhard, *Guidebook*, 148.

98 John R. Davis, *Soil Survey of the United States Virgin Islands* (Washington D.C.: United States Department of Agriculture, Natural Resources Conservation Service in Cooperation with the Virgin Islands Department of Planning and Natural Resources, the Virgin Islands Cooperative Extension Service, and the United States Department of Interior, National Park Service. United States Dept. of Agriculture, Natural Resources Conservation Service, 2002), 12–13, www.mo15.nrcs.usda.gov/technical/surveys/caribbean/VI.pdf (accessed 30-05-2011).

99 1 square foot = 0.0985 m².

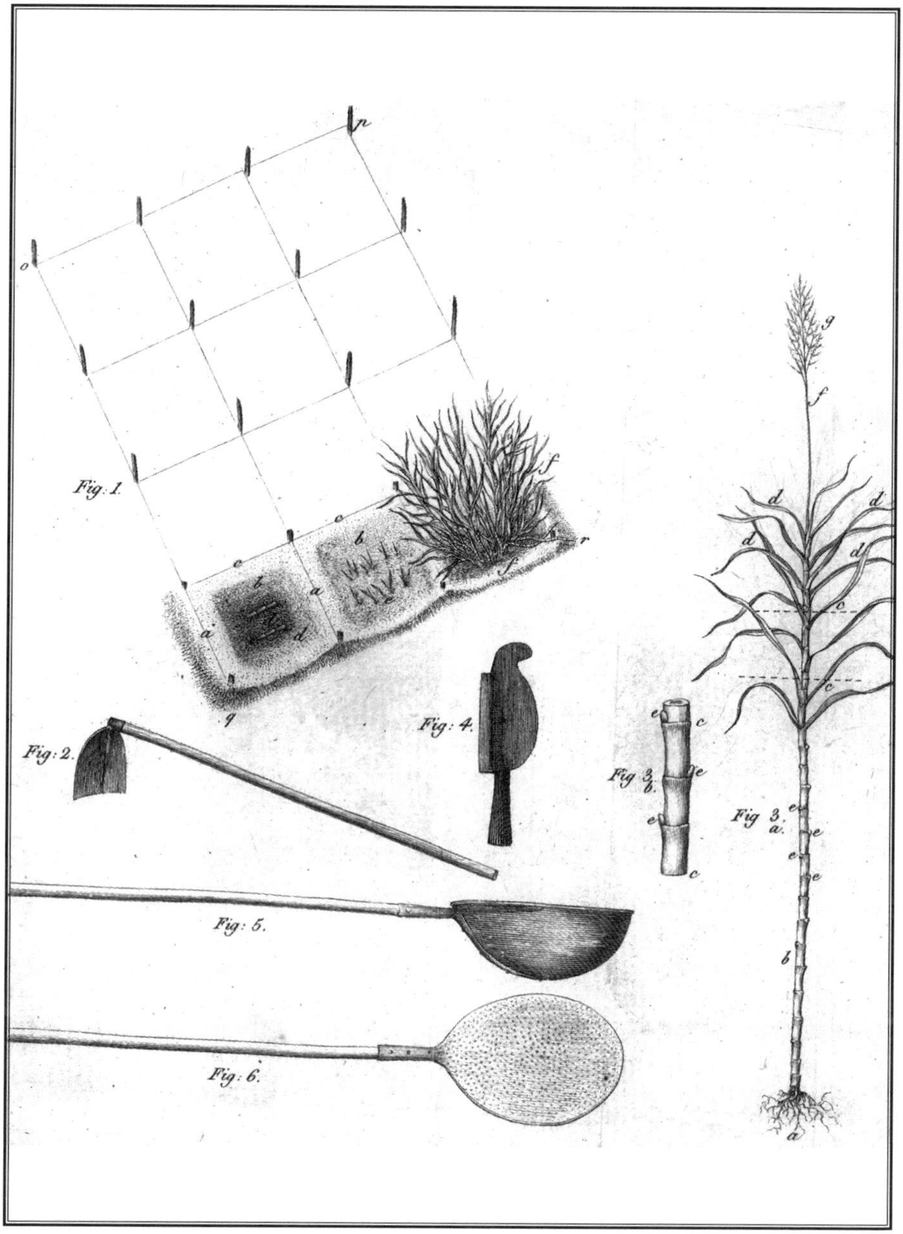

Fig. 2.4: Illustration showing a cane field divided into squares of 4 × 4 feet, the stages in the growth of the sugar cane and the form of the ripe sugar cane. In addition, various tools: the cane knife and the hoe used for the agriculture of sugar, and the scoop and the skimmer used during the boiling process. Oxholm, *De danske Vestindiske Øers Tilstand* (1797), Plan II.

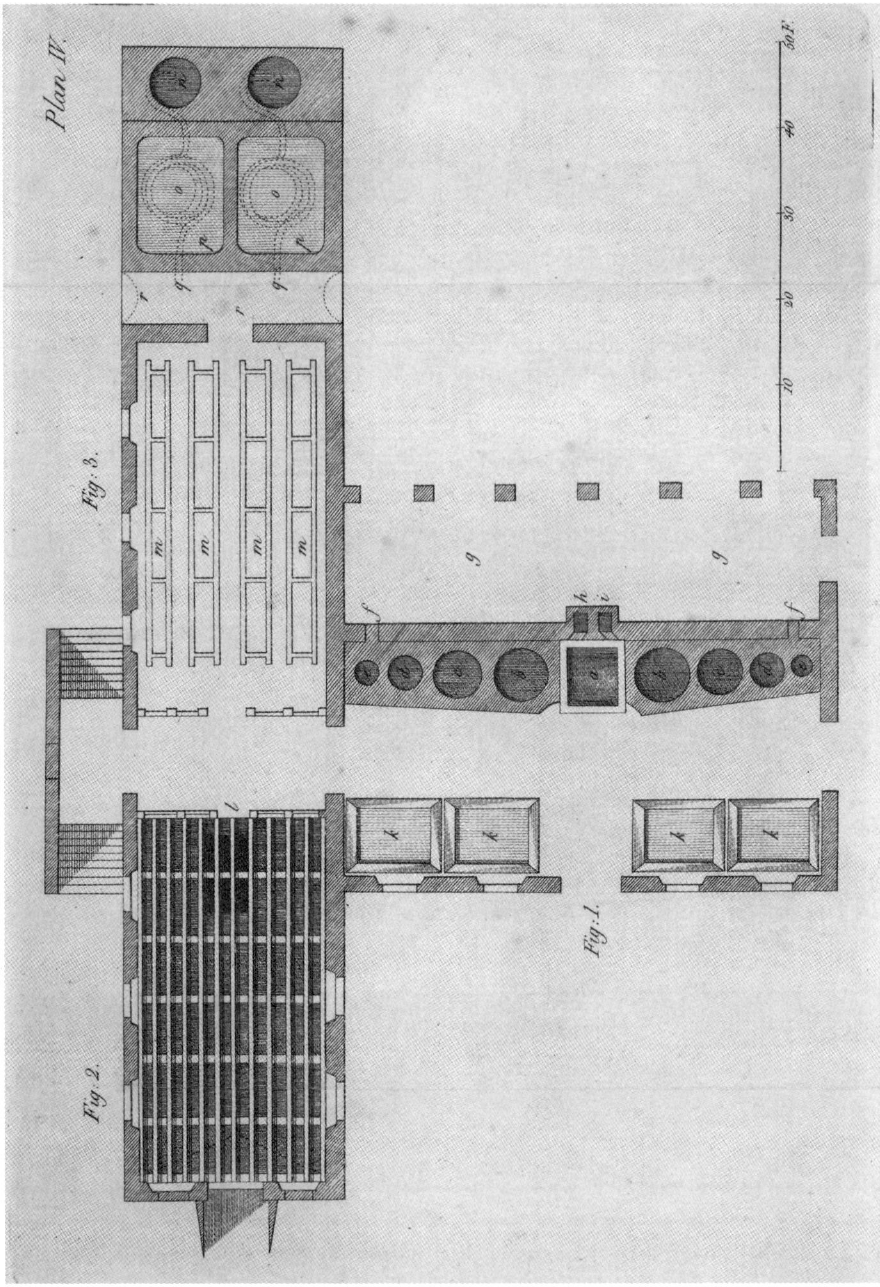

Fig. 2.5: Illustration of a boiling and distillation house with kettles (b, c, d, e), cooling pans (k), the molasses cistern (fig. 2) and distillers (o). Oxholm, *De danske Vestindiske Øers Tilstand* (1797), Plan IV.

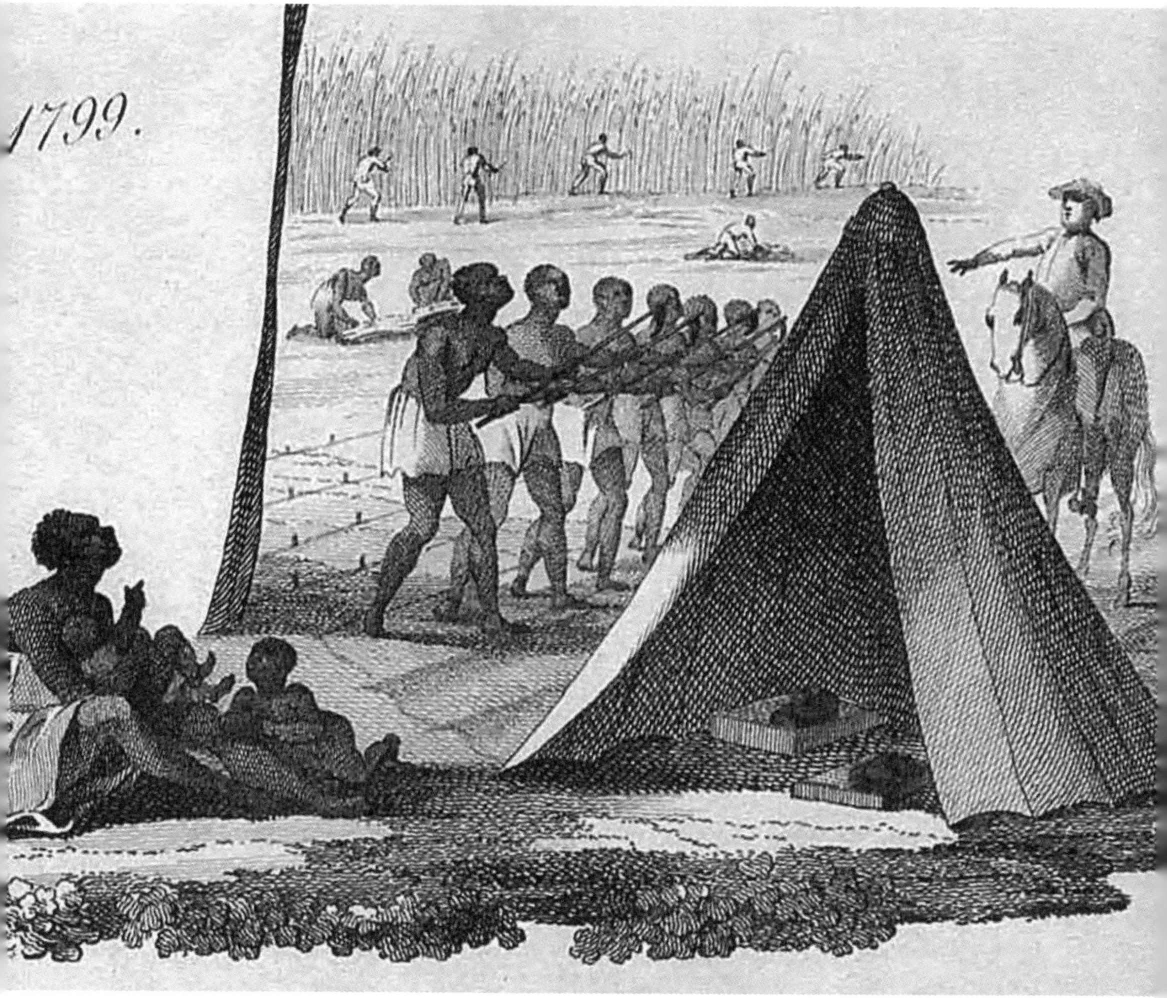

Fig. 2.6: Detail of Fig. 2.3. In the background enslaved workers harvesting sugar cane, in the middleground enslaved holing the field under supervision of a Euro-Caribbean overseer on horseback, and in the foreground an enslaved woman nursing the small children while their mothers are working the fields.

here the cane was crushed twice between the rotating rollers. From the mill, the cane juice was led to the first and largest of the kettles in the boiling house where the processing began. The fire under the kettles was fuelled by bagasse or megasse (dried cane refuse left over after the milling). After being boiled in several kettles of decreasing size and cooled in a special pan, the crystallised brown sugar (called muscovado) was shovelled into perforated barrels for draining. The syrup that drained off the sugar, called molasses, was collected with the scum removed during boiling and put aside for fermentation and later distillation into rum. After draining, the sugar barrels were sealed and carted for shipment from one of the harbours. The rum was also sold or consumed on the plantation.[100]

The annual rhythm of the sugar production to a large extent determined the life and health of the enslaved plantation workers. On St Croix, in the period 1803–48, the heavy work during holing was normally carried out from September to December but occasionally holing also took place from February to April.[101] The full duration of the harvest season was from January to August, when the enslaved workers harvested the sugar cane that had been planted the previous year.[102]

The British and French West Indies: History, Geography, and Ecology

The conditions in the various West Indian colonies in relation to history, geography, ecology, economy and so on were very diverse but of great importance for the health of the enslaved workers in these colonies and the health policy carried out by their governments. Geographically and ecologically the British West Indies ranged from the mainland colonies of British Honduras and British Guiana (Demerara-Essequibo and Berbice), through larger island colonies like Jamaica and Trinidad to many smaller islands like Barbados. In the mainland colonies, the settlements were located along the coast and rivers, while the inland was covered with impenetrable rainforest. In British Guiana,

100 Peter Lotharius Oxholm, *De danske Vestindiske Øers Tilstand i henseende til Population, Cultur, Finance-Forfatning i Anledning af nogle Breve fra St Croix, indrykkede i det Politiske og Physiske Magazin for Marts og April Maaneder 1797, hvortil er føiet Beskrivelse om Sukkerets Fabrikation, med 4 Planer* (Copenhagen, 1797), 42–47.

101 See for instance the plantation records of the royal plantations North Star and Longford, which cover the period 1830–35, Danish National Archive (DNA), West Indian Local Archives (WILA), no. 46.17.46 and 46.17.55.

102 Highfield, *Observations*, 31–32 (original: Brady, 1829).

the arable land was protected by embankments and intersected by canals for irrigation. On the larger islands like Jamaica, there were high mountain ranges, occasionally volcanic, but also large areas of cleared farmland. The same pattern was found on the smaller islands, for instance Dominica, St Lucia, and St Vincent. Other of the smaller islands were made up of low-lying limestone beds with sandy, infertile soil and surrounded by mangroves and coral reefs like for instance the Bahamas and Cayman islands.

In terms of meteorology, these colonies were also quite diverse. Of course, the temperature was uniformly tropical with limited seasonal variations, but the amount of precipitation varied greatly. The islands with the lowest elevations received the least amount of rain and experienced the longest droughts, whereas the high mountains in other islands acted like condensers and provided larger amounts of rain. However, within each colony the water could be distributed very unevenly because of the geography of the mountains.

The British West Indian colonies also had different histories, which determined their level of development in terms of economy and production. The British colonisation in the Caribbean took place in three stages. The first stage between 1650 and 1700 saw the colonisation of St Kitts, Barbados, Nevis, Antigua, Montserrat, Jamaica, Virgin Islands, Anguilla, Barbuda, Bahamas, Cayman Islands, and British Honduras. The colonisation was a private enterprise, which caused these colonies to form their own legislative assemblies, and accordingly they achieved a greater independence from the central authorities in London. The islands of Barbados, St Kitts, Nevis, Antigua, Montserrat, and Virgin islands quickly developed a monoculture of sugar producing plantations, while the remaining colonies took up other kinds of production. Accordingly, these last colonies can be considered marginal and not comparable to the Danish West Indies. The second stage of the colonisation took place in the 1760s through the acquisition of existing colonies from other European powers. In this group were Dominica, St Vincent, Tobago, Grenada, and the Grenadines. These colonies never became completely dominated by sugar production, but they also established their own legislative assemblies. In the third and final stage of colonisation, the British acquired the colonies of Trinidad (1797) and St Lucia, Demerara-Essequibo and Berbice (1803). These colonies were dominated by sugar production but they were not granted their own legislative assemblies because the British government wanted to control the slave trade and the treatment of the enslaved in the new colonies. The emancipation of the enslaved workers in the British West Indies took place in 1834.[103]

It is evident that the health conditions of the enslaved in the various British West Indian colonies had to be very diverse because of the geographical and climatological differences, but also because a long history of sugar production had exhausted the soil in some colonies, whereas in others the sugar production had only recently begun. This created very different working and living conditions for the enslaved workers. Furthermore, the differences in governmental structures decided what effect the initiatives of the central government could have in the colonies, for instance in relation to health.

In 1804, the French colony of St Domingue declared itself independent of France as the republic of Haiti. Consequently, the French West Indian possessions in the period in question here were limited to the islands of Guadeloupe and Martinique.[104] These islands were far more similar geographically, topographically and ecologically than the many different colonies that made up the British West Indies. Both islands are of volcanic origin and dominated by mountains above 1,400 metres. The mountains influence the rainfall, which is very diverse depending on the locality. Generally, the rainfall is most plentiful on the eastern side of the mountains and the greater the altitude. The western side and the low-lying areas receive less rainfall, but not below the average of St Croix. The temperature is tropical, stable all year round and about the same as on other Caribbean islands. Both islands are located in the tropical hurricane zone and they are regularly affected by hurricanes. In terms of ecology, both islands are forested in their natural state, yet the type of forest varies with the rainfall from rainforest to dry, deciduous forest. In several places, the soil is extremely fertile because of the volcanic origin but other zones are dry and rugged. Finally, the islands also contain coral reefs, lagoons, and mangroves.[105]

Guadeloupe and Martinique were colonised by France in 1635, and from 1674 the French Crown gained direct control of the colonies through a local governor. In 1787, the colonies received local legislative assemblies and under the French Revolution they obtained representation in the National Assembly. When the French monarchy was restored in 1815 after the Napoleonic Wars, both of these systems were abolished and the central government in Paris took

103 Higman, *Slave Populations*, 40–45.

104 Since 1664, France also possessed the colony of French Guiana; however, as it is normally not perceived as belonging to the West Indies it has been left out of this investigation.

105 Pierre Pluchon, ed., *Histoire des Antilles et de la Guyane* (Toulouse: Edouard Privat, 1982), 19–26.

over the direct control of the islands. In 1834 the local assemblies were reinstated but with limited authority. Following the revolution in 1848, the colonies again obtained representation in the National Assembly and their connections with France were strengthened. The year 1848 also saw the emancipation of the enslaved workers in the French West Indies.[106]

From the above it is evident that the Danish, British, and French West Indian colonies had a lot in common, but that the geographical, ecological, and historical differences were large enough to create considerable differences in the living conditions of the enslaved workers.

Demography in West Indian Enslaved Populations

Until emancipation enslaved populations in most sugar producing West Indian colonies suffered a negative demographic development. With the bans on imports of new enslaved workers from Africa (1803/1807/1818) this became a vital problem that stimulated European and Euro-Caribbean interest in the health of enslaved workers. In the following, I will examine the main problems in the demography of the enslaved of the British, French and Danish West Indies.

According to Barry W. Higman's authoritative study *Slave Populations of the British Caribbean, 1807–1834,* the British West Indian colonies experienced a continuous decline in the enslaved population from the British prohibition of the slave trade in 1807 to the emancipation of the enslaved in the British possessions in 1834.[107] In total, the decrease amounted to around 14 per cent, i.e. about 0.5 per cent annually. However, the development was far from the same in all colonies. Some experienced an increase in the enslaved population, while some experienced a drastic decline.[108] If we focus specifically on the sugar producing colonies and on the part of the development caused by natural increase, i.e. the number of births in proportion to the number of deaths, only the colony of Barbados maintained positive natural growth throughout the period from 1810 onwards (see Fig. 2.7). The old sugar colonies from the first phase of colonisation generally maintained positive natural growth throughout most of

106 Isaac Dookhan, *A Pre-Emancipation History of the West Indies* (London: Longman, 1976), 121–22.

107 The following section is based on B.W. Higman, *Slave Populations of the British Caribbean, 1807–1834.* In this book, Higman undertakes the most thorough comparative demographic study of any enslaved population to date. Accordingly, his book is indisputably at the centre of historical research on the demography of West Indian enslaved workers. See also Scarano, 'Slavery and Emancipation', 267, 269.

108 Higman, *Slave Populations,* 72–76.

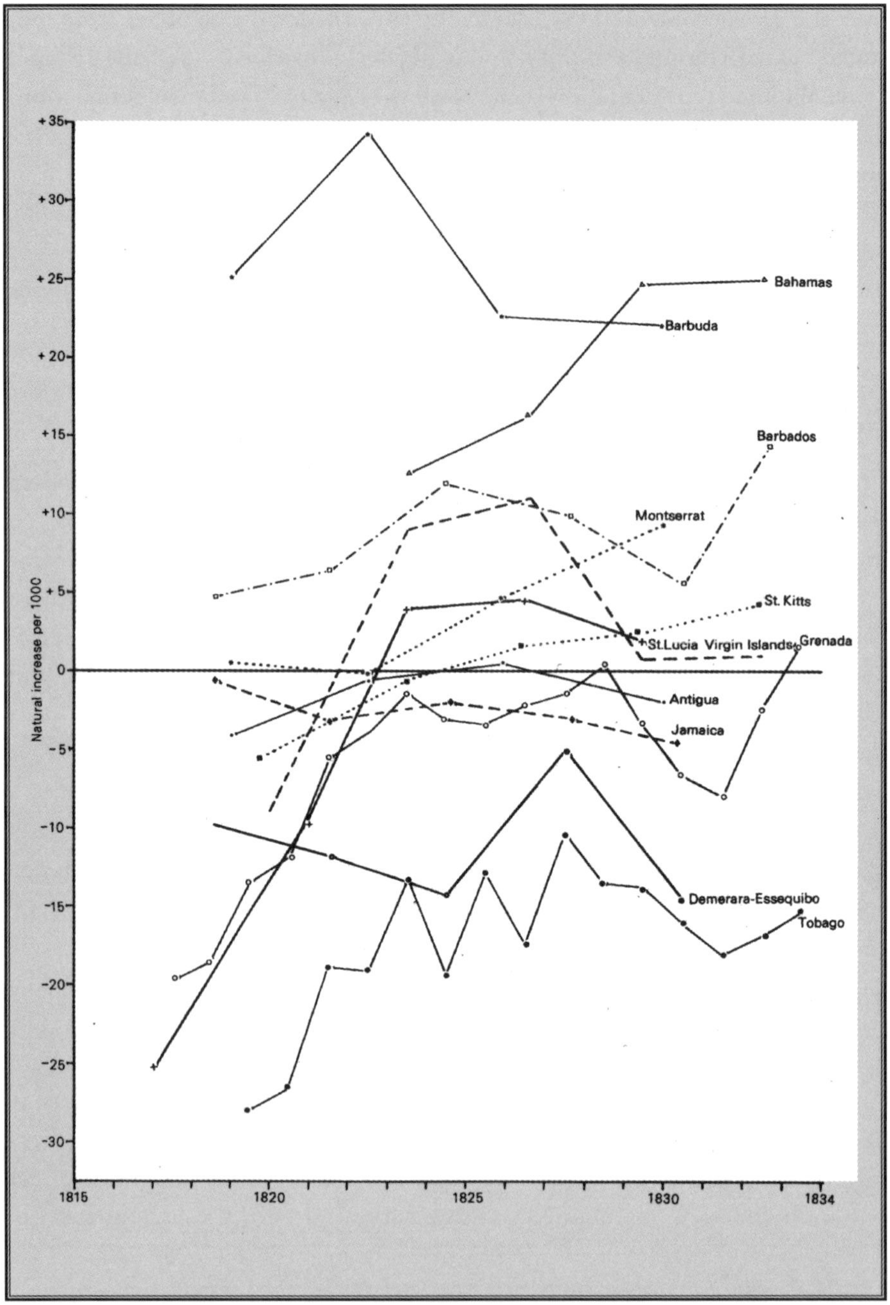

Fig. 2.7: The natural increase per 1,000 individuals in the enslaved populations of the British West Indian colonies, 1815–34. Higman, *Slave Populations of the British Caribbean, 1807–1834*, 312.

the period, while the younger sugar colonies from the second and third phase experienced a constant negative natural growth, which, however, was gradually reduced through the period.[109]

The fundamental reasons for the decline in the enslaved population can be found in two factors: the mortality and the fertility. According to Higman, the mortality of the enslaved workers was influenced by several circumstances. First and foremost, there was a strong correlation between sugar production and high mortality among the enslaved workers – a crucial relationship which was known at the time, and which has been confirmed by other researchers in other geographical areas.[110] All other crops raised in the British West Indies correlated to lower levels of mortality. Additionally, there was a marked difference between the mortality of the different occupations on the plantations, as the majority of the enslaved working in the fields had a higher mortality than enslaved artisans and domestics. However, it was not only a question of the nature of the work but also of the working hours, living conditions, and nutrition. Higman concludes that the higher mortality of the enslaved working in the fields was caused by a combination of hard work, the unhygienic conditions under which they lived and seasonal problems with the food supply.[111] Unfortunately, Higman's material does not offer any information on child mortality, which played a significant role in the overall mortality rate among the enslaved workers of St Croix (on which, more below).

The fertility of the enslaved workers was also influenced by several factors. First, the different age and sex distributions in the various enslaved populations were important. Both of these factors depended on when the import of enslaved workers from Africa had stopped and how intense it had been until then. Colonies which had imported many enslaved workers right up to the enforcement of the ban on imports in 1807 (i.e. the young sugar colonies) had a young enslaved population with high fertility. However, they also had an uneven sex distribution because the British planters, like most West Indian planters, preferred to buy young, male enslaved workers. In these populations, the high mortality

109 Higman, *Slave Populations*, 307–11.

110 Higman, *Slave Populations*, 324–29, 374–75. Concerning enslaved mortality and sugar production in Louisiana (USA) see Michael Tadman, 'The Demographic Cost of Sugar: Debate on Slave Societies and Natural Increase in the Americas', *The American Historical Review* 105, no. 5 (2000). For a similar investigation of Surinam (Dutch West Indies), see Alex van Stipriaan, *Surinaams Contrast, Roofbouw en overleven in een Caraïbische plantagekolonie, 1750–1863* (Leiden: Koninklijk Instituut voor taal-, land- en volkenkunde, 1993), 316–18.

111 Higman, *Slave Populations*, 324–29, 333–35, 347.

only caused a small decrease in the years after 1807, since fertility was still quite high, yet from around 1820 fertility began to decrease with the increasing age of the enslaved, which accelerated the population decline.

In contrast to this situation, the import of enslaved workers in the old sugar colonies had long been minimal, which caused the sex and age distributions in these enslaved populations to level out even before 1807. This also meant that they had only very few African-born individuals in their enslaved populations after 1807 and since Creole enslaved workers (i.e. enslaved workers born in the West Indies) were always more fertile than African-born ones, this had a positive effect on population growth. The best example of this is Barbados, which had positive natural growth after about 1810.[112]

In the French West Indies, here represented by the island of Martinique, slavery was abolished as early as 1794 as an effect of the French Revolution. Nonetheless, slavery was restored in 1802 when the French recaptured the island from the British. In the following years, the fighting continued in connection with the Napoleonic Wars and accordingly we have no useful data on the demography of the enslaved population of the island from this period. After the end of the war, in 1818, the slave trade was abolished, yet continued illegally and on a considerable scale until about 1830.[113] Between 1814 and 1831, Martinique imported around 25,000 enslaved workers.[114] The slaves imported illegally were of course not recorded and accordingly the records for this period are less reliable than one would wish. Generally, it is safe to say that despite the illegal imports there was a massive decline in the enslaved population during this period. For the years 1832–47, the records are relatively reliable and they show a fall in the total enslaved population on Martinique from 86,000 to 74,100 individuals. It is not known what percentage of this decline was caused by manumissions. Based on these numbers the actual annual mortality among the enslaved workers between 1837 and 1847 has been calculated to have been around 30.4 deaths per 1,000 slaves.[115]

As to the fertility among the enslaved population on Martinique, calculations for the entire period 1660–1847 have shown an average of 29.9 births

112 Higman, *Slave Populations*, 78, 123, 142.

113 Geneviève Leti, *Santé et société esclavagiste à la Martinique, 1802–1848* (Paris: L'Harmatan, 1998), 7–9, 23–27.

114 Stanley L. Engerman and Barry W. Higman, 'The Demographic Structure of the Caribbean Slave Societies in the Eighteenth and Nineteenth Centuries', in *General History of the Caribbean* III, ed. Franklin W. Knight (London: UNESCO Publishing, 1997), 62.

115 Leti, *Santé et société*, 25, 30.

per 1,000 enslaved per year. However, in the period 1834–47 the average was around 32 per 1,000 enslaved per year.[116] Accordingly, the growth in the entire enslaved population on Martinique was generally positive in the period 1834–47, because the average fertility was higher than the mortality. Nonetheless, the growth was not positive among the enslaved workers on the island's sugar plantations. The very incomplete material available from sugar plantations show a mortality averaging 42.49 per 1,000 enslaved per year and a fertility of 28.96 per 1,000 enslaved per year.[117] So, the demographic development was negative among the enslaved workers on sugar plantations, and again we have reason to believe that the cause was specific factors related to the production of sugar.[118] With the French revolution of 1848, the enslaved workers in the French West Indies were emancipated.

Returning to the Danish West Indies, the number of enslaved workers on the island of St Croix generally grew after the takeover by the Danish state in 1755 until the abolition of the (external) slave trade in 1803. After a period of stagnation beginning around 1780, the imports increased dramatically from 1792 to 1803 because of special state-funded credit facilities for the purchase of enslaved workers in anticipation of the enforcement of the abolition law. It was only this import of new enslaved workers from Africa that caused the increase in the number, since the natural increase of the enslaved population in the Danish West Indian was about minus 1.1 per cent annually in the years 1780–1804.[119] This general negative trend for the whole of the Danish West Indies continued more or less unchanged after the abolition of the slave trade, and in 1846 the enslaved population on St Croix had decreased to around 70 per cent of its 1804 level.[120] Part of the decline was caused by manumissions but even when they are excluded, the population decreased by on average 107 enslaved individuals per year between 1804 and 1846 (see Fig. 2.8).[121]

116 Myriam Cottias, 'La Martinique: Babylone fertile ou terre stérile? Des discours sur la fécondité aux indicateurs démographiques et sociaux (XVIIe-XIXe siècle)', *Annales de démographie historique* (1992), 207.

117 Leti, *Santé et société*, 28, 258–60.

118 Engerman and Higman, 'The Demographic Structure', 72.

119 Svend E. Green-Pedersen, 'Slave Demography in the Danish West Indies and the Abolition of the Danish Slave Trade', in *The Abolition of the Atlantic Slave Trade: Origins and Effects in Europe, Africa, and the Americas*, ed. David Eltis and James Walvin (Madison: University of Wisconsin Press, 1981), 234–35, 238–39.

120 Asmussen, *Slavedemografi*, 35–36.

121 The increase of free coloured in the period 1792–1834: 3411 – 1164 = 2247 free coloured. The annual increase (42 years): 2247/42 = 53.5 new free coloured per year. Decrease in the number of enslaved workers in the period 1804–46: 22076 – 15310 = 6766 enslaved. The annual decrease (42 years): 6766/42

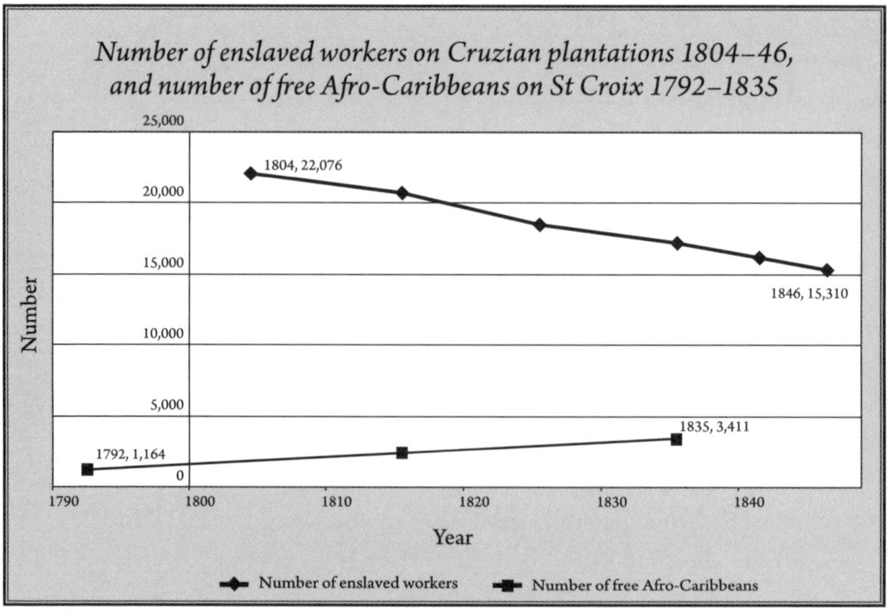

Fig. 2.8: Source: Table 2.1 and 2.2.

Because the principal industry of St Croix was sugar production, most of the enslaved worked in the fields and lived in the area with the largest plantations and the most intensive agriculture, which was the level central plain in Queen's, King's and Prince's Quarters (see Fig. 2.9).[122] In 1804, the sex distribution among the enslaved workers on plantations was 109 men per 100 women. This was a consequence of the traditional purchasing strategy of the planters, because they had preferred to buy male workers for the hard work in the fields. During the years up to 1848, the distribution gradually changed to a predominance of women so that in 1848 there were 94 men per 100 women.[123] The population's age distribution was also marked by the purchase strategy of the planters, because the distribution did not form a normal age pyramid, but showed a disproportionately large percentage of people of working and fertile age (aged roughly between 20 and 40), which the planters had preferred in their purchases. In 1846, the age distribution had changed, so that the percentage of

= 161.10 enslaved per year. Estimated real decrease in the number of enslaved workers in the period 1804–46 due to mortality: 161.10 – 53.5 = 107.6 enslaved per year. See Asmussen, *Slavedemografi*, 37.

122 Asmussen, *Slavedemografi*, 38–39.

123 Asmussen, *Slavedemografi*, 40–41.

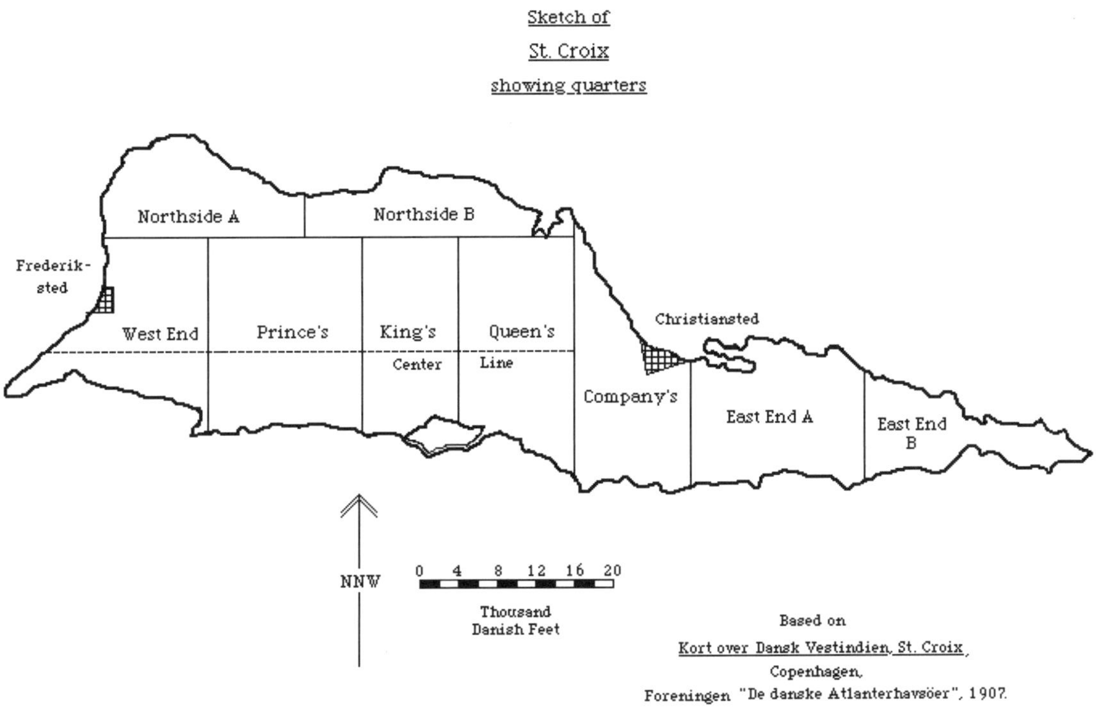

Fig. 2.9: The nine quarters of St Croix. Sketch by Daniel Hopkins et al., http://cas.umkc.edu/StCroix/ (accessed 30-05-2011).

enslaved workers either younger than 20 or older than 40 had increased, yet the percentage of children was still remarkably low. Of this population, the Creole enslaved workers made up the largest part.[124]

As mentioned above, the reason for the negative demographic trend was not manumissions, but a deficit of births compared to deaths. The mortality rate among the enslaved plantation workers was high throughout the period and at no time did the number of births surpass the number of deaths. In 1804, the annual death rate amounted to around 38 per 1,000 enslaved workers and in 1846 to around 44 per 1,000 enslaved. In comparison, the death rate in Denmark in the period 1850–60 was around 21 per 1,000 inhabitants. The decisive factor among the enslaved was child mortality, as up to 40 per cent of those who died

124 Asmussen, *Slavedemografi*, 43, 47, 49.

were under 5 years of age. About 25 per cent of all those who died under the age of one died within the first fourteen days, which amounts to between 10 and 15 per cent of all deaths. In Denmark, infant mortality was at about the same level, but from the age of one, the mortality of the enslaved children greatly exceeded the level in Denmark. The lowest mortality rate amongst the enslaved population was for those between 10 and 20 years of age, after which it increased again. Finally, there was a significantly higher rate of mortality among male enslaved than among females, which explains the change in the sex distribution from a surplus of men to a surplus of women.[125]

The fertility of the enslaved population is difficult to calculate because of the incompleteness of the source material. However, it does seem to have increased slightly during the period, from under 30 births per 1,000 enslaved workers per year in 1804 to around 34 births per 1,000 in 1846. In Denmark at that time the birth rate was between 30 and 32 per 1,000 inhabitants, and so fertility among the enslaved plantation workers was not as low as claimed by many contemporaries.[126]

To sum up, we can conclude that the reason for the negative demographic development among the enslaved plantation workers in the Danish West Indies in the period between 1804 and 1848 was not low fertility, but a high mortality rate during childhood and adulthood.[127] The reason for this pattern does not seem to be demography, but it could have been caused by the nature of the work carried out, at least for enslaved over 10 years of age who were regarded as old enough to participate in the hard work. Nevertheless, as previously mentioned child mortality made up a substantial part of the excess mortality and this cannot be immediately explained by the detrimental effects of hard work in the sugar production. Here factors like inadequate nutrition, deficient hygiene and other physical factors must have played a larger role. In that context, it is relevant to pay attention to how the population developed after 1848. It turns out that the high mortality rate continued in the Cruzian countryside up until the 1880s, when improvements in the system of midwives finally managed to reduce infant mortality, which was still of disastrous proportions. In the period 1872–87, the average mortality in the rural population of former enslaved work-

125 Asmussen, *Slavedemografi*, 53, 58–59, 61, 63–64.
126 Asmussen, *Slavedemografi*, 66–67, 69.
127 Regarding this question, Asmussen's results are in accordance with those of Hans Christian Johansen, yet more precise because they only deal with St Croix. See: Hans Christian Johansen, 'Slave Demography of the Danish West Indian Islands', *The Scandinavian Economic History Review* 29 (1981).

ers was 1433 deaths per 1,000 births, while in the period 1888–99 it decreased to an average of 933 deaths per 1,000 births.[128] In other words, it does not seem as if the reduction in workload that followed emancipation, and the freedom to acquire their own food, in itself had a sufficiently positive impact on infant mortality, and so on the negative demographic development on the sugar plantations. Accordingly, there is even more reason to believe that the workload of the enslaved plantation workers in sugar production was not the only cause of the excess mortality, but that it was more likely caused by a larger complex of factors surrounding the health of the enslaved and later the emancipated workers.

To sum up, the general demographic developments among the enslaved workers in the British, French and Danish sugar colonies were very much alike. In the vast majority of the colonies, the natural increase was negative. Everything seems to indicate that the main reason was the sugar production, but that the workload was not the only factor. In his study of the British West Indies, Higman has pointed to living conditions and nutrition as other important factors. Similarly, the material from the Danish West Indies suggests that the excess mortality was caused by a larger synergic complex of factors surrounding the sugar plantations.

The Development of Western Medicine and the Health Service on St Croix

Euro-Caribbean medical perceptions, treatments and prophylactic initiatives concerning enslaved workers were rooted in European medicine. To establish this important context for the contested management of the health of the enslaved, I will explore the state of European medicine in the first half of the nineteenth century, its perceptions of the Caribbean (tropical) environment and the health service on St Croix compared to those of the British and French West Indies.

Western Medicine: Development and Perception of Illness

Between 1803 and 1848, Western medicine experienced a rapid development. From antiquity until about the middle of the nineteenth century, the foundation of Western medicine was the so-called theory of humoral pathology. In brief, this perception of illness specified that disease was caused by an imbal-

128 Hoxcer Jensen, *From Serfdom*, 88–89n 25, 202–3.

ance between the four humours, blood, phlegm, yellow bile and black bile. The imbalance could be corrected by removing the excess humour and/or increasing the amount of the other humours. In a holistic sense, the four humours were connected to the four 'qualities' (warm, cold, dry, wet), the four corners of the world (North, South, East, West), the four tempers (sanguine, choleric, phlegmatic, melancholic) etc. These qualities were also present in the many different factors that had the potential of bringing the four humours out of balance. Two of the most important factors were wrong diet and the local environment, i.e. geographical, topographical, and meteorological conditions.[129]

One environmental factor, which had been known since antiquity to influence health but became the focus of many discussions in the period in question, was 'miasma'. The word meant 'bad air' in every sense of the word, especially when caused by pollution in the form of rotting biological matter, as it was known from latrines, churchyards, stagnant ponds, swamps, jungles and other places with dirt and impurities.[130] The bad air was detectable through the smell and was according to the theory the cause of epidemic diseases, because it contained seeds of disease generated by the decay of filth. However, it was not clear exactly how miasma caused infection. Furthermore, the miasma theory was not the only explanation for epidemic diseases. Parallel to and in competition with this theory, there was another equally old theory, which stated that infection was contagious, i.e. that it went directly from person to person. This theoretical dispute had a great impact on the efficiency of quarantine systems, which were founded on the principle of contagion. Nevertheless, the supporters of both theories did agree that generally infection could be prevented by removing garbage, filth, and dirt.[131]

In the latter part of the humoral pathologic period, the end of the eighteenth and the first half of the nineteenth centuries, the doctor's[132] diagnosis was still carried out using the five senses. This meant to feel the patient's pulse and tem-

129 Vivian Nutton, 'Humoralism', in *Companion Encyclopedia of the History of Medicine*, vol. 1, ed. W.F. Bynum and Roy Porter (London: Routledge, 1993).

130 Caroline Hannaway, 'Environment and Miasmata', in *Companion Encyclopedia of the History of Medicine*, vol. 1, ed. W.F. Bynum and Roy Porter (London: Routledge, 1993).

131 Nick Nyland, *De praktiserende læger i Danmark, 1800–1910: Træk af det historiske grundlag for almen medicin* (Odense: University of Southern Denmark, 2000), 235–36.

132 Throughout this book the term 'doctor' functions as a collective designation for men trained in and working under authorisation within the European medical tradition. This means that the term covers both proper doctors (physicians) and surgeons. Traditionally, a 'doctor' had a theoretical education from a university, whereas a surgeon had received practical training in the craft of surgery. At the beginning of the nineteenth century, the dividing line between the two had been eroding for a long time.

perature, smell for putrefaction, taste the urine, listen for irregularities in the respiration and to observe the colour of the skin and the eyes. Normally, a closer physical examination was only performed in external illnesses because of the social etiquette at the time. Therefore, the patient's own description of the duration of the disease, the symptoms, and so on was a very important tool for the doctor.[133] The investigation of enslaved patients was probably less hampered by etiquette, but we have very little information on this aspect. In this period, therapy consisted mainly of diets, bloodletting, purges and plasters. The purges were induced and supported by more or less effective drugs in the shape of pills, powders, elixirs, and syrups. The time was characterised by a strong focus on these drugs, some of which contained very powerful ingredients, for instance mercury, opium, and quinine.[134]

The rapid development in medicine happened primarily on the level of diagnosis because of a gradual shift in paradigm from the humoral pathological perception to a new anatomical-pathological perception. After the French Revolution, France, and especially Paris, became the centre of this new medicine, which was based on the inexhaustible amount of research material (patients) in the large public hospitals of Paris. Here new knowledge about diseases was founded only on direct observation of patients, while old theoretical systems were put aside. Less emphasis was put on the patient's personal case story and more on the physical signs of the body, especially the signs visible through autopsies of the thousands of diseased patients. By comparing the clinical symptoms of the living patient with the damage to internal organs discovered during the autopsy of the same patient, the French doctors were able to define specific diseases and separate them from each other. Another important tool in this research was the so-called 'numerical method', which used statistics to compare specific diseases with the efficiency of various therapies. Through this method, the doctors discovered which drugs in the traditional pharmacopoeia were effective against specific diseases. However, the ability of this so-called Parisian Medicine to diagnose diseases was not accompanied by a comparable ability to treat diseases. This created a vacuum in therapy, in which the old humoral pathological therapies were often retained for want of better methods.[135]

133 Roy Porter, *Ve og Vel – Medicinens historie fra oldtid til nutid* (Copenhagen: Rosinante, 2000), 256–57.
134 Porter, *Ve og Vel*, 266–70.
135 Kenneth F. Kiple, ed., *The Cambridge World History of Human Disease* (Cambridge: Cambridge University Press, 1993), 16–17.

The focus of the Parisian Medicine on the bodily functions also generated developments in the field of obstetrics. The anatomy of the pelvis and mechanisms of birth became the focus of increasing attention. New devices were invented, for instance to measure the pelvis and to enlarge the uterine cervix in order to make births easier. Simultaneously, doctors developed the existing forcipes into an arsenal of specialised instruments, and they began to use the oxytocic drug *Secale cornutum* (from ergot, a fungus growing on rye).[136]

In the 1830s a new development began, which was eventually to overtake the French school. This was the so-called German scientific medicine, whose results came from laboratories and dissection rooms in the German universities. Based on a reductionist philosophy in which all biological phenomena had to be explained through physics and chemistry, research now focused on physiology, microscopic anatomy, embryology, comparative and pathological anatomy etc. When the French school's methods and knowledge about morbid changes and human physiology were combined with the microscopes and knowledge of the causes of disease emerging from the German labs, the results were revolutionary.[137]

As mentioned above, this first period under the new medical paradigm, which lasted until the middle of the nineteenth century, was characterised by a lack of efficient therapies. However, over time the intensive research did result in new drugs. The field of pharmacology presented a few powerful drugs prepared by isolation of the active substances in old herbal medicines, for instance quinine, strychnine, caffeine, nicotine, and morphine.[138] Of these drugs, at least quinine sulphate was used against fever on St Croix in the 1830s. Furthermore, anaesthesia also saw enormous improvements, because of the introduction of ether and chloroform in the last years of the period in question.

In the last years of the period, the science of nutrition also developed as a separate discipline founded on research in chemistry.[139] Of course there already existed plenty of experience and even strict guidelines as to what certain groups supported by the government should be fed, for instance soldiers, seamen, patients, and paupers. Similar kinds of knowledge existed pertaining to the

136 Philip Rhodes, *A Short History of Clinical Midwifery: The Development of Ideas in the Professional Management of Childbirth* (Cheshire: Books for Midwives Press, 1995), 62–69.

137 Kiple, *History of Human Disease*, 17–18.

138 Porter, *Ve og Vel*, 333–34.

139 Kenneth J. Carpenter, *Protein and Energy: A Study of Changing Ideas in Nutrition* (Cambridge: Cambridge University Press, 1994), 1–54.

nutrition of the enslaved workers,[140] but this was the knowledge and calculations made by planters, managers and doctors founded on economical considerations and not on the science of nutrition.

Medicine, Health and Diseases in the West Indies

The focus of humoral pathology on the influence of geographic, topographic, and meteorological conditions on health was especially pronounced in the tropical colonies. They often had a more extreme environment than Europeans were used to, and they were afflicted with foreign lethal diseases, the cause and treatment of which was deduced from the special local circumstances. From the beginning of the eighteenth century and well into the period dealt with here, European doctors perceived the tropical environment as so fundamentally alien to the constitution of Europeans that they were not capable of adjusting to it. Europeans were vulnerable to the strange and dangerous environment and premature death caused by disease was a probable result. Consequently, Europeans who travelled to and inhabited the tropics put their lives on the line. By contrast, 'natives', including imported enslaved workers from Africa, were perceived as constitutionally fit for the tropical climate, for which reason their ability to work and be productive in this environment was perceived as much better than that of Europeans. Regarding the enslaved workers, some hereditary resistances may have contributed to this perception.[141] However, there were a number of illnesses that afflicted the enslaved workers much more frequently than Europeans, for instance, leprosy, elephantiasis, yaws, hernia, scabies, respiratory diseases, tetanus, dropsy and a variety of sores and work related injuries.[142] Important tools used for the definition of the dangerous tropics were the previously mentioned medical statistics and medical geography, topography and meteorology (rainfall, wind direction etc.).[143] In the Danish West Indies, the awareness of the influence of the environment, and especially of the weather, on the health of both the enslaved workers and Euro-Caribbeans was also very prominent among doctors.

140 See for instance: Collins, *Practical Rules for the Management and Medical Treatment of Negro Slaves in the Sugar Colonies* (New York: Books for Libraries Press, 1971 [original: London, 1811]).

141 David Arnold, ed., *Warm Climates and Western Medicine: The Emergence of Tropical Medicine, 1500–1900* (Amsterdam: Rodopi, 1996), 6–10.

142 James Grainger, *An Essay on the More Common West-India Diseases; and the Remedies which that Country itself Produces; to which are added, some Hints on the Management of Negroes. With practical Notes, and a Linnæan Index by William Wright, M.D.F.R.S* (Edinburgh: Mundell and Son, London: Longman and Rees, 1802[1764]).

143 Arnold, *Warm Climates*, 6–10.

The disease environment of the Danish West Indies during this period presented a mixture of diseases from three continents: Africa, Europe, and America. The immigrants from Europe and the enslaved workers from Africa brought their local diseases with them, diseases that those indigenous to the Caribbean had not experienced before and so did not have any defence against, neither immunologically nor medically. In addition, both parties enountered the diseases originating in America.[144] The result was an aggressive disease environment, which took its toll of both Euro-Caribbeans and Afro-Caribbeans.

The Health Service on St Croix

From the takeover by the Danish state in 1755 until about 1800, the Danish West Indies developed a complete health service designed after the health service in Denmark. Because of its origin, this system was fundamentally designed to take care of the needs of Euro-Caribbean inhabitants, but it also participated in and controlled several parts of the management of the health of the enslaved workers. The health service was structured as a hierarchical pyramid with the landfysikus, i.e. the royally appointed and state-employed doctor, at the top (the first official landfysikus was employed in 1780). Below him, the St Croix part of the pyramid had two garrison surgeons (from 1755), likewise royally appointed and state employed, one in each of the two towns of Christiansted and Frederiksted. Below them was the group of government-authorised doctors in private practice. At the bottom of the pyramid, we find the royally appointed and state-employed midwives (from 1768) and the royally privileged apothecaries (the first in 1770, continually from 1826).[145]

In addition to these groups of healthcare professionals, the Danish West Indian health service contained a number of public state institutions. There were royally privileged pharmacies and garrison hospitals, one in each of the towns (1759). The hospitals were intended primarily for army and navy personnel, but also received civilians and can so be regarded as public hospitals.[146] In addition, the towns each had a Health Commission (1816) responsible for the quarantine of ships and by extension for the quarantine of the entire island in the event of imminent epidemics, for instance smallpox or cholera.[147] Finally,

144 Sheridan, *Doctors and Slaves*, 1–5.
145 Jensen, *En verden til forskel?*, 41–42, 45–46.
146 Jensen, *En verden til forskel?*, 43–46.
147 DNA, WILA, no. 3.81.599 and no. 2.1.6. Regulations of 4 March 1833, p. 209: Regulations for the fight against cholera.

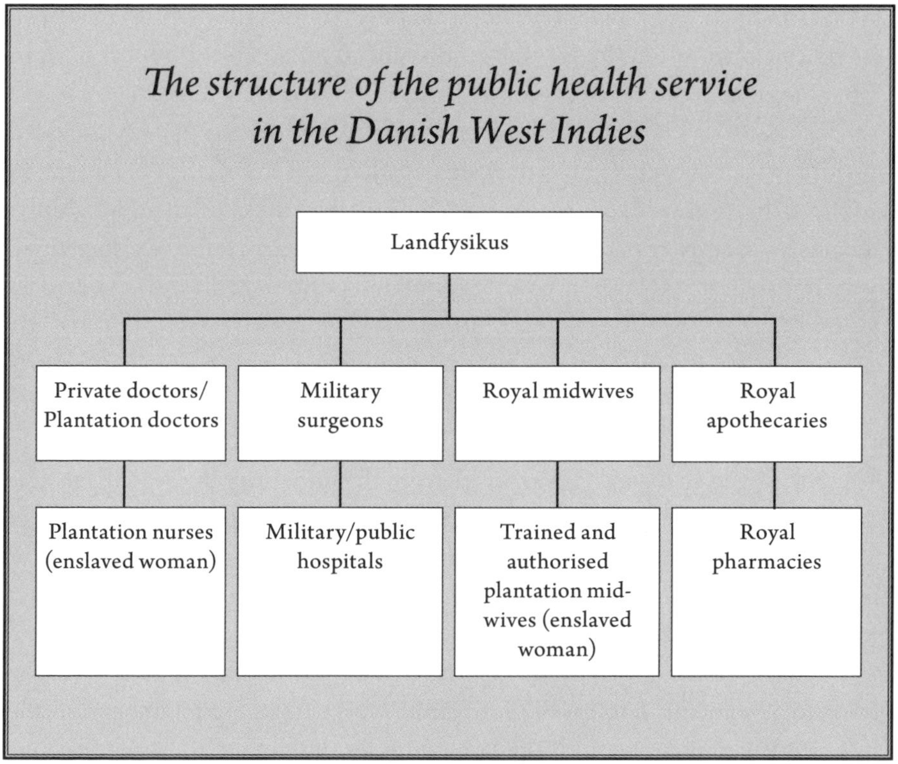

Fig. 2.10: Organisation diagram of the public health service in the Danish West Indies.

there was a system handling vaccination against smallpox, normally managed single-handedly by the landfysikus.

The hierarchical structure of the health service was clearly defined in the royal instructions and licences of the state-employed groups in the system. According to the instructions of the landfysikus, his primary function was to supervise the general state of health in his district.[148] It was his duty to attend to any patient who sent for him, rich or poor, and to monitor the quality of foods and water, as well as the cleanliness of the district. Further, he was obliged to undertake autopsies in the event of unnatural deaths (suicides, poisoning etc.), and to supervise the services of midwives and apothecaries. He was also required to be a member of the Health Commissions, promote the vaccination

148 The geographical area for which he was responsible, in this case the three Danish West Indian islands.

against smallpox, fight quackery and to that end control the licences of all doctors on the islands. Finally, he was required to send an annual report back to Copenhagen concerning all the above matters.[149] According to the instructions of the garrison and regimental surgeons, their sphere of activity only included the military personnel,[150] yet as they were in charge of the semi-public garrison hospitals, they were also concerned with the health of the civilian population.[151] The spheres of activity of the royal midwives and apothecaries were also defined by their instructions.[152] These royally appointed posts were always occupied by Danes.

Alongside their official duties the state-employed doctors also had private patients, which made them part of the much larger group of doctors in private practice. This group was also regulated by legislation to the extent that from 1818 they all had to have either an exam from the university in Copenhagen (or Kiel), which would automatically license them to work as doctors in all parts of the Danish monarchy, or a dispensation to practise in the Danish West Indies.[153] The reality behind this requirement was that the majority of doctors in private practice originated in the Anglophone world (Britain with its colonies and the USA) and had been trained there.[154] Furthermore, the doctors were required to attend to all patients, not just because of the Hippocratic Oath but because the law explicitly demanded it.[155] The large number of doctors in private practice made the ratio of people per doctor much lower than in contemporary Denmark (Fig 2.11). The reason for the relatively large number of doctors in private practice was primarily the enslaved workers. Their labour was the foundation of the sugar production and so of the economy, and made up a large part of the planters' investments. Since it was no longer possible to import new enslaved workers from Africa and the enslaved population continued to decrease, the planters had

149 Christian Poulsen Nørbom Petersen, *Den Danske Medicinal - Lovgivning eller Samling af de Forordninger, Placater, Kongelige Rescripter og Resolutioner, Reglementer og Instruxer, Fundatser, Collegialbreve og andre offentlige Aktstykker, som vedkomme Læger, Apothekere og Gjordemødre i Danmark* (Copenhagen, 1834), part 2, vol. 1, 259–70. *'Instruction, hvorefter samtlige Stifts- og Landphysici i Danmark sig i deres Embeder skal rette og forholde'*, 4 March 1818.

150 Regimental surgeons were subject to a large number of regulations. See for instance Petersen, *Den Danske Medicinal-Lovgivning*, regulation of 19 April 1747 with later additions.

151 Niklas Thode Jensen, 'Sundhed, citroner og slaver', *1066 – Tidsskrift for Historie* 33, no. 1 (2003).

152 National Archives and Records Administration (NARA), Washington DC, Record Group (RG) 55, Entry 82, Box 315. Doctor's License, P. Eggert Benzon, 1826.

153 Niklas Thode Jensen, 'En verden til forskel? Undersøgelser af lægerne og sundhedsvæsenet i Dansk Vestindien mellem 1755 og 1830', *Bibliotek for Læger* 194, no. 4 (2002), 281–86.

154 Jensen, *En verden til forskel?*, 37–40, 50–66.

155 DNA, WILA, no. 2.1.6. Proclamation of 24 November 1841, p. 308: 'Angaaende at det paalægges Lægerne at yde Assistance der, hvor deres Hielp er fornøden m.m.'

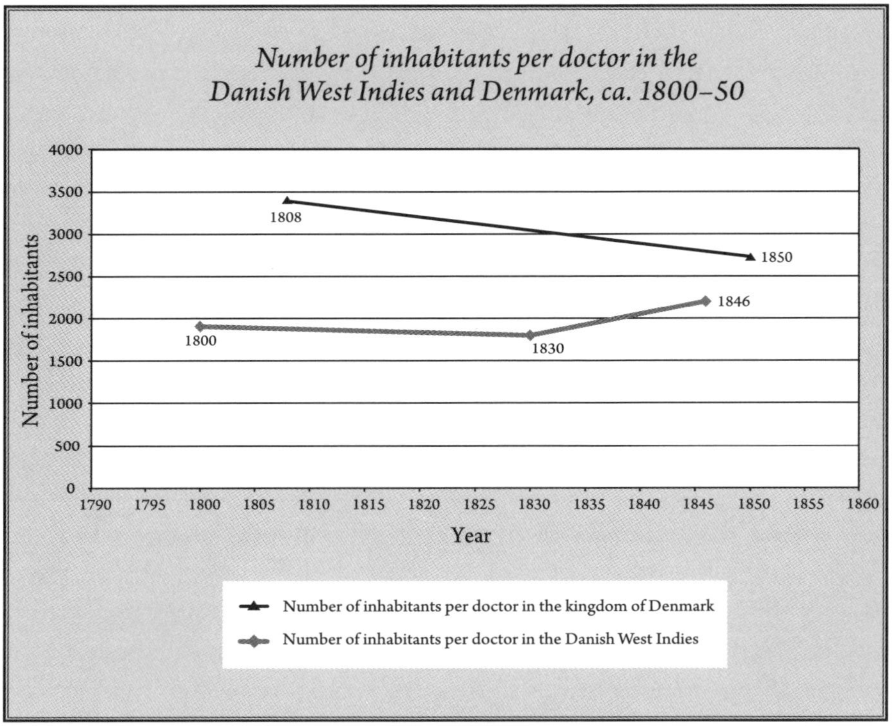

Fig. 2.11. Source: Table 2.3: Inhabitants per doctor in the Danish West Indies and Denmark.

a great self-interest in keeping their workers alive. Another important reason for the high number of doctors was the health of the Euro-Caribbeans themselves, which was perceived to be threatened by the tropical environment.[156]

The Health Service on the Plantations

It was the custom for all plantations to employ a doctor in private practice on an annual contract but it was not legally required. However, in the few instances when a manager chose not to employ a doctor, the reactions of the colonial administration and the other doctors show that such behaviour was unusual, and that the administration tried to prevent it.[157] According to the terms of the leases for royal plantations (1834), every plantation had to contract a doctor,

156 Jensen, *En verden til forskel?*, 58.

157 DNA, Sundhedskollegiet (Board of Health, BH), archive no. 1252, Medicinalindberetninger (Medical reports, Med. rep.), Vestindien (Danish West Indies), 1839. Surgeon J. Roebuck from the island of St

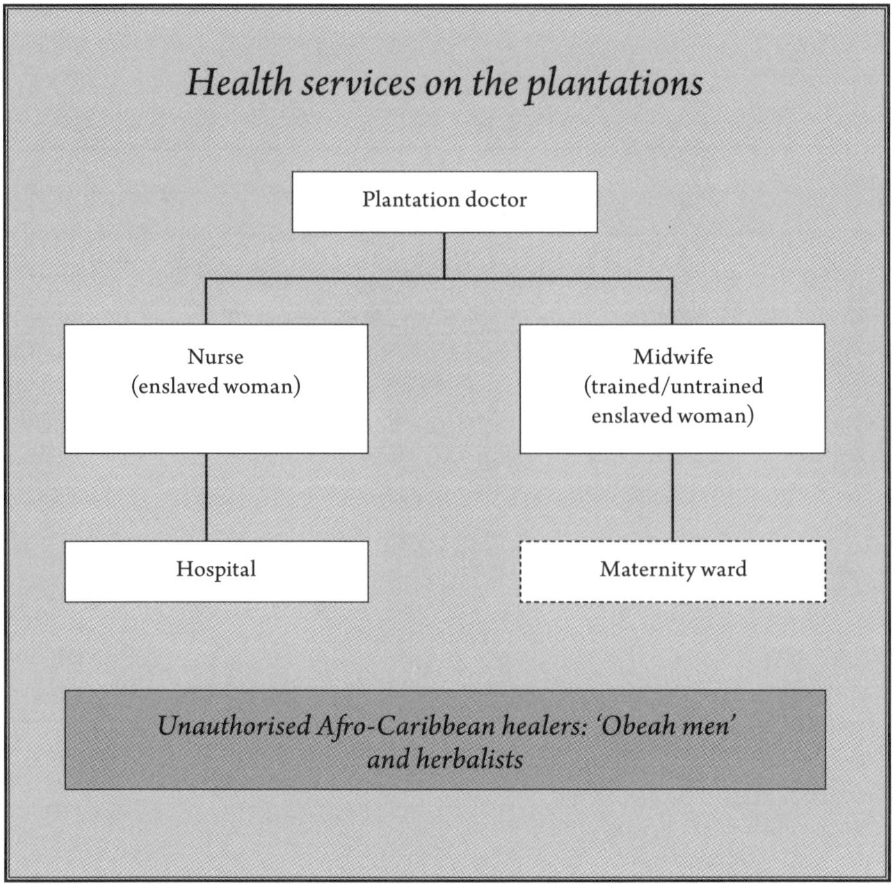

Fig. 2.12: Organisation diagram of health services on Cruzian plantations.

who was to be paid directly by the government agency in charge of the royal plantations, the so-called Liquidations Commission, and not by the leaseholder. This contracted doctor received a fixed annual salary per enslaved worker, usually 1 Peso per head, and he usually visited the plantation once or twice a week.[158]

John complained that five of the island's 15 plantations did not have a contract with a doctor. This was unheard of on St Croix.

158 The monetary system in the Danish West Indies was complicated because the currencies of many countries were used concurrently. In the period 1803–48, the most common monetary standard was Pesos or Pieces of eight (Ps.). One Ps. was subdivided into eight reales and each real into six stivers. Other common currencies were US dollars, Rigsdaler (Rix-dollars) in 'Danish West Indian Currency' (abbr. *rdl.v.c.*) and Danish Rigsdaler (abbr. *rdl.*).

If the doctor was summoned for acute diseases or if he had to perform operations or use special drugs or equipment, he charged extra following an officially approved tariff.[159] It was not unusual for a doctor to be in charge of several plantations. Dr William Stevens (1789–1862), for instance, had thirty plantations in his care in 1822 (although he probably also had an assistant).[160]

When the doctor visited the plantation, his primary place of work was the plantation hospital. Nearly all sick enslaved workers were admitted to the hospital when they presented themselves to the manager. In the period in question, all plantations on St Croix seem to have had a hospital, even though it was not legally required.[161] However, the plantation hospitals were very different in size and quality depending on the means of the planter and the size of the enslaved population. From the royal plantations, we have detailed descriptions of what the hospitals looked like and how they were furnished. For instance, the 'sick house' on the North Star plantation was described in the following way in 1831:

> The plantation does not have a sick house but instead they use one of the Negro houses. The manager is forced to keep all the sick, men and women, together in this small house of only 12 feet square. Furthermore, the so-called stocks, which is allegedly necessary and found on all plantations, is housed in the same room, yet generally in a compartment of its own. There is no latrine or other conveniences.[162]

This situation was regarded as appallingly poor and nothing similar was found on any other royal plantation. Consequently, the Liquidations Commission immediately decided to commission the construction of a new hospital, which was finished the following year. This new hospital was designed according to a layout that was later copied for hospitals on other royal plantations (see Fig. 2.13).

159 DNA, WILA, no. 3.81.592. 'Reglement over Lægernes Fordringer for Medicamenter og Oppassning' (Rules for doctors' claims for medicine and care), by landfysikus John Gordon, 1786. These rules or tariffs seem to have been the basis for doctors' bills in the period.

160 DNA, BH, Med.rep., 1803–1958. 1822.

161 DNA, WILA, no. 3.81.690. Inventories for a large number of plantations from the years 1805–25. They all had a hospital.

162 DNA, WILA, no. 46.17.53. Original text in Danish: 'Der findes på Plantagen intet Sygehus, men afbenyttes hertil eet af Negerhusene. I dette lidet, kun 12 fod i qvadrat store Hus er Forvalteren nødt til at holde alle Plantagens Syge, Mænd og Qvinder sammen, desuden er i samme den saakaldte Stocks, der vistnok er nødvendig og findes paa enhver Plantage, men i almindelighed i et eget Aflukke af Sygehuset. Der findes intet Locum eller andre Beqvemmeligheder.' 12 feet square is 12 × 12 Danish feet = 144 square feet = ca. 14.2 m^2 (1 Danish square foot = 0.0985 m).

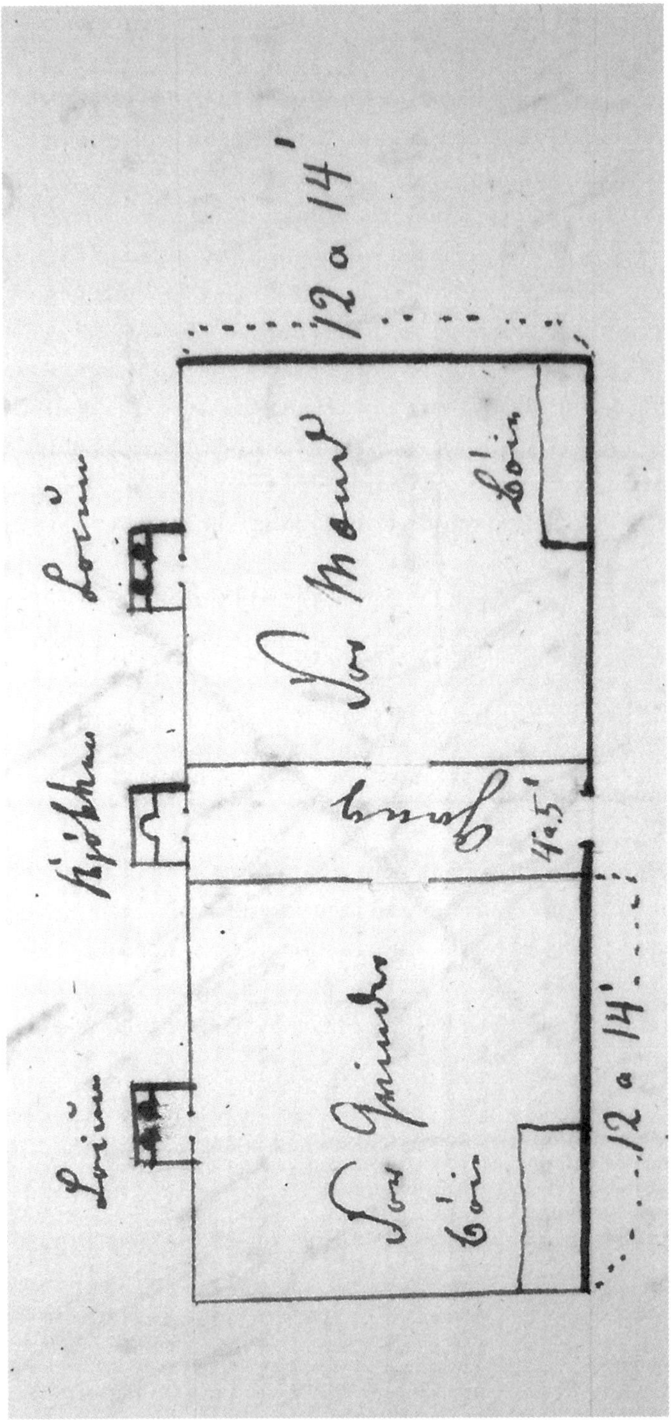

Fig. 2.13: Hospital on the royal plantation North Star, ca. 1831. DNA, WILA, no. 46.17.53, case no. 450 and 509, 1831. Photo: Niklas Thode Jensen, June 2011. Courtesy of the Danish National Archives.

As can be seen from the sketchy plan, the building was divided into separate wards for male and female slaves. The 'sick-nurse' (see below) resided in the central corridor near the kitchen where she could monitor all traffic in and out of the building. Each ward had a latrine ('locum') and the stocks ('boie'). The presence of the latter instrument shows the double function of the plantation hospital both as a clinic and a repository for the sick, but also as a correctional facility. To further facilitate the latter function, the house was buildt entirely of brick and the windows were barred. The intention was that 'all the convalescents locked up in there, or others who were locked up there for some minor misdemeanour, could not escape at night.'[163] Later a small annex containing a jail cell was added to the building. The plantation hospital on North Star was somewhat longer than shown on the plan, in fact 39 feet, which amounted to a total floor area of around 54 square metres.[164]

The only furniture in the wards apart from the stocks seems to have been 'cabans' and 'benches', i.e. some sort of beds.[165] Such furniture seems to have been standard in plantation hospitals in general, but some had far more advanced equipment. The most curious example originates from the royal Hermon Hill plantation, which in 1825 possessed a machine for steam bathing of North American manufacture, bought specifically to be used in the hospital.[166] Perhaps the intention was to treat the skin diseases of the enslaved workers, since vapour therapies for such ailments were fashionable at the time.[167] Unfortunately, it is not known exactly how the machine and the special herbs that came with it were used, but the very existence of the machine illustrates the efforts made by some planters to keep their enslaved workers healthy.

In the following years, the above layout was used for hospitals on other royal plantations. The buildings were not always made entirely of brick but they had the same facilities and occasionally an extra ward for female enslaved who had come to give birth.[168] On some royal plantations, the hospital was located on the

163 DNA, WILA, no. 46.17.53. Letter, 1831. Original Danish text: '[...] alle de deri indelukkede Rekonvalescenter eller nogen der for en eller anden liden Forseelse maatte være indelukkede om Natten ei kunde undløbe'.

164 1 Danish foot = 0.3141 metre (see: Knut Birkeland, *Mål & Vægt* (Copenhagen: Høst og Søn Forlag, 1970), 14 × 39 feet = 4.4 metres × 12.2 metres = 53.7 m².

165 DNA, WILA, no. 46.21. North Star, report 1834 and 1838.

166 DNA, Direktionen for Statsgælden og den Synkende Fond (The directorate of the state debt and the decreasing fund, hereafter DSD), no. 1128. Hermon Hill, 31. December 1825.

167 On Martinique, steam bathing against skin diseases was introduced in 1818. See: Leti, *Santé et société*, 385.

168 For instance: DNA, WILA, no. 46.17.6 and no. 46.21, Estate Work and Rest, report 1833.

first floor of larger buildings with storerooms on the ground floor. These sizable buildings often had a gallery at the front, which gave the patients access to the cooling wind even when it rained. In relation to the perceptions of the causes of disease in contemporary Western medicine, this focus on fresh air makes good sense.[169] Hospitals of similar size and design existed on the private plantations (see Fig. 2.14).

The plantation hospital usually had a 'sick-nurse',[170] i.e. an enslaved woman who worked as a nurse and was responsible for the care of the sick and the daily management of the hospital.[171] Presumably, this job included cleaning and cooking, as well as dispensing the medicines prescribed by the plantation doctor during his visits.[172] The sick-nurse was often an older woman and sometimes she was also an invalid, which may have been the reason why she was given the job (see Table 2.4). However, the reason could also have been her knowledge of herbal medicine, though no source materials exist to reveal what kind of healing the plantation sick-nurses performed.

As mentioned, one of the responsibilities of the sick-nurse was the hospital food. It seems to have been a relatively good and varied diet compared with the food that was normally handed out to the enslaved workers. According to accounts from both private and royal plantations, the sick enslaved received fresh meat from sheep and chicken, Madeira wine, pearl barley and special starchy foods like arrowroot (*Maranta arundinacea*) and tapioca (*Manihot esculenta*).[173] This of course depended on which diet the doctor or the manager had prescribed and ordered the sick-nurse to prepare for the patient as part of the therapy.

Finally, the planter also played a central role in taking care of the health of the enslaved workers on a daily basis. Since the doctor was only present once or twice a week, usually the planter decided if an enslaved worker had to be admitted to hospital or if the illness was so serious that the doctor had to be called in. Sometimes the planter dispensed medicine for the enslaved on his own. It was legal to import drugs for the consumption in one's own household[174] and the

169 DNA, WILA, no. 46.21, Estate Rust up Twist, report 1838.

170 Not to be confused with the ordinary nurse, i.e. the child nurse, who took care of the master's children.

171 See Table 2.4. There is no reason to assume that the private plantations differed from the royal ones in this respect.

172 Highfield, *Observations*, 24 (original: Brady, 1829).

173 DNA, WILA, no. 46.17.43, alphabetical index of account, 1828. DNA, WILA, no. 46.17.33, Pro memoria, 4 January 1842 and 7 January 1843. DNA, WILA, no. 41.6.6, accounts of the private plantations Upper Bethlehem and Fredensborg.

174 NARA, RG55, Entry 82, Box 315, records concerning trade in medicine and poisons, 1829.

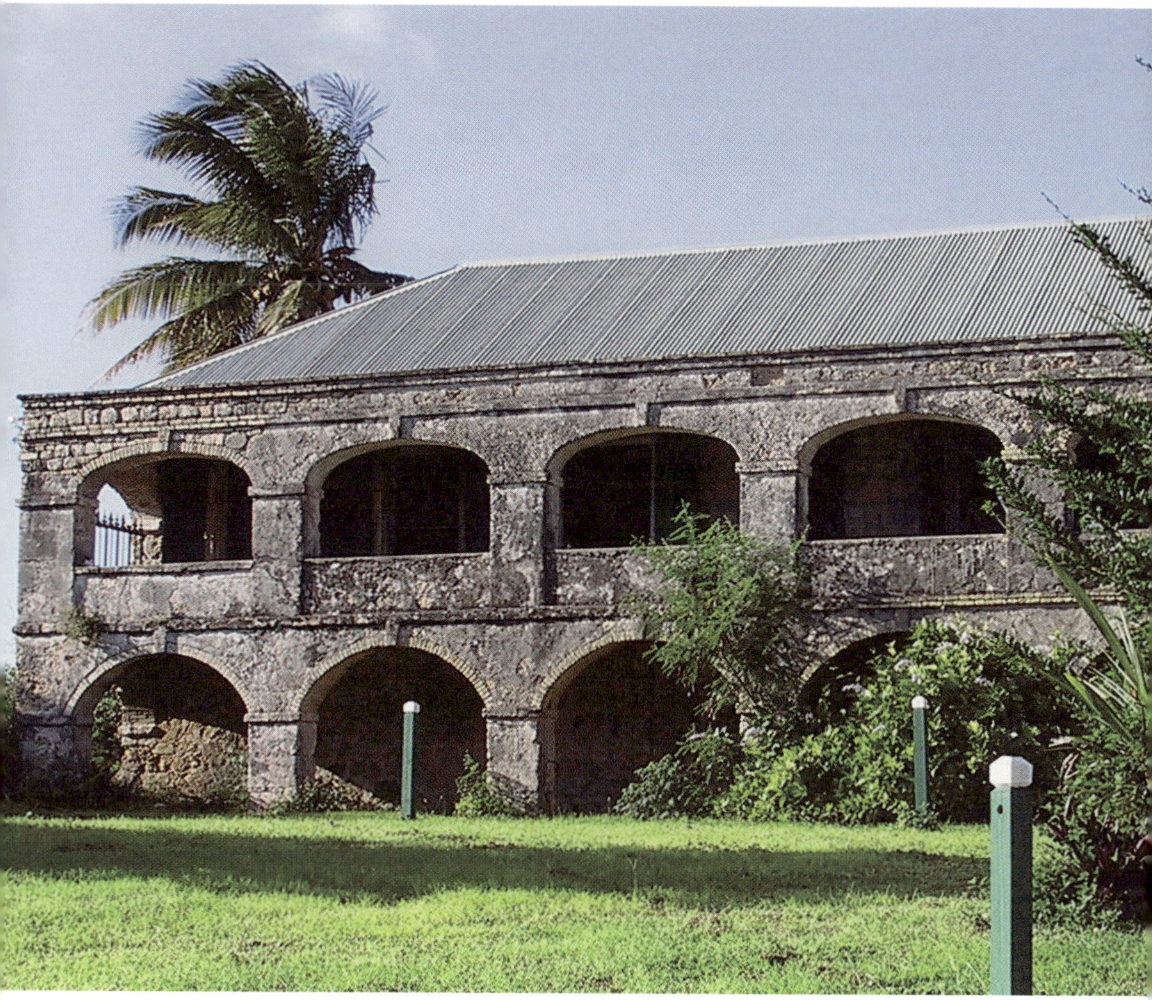

Fig. 2.14: An example of a plantation hospital with a front gallery can still be seen today at what was formerly the private plantation Little Princess. Constructed in the last part of the period 1803–48, it was most likely among the largest and finest of its kind on St Croix. The ground floor contained storerooms while the first floor contained wards for the sick enslaved workers. Photo: Niklas Thode Jensen, November 2004.

Euro-Caribbean community had a longstanding tradition of self-medication.[175] Accounts from a number of plantations show that apart from special foods and beverages purchased specifically for the sick enslaved workers, the planter also purchased some common remedies like castor oil and white mustard (for mustard plasters).[176]

The Health Service in Comparative Perspective

In the British West Indies, planters also contracted doctors, who visited the plantations on a weekly basis and treated the enslaved workers. For this purpose, larger plantations usually had a hospital, equipped with wards for men, women, and lying-in women. The daily care and treatment at the hospital was managed either by a female enslaved working as a sick-nurse or by a male enslaved working as so-called 'slave doctor'.[177] Here too, the plantation hospitals often doubled as correctional facilities with stocks and barred windows. Only a few of the British West Indian colonies had laws that prescribed hospitals and medical attention for the enslaved workers and in these cases the laws were very general.[178] Accordingly, the situation in the British West Indies was very similar to the situation on St Croix; however, the colonial administration's role in relation to the health service was different. Only in a few of the British West Indian colonies did the authorities control the credentials of the doctors and maintain a licensing system. This was true for Demerara from 1810, Trinidad in the period 1818–24, Grenada from 1821 and Jamaica after 1833. Significantly, the three first were Crown colonies or had a strong connection with the central government in London, whereas Jamaica had its own legislative assembly, yet only enacted a licensing system just prior to emancipation.[179] The other British West Indian colonies did not establish anything similar in the period in question. The only government-funded and supervised form of medical service in the British West Indies provided for the army and navy personnel, and the hospitals were part of this system. Beyond this, the health service in the British West Indies operated along the lines of

175 DNA, BH, Med. rep., Danish West Indies, 1844 and 1846. Herman Barclay, *Bidrag til Kundskab om vestindiske Sygdomme med didhørende Bemærkninger, Samlede paa St Thomas i Aarene 1823–1827 af Garnisons- og Distriktslæge H. Barclay* (Copenhagen and Schleswig, 1829 and 1830), 197.

176 NARA, RG55, Entry 1109, Box 2438, Estate Mount Victory. Entry for 2 June, 29 August and 6 November, 1827.

177 Jensen, *En verden til forskel?*, 94–98.

178 Higman, *Slave Populations*, 267–68.

179 Higman, *Slave Populations*, 44–45, 265–66.

the same laissez-faire philosophy as the health service in Britain and in the USA. Medical assistance was a service that had to be purchased in the free and uncontrolled medical marketplace.[180]

On the island of Martinique, here representing the French West Indies, it was not until the 1845 slave law (the so-called Mackau Law) that every plantation with a workforce of more than twenty enslaved workers was required to employ a doctor. The doctors who undertook the inspections were employed on a contract and had contracts with several plantations. The medical examinations, treatments and so on were carried out in the plantation hospital, which had been made mandatory for all plantations with more than twenty enslaved workers by the slave law of 1786. However, there was no sanction against planters who did not obey the law. With the law of 1845, these existing rules were reinforced, as well as the fact that it was the duty of the planter to take care of sick enslaved workers. In addition, the hospital had to have separate wards for each sex, beds, and bed linen. However, the demands of the law do not seem to have been followed. The larger, privately owned plantations did have a hospital and the doctor did visit on a weekly basis, but the hospitals were very diverse in size, build, and equipment. The daily management of the hospital was in the hands of the sick-nurse. On the smaller plantations, the enslaved workers were treated in their own houses or huts, but not always by doctors. The first treatment was carried out by the manager or the plantation owner himself, or an unauthorised slave doctor was called in. Only if this was not enough was the Euro-Caribbean doctor called in. On the state-owned plantations there were several rules for the layout, equipment, cleaning and cooking in the hospitals, yet it is not known if these very elaborate and, consequently, costly rules were followed. Regardless of what kind of plantation the hospital was on, it often doubled as a prison and housed various instruments for punishment.[181]

The structure of the health service in the French West Indies was pyramidal and hierarchical just as in the Danish West Indies. Throughout the period in question, it was presided over by a royal physician, who was responsible for the military personnel, for checking the licences of the surgeons, midwives and apothecaries, and for supervising health on the visiting ships. Furthermore, there was a royal surgeon and a royal apothecary. Among the duties of these three officers was the supervision of health in prisons and schools, and as mem-

180 Jensen, *En verden til forskel?*, 103.
181 Leti, *Santé et société*, 301–8, 352–60.

bers of the local Board of Health (1816) to promote vaccination against smallpox. From 1823, health officers (*Officier de santé*)[182] had to pass an exam before a jury of doctors before they could obtain their licence to practise in the colony. The navy had its own medical corps.[183]

In conclusion, the part of the Cruzian health service that dealt with the enslaved workers had a lot in common with similar systems in the British and French West Indies. In all three colonial systems we find plantations supervised by contracted doctors, plantation hospitals that doubled as correctional facilities and staffed with enslaved, female sick-nurses who managed the daily care of the patients. These systems were rarely sanctioned by law, but in the French and Danish West Indies doctors were licensed by the local medical authorities, which was only the case in a few of the British colonies. The reason for the more extensive control seems to be the hierarchical structures that the health services in the Danish and French West Indies had received from their mother countries. Furthermore, it is possible that the medical supervision on St Croix starting in 1818 was generally characterised by a stronger control than in the British and French West Indies. For instance, the use of unauthorised enslaved healers does not seem to have been as common on St Croix, in view of the fact that the doctors did not perceive quackery to be a problem (more on this below). It is possible that there was a connection between the smaller size of St Croix and the tighter control, but the example of the health service in Denmark must also have been important.

The Medicine of the Enslaved: Obeah and Herbs

Parallel to the authorised Euro-Caribbean health service and the prophylactic initiatives of the colonial administration, the enslaved workers practised their own medicine with their own healers and a perception of disease very different from the European one. In the following, I will explore these beliefs and practices in order to complete the picture of the medical world on St Croix.

182 A special group of healthcare professionals who had a shorter practical or academic training than the doctors did and hence not the same rights and obligations.

183 Leti, *Santé et société*, 319–23, 329, 335.

The Enslaved Workers' Perception of Disease and Obeah: The General Picture

The perception of disease and therapy among the enslaved workers in the Caribbean, their 'illness' perception, was part of the cultural heritage they had brought with them from Africa. Of course, there were tremendous variations in the perceptions of disease between the various regions of the African continent, yet there seems to have been a common basis, which became characteristic of the disease perceptions of the enslaved workers in the West Indies. In general, this was a belief in a connection between disease and powers in the spirit world where the ancestors lived. Accordingly, there was no great divide between body and mind/spirit, which meant that therapy was not just aimed at the physical body of the patient, but at the individual's entire social and spiritual environment. Therapy often consisted in more or less collective rituals, which were meant to re-establish the damaged balance in both the magico-religious universe and the social universe. Alongside the ritual therapy, herbal medicine was an important form of treatment, which however seems only to have addressed the symptoms, since the reason for the disease was perceived to be magico-religious and so could only be removed by magical and ritual means.[184]

This magico-religious manipulation of primarily the spiritual but also the physical world was referred to as 'Obeah' (Obi, Obiah) and the practitioners were generally called 'Obeah-men', even though there were also women among them. The enslaved workers honoured and feared the Obeah-man because of his power not only to heal but also to use black magic. In the period in question, Euro-Caribbeans regarded Obeah as pure superstition and persecuted the practitioners because they allegedly tried to 'deceive' the 'ignorant' enslaved workers with their 'arts'. However, the reaction was severe when Obeah caused the death of an enslaved worker, because the victim was convinced he was under a curse and consequently lost the desire to live. In the first half of the nineteenth century, the British colony of Barbados several times saw the introduction of harsh punishments for the practice of Obeah, because Euro-Caribbeans regarded it as harmful to other enslaved workers – not least if it involved the use of poison.[185]

Apart from the practitioners of Obeah, the sphere of enslaved therapists also

184 Jerome S. Handler, 'Slave Medicine and Obeah in Barbados, circa 1650 to 1834', *New West Indian Guide / Nieuwe West-Indische Gids* 74, nos. 1+2 (2000), 59–62.
185 Handler, 'Slave Medicine', 65–77.

seems to have contained a group of specialists focusing on the physical treatment of one particular disease. Here the mode of therapy was usually herbal.[186]

Obeah and Herbal Medicine on St Croix

The attitude of the Danish administration towards Obeah was consistently negative. Since 1733, the draconian slave law of Governor Phillip Gardelin had mandated flogging as the punishment for the practice of Obeah. However, if the practice of Obeah had included the use of poison, which was perceived to be a related practice, then the enslaved worker was to be pinched with red-hot tongs, broken on the wheel and burned alive.[187] The latter severe punishments were no longer used in the period in question, but the perception of the connection between Obeah and poison still existed. Whereas poisoning was regarded as a real threat to the Euro-Caribbeans themselves, and so viewed with the utmost gravity, Obeah was regarded more as a stupid superstition, which mainly had to be prevented because it could make enslaved workers harm themselves and by extension their owners.

This more lenient attitude to Obeah is illustrated in the book by Lieutenant Brady from the end of the 1820s. Here, by way of introduction, Brady explains that Obeah was a crime, which often led to other crimes, and that almost all enslaved workers believed in Obeah. Further, Brady described how an Obeah séance was discovered on the Mannings Bay plantation, and how the enslaved workers involved were punished. One enslaved worker, who belonged to another plantation, was sent home to receive his punishment there, which probably meant that the punishment would of course be hard (flogging, imprisonment) but not life-threatening. If that had been the case, the authorities and the courts would have been involved. However, two female enslaved workers, who had taken part in the séance and both belonged to Mannings Bay, could not receive a similar physical punishment because they were too weak. Consequently, the manager chose to punish them in a way that shows the perception of Obeah as mainly a religious problem. The manager reported the incident to the priest of the church of the two enslaved women (the Moravian Church), which would entail that they were demoted

186 Handler, 'Slave Medicine', 63–68. See also: Juanita de Barros, '"Setting Things Right": Medicine and Magic in British Guiana, 1803–38', *Slavery and Abolition* 25, no. 1 (2004).

187 Neville A.T. Hall, *Slave Society in the Danish West Indies: St Thomas, St John, St Croix,* ed. Barry W. Higman (Jamaica: The University of the West Indies Press, 1992), 58.

in the internal hierarchy of the church or expelled from it altogether.[188] At first, it may seem paradoxical that two members of a church also took part in the practice of Obeah. However, this was by no means unusual, since by that time the overwhelming majority of the enslaved population on St Croix belonged to one of the many congregations on the island. In 1835, 99 per cent of the enslaved workers were baptised.[189] It appears that the pervasive affiliation to the churches slowly weakened the belief in and practice of Obeah during the continuous process of creolisation.

Occasionally, cases concerning the practice of Obeah were not just dealt with on the plantations but ended up in the judicial system. One example is the case against an enslaved man named Jacob in 1831. Jacob belonged to the Fountain plantation and he must have been high ranking, since his nickname was 'Bosen', i.e. boss or driver of the enslaved workers in the field. He was caught red-handed on the Jealousy plantation, where he was engaged in the act of curing an enslaved woman called Nancy. With him, Jacob had some of the common tools for the practice of Obeah: nails, pieces of broken glass, pebbles, feathers, and hair. In court, he claimed that he had previously cured other enslaved workers, for instance delivering a pregnant woman on River plantation, and the pebbles in his possession he claimed to have 'taken out of the stomach' of a woman on Montpellier plantation. Jacob refused that he had used his 'arts' to hurt anyone, yet the court had a more overarching agenda, as it held that

> his conduct is culpable, because it is always dangerous to strengthen the superstition among the weak and ignorant class of Negro slaves, which always regard such a charlatan as a person in possession of supernatural powers. Accordingly, it is all the more culpable, since such a person knows full well that he cannot accomplish anything with his tricks and so the only reason for them is his own interests or possibly the intention to inspire fear.[190]

188 Highfield, *Observations*, 40–41 (original: Brady, 1829).

189 Hall, *Slave Society*, 46.

190 DNA, WILA, no. 2.27.6. Case no. 231. Original Danish text: '[...] så er dog hans Adfærd strafværdig, da det altid er farligt at bestyrke Overtroen hos den Svage og uvidende Klasse af Negerslaver, hvilke stedse betragte en saadan Gøgler, som een der besidder overnaturlige Evner. Saa bliver det og saa meget mere strafværdigt, som en saadan Person selv ret vel veed at han med sine Gøglerier intet kan udrette, og har altsaa kun egen Interesse til Grund og Årsag, eller og maaskee den Hensigt at indjage Frygt.'

In other words, the practice of Obeah was not a crime because it might harm the enslaved workers directly, but because it was founded on a 'superstition', which through fear might give the practitioner some power over other enslaved workers that the Euro-Caribbeans could not control. As Brady remarked, Obeah might lead to other crimes, i.e. Obeah could produce transgressions of the laws, by which the Euro-Caribbean tried to control the enslaved population. Jacob was punished with ninety lashes and forced to wear an iron plate with the inscription '*Gøgler*' (charlatan).

In contrast to Obeah, neither the colonial administration nor the Euro-Caribbean population on St Croix harboured any noticeable concern regarding the enslaved workers' attempts to cure each other with physical means (herbal medicine etc.). It is evident from the medical reports that there were healers among the enslaved with great powers in this field, and that the enslaved workers treated each other extensively – at times with better results than the doctors. Apparently, no one saw this as a problem, not even the doctors, or at least no one tried to prevent it. On the contrary, doctors were very interested in investigating and discovering the medicines used by the enslaved healers, though they rarely succeeded.

At the beginning of the period, the doctors' attention was attracted to the behaviour of the enslaved workers in regard to a particular kind of disease: venereal diseases. It appears that enslaved workers with venereal diseases were particularly reluctant to approach the doctors, but preferred to consult their own healers. This is interesting because it accords with research from the USA which shows that enslaved workers on the plantations in the South were dismissive of the doctors' treatments and especially their treatment of venereal diseases. The enslaved workers regarded the treatment as a violation and as sexual control, and as an inseparable part of the Euro-Caribbeans' perception of the enslaved as property and workforce.[191] The behaviour of the enslaved workers in the Danish West Indies gives reason to believe that they held similar views, particularly of the treatment of venereal diseases, which is, of course, very intimate by nature. Perhaps an attempt to solve this problem can be gleaned from a couple of incidents in the period just prior to the one dealt with there, where the planters paid enslaved healers or free Afro-Caribbean specialists to cure individual enslaved workers of venereal diseases.[192] To pay

191 Fett, *Working Cures*, 34.

192 DNA, WILA, no. 3.42.30. Case no. 299, 1790. An old enslaved woman healed a wound, which the doctor had given up on. DNA, WILA, no. 3.81.685. In the accounts of Estate Wheel of Fortunes of 1792 it says:

an unauthorised person, enslaved or free, to treat one's enslaved workers was illegal, and punishable as quackery.[193]

Broadly speaking, there exists no source material to describe the medicinal plants used on St Croix in the period in question, let alone what plants the enslaved workers used and for what. However, we can assume that the majority of the medicinal plants in existence today in the Cruzian environment, which are regarded as authentic by botanists, were also present on the island in the period. Accordingly, an investigation of the 'traditional' use of these plants among more recent inhabitants of St Croix could give a very tentative picture of what the pharmacopoeia of the enslaved workers contained, which therapies were used and which ailments were treated. In 1979, Ronald L. Kuby conducted such an ethno-botanical investigation of the 'folk medicine' on St Croix. He concluded that the pharmacopoeia of the folk medicine primarily consisted of local plants, called 'bush medicine'. The most typical therapy was to drink a decoction of the leaves from a plant or mixture of plants called 'bush tea'. Other therapeutic forms could be herbal poultices or a medical bath, a 'bush bath', in hot water with various herbs. Kuby identified 109 different medical plants and 182 different therapies utilising the 109 plants. This is not the place to give a closer account of the use of this virtual pharmacy, but one example could be the plant called Cane-Piece Balsam (*Justicia pectoralis*). The leaves of this plant were used to heal wounds and for a cough-suppressant drink.[194] Modern medicine has shown that the plant contains active substances that inhibit inflammation, assist the healing of wounds, have an anaesthetic effect and are hallucinogenic.[195] The effects of many of the other plants have also been scientifically proven, yet just as many do not seem to have the effects ascribed to them. Some of the plants have turned out to be extraordinarily poisonous, but according to the folk medicine, they were used in ways that protected the patient against poisoning.[196]

'Paid Adjuba for curing Adam of a venereal complaint' and 'Cash paid free wench Merotta for curing Negroe Frederic of a venereal.'

193 Rescript of 26 October 1764, see: Laurids Fogtmann, *Kongelige Rescripter, Resolutioner og Collegialbreve for Danmark og Norge udtogsviis udgivne i chronologisk Orden* (Copenhagen, 1786–1890), vol. 2, part 5, 1754–1765. Rescript of 25 August 1818, see: Petersen, *Den Danske Medicinal-Lovgivning*, vol. 2, part 1, 198.

194 Ronald L. Kuby, *Folk Medicine on St Croix: An Ethnobotanical Study* (unpublished thesis, Department of Anthropology, University of Kansas, 1979), 27–30, 32, 64.

195 Toni Thomas, *Traditional Medical Plants of St Croix, St Thomas and St John: A Selection of 68 Plants* (St Croix: University of the Virgin Islands Cooperative Extension Service, 1997), 67.

196 Kuby, *Folk Medicine*, 81–97.

Table 2.5: Therapeutic categories and preparations in the folk medicine of St Croix

Therapeutic categories	Number of preparations
Treatments for 'colds'	20
Treatments for digestive disorders	18
Treatments for injuries	15
Treatments for high blood pressure	10
Cough suppressors and expectorants	10
Treatments for skin problems	10
Treatments for 'fevers'	9
'Obeah' (healing, protecting ritual etc.)	9
'Bush bath'	8
Treatments for intestinal parasites	6
Treatments that 'clean' the 'body' and the 'blood'	6
Treatments that produce internal 'cooling'	4
Abortifacients	4
Treatments for 'strains'	4
Treatments for 'gonorrhoea'	3
Treatments for 'abcesses'	2
Treatments for 'earache'	2
Treatments for 'headache'	2
Treatments for 'toothache'	2
Treatments for 'pains'	2
Treatments for 'kidney trouble'	2
Treatments for 'measles'	2
Other ailments: Treatments for 'animals born blind', 'asthma', 'backache', 'bad legs', 'bedwetting', 'chicken pox', 'dandruff', 'delayed menses', 'diabetes', 'fish poisoning', 'flu', 'heart trouble', 'impotence', 'poor circulation', 'sugar diabetes', 'TB', 'pain caused by exposure to stinging nettle', 'purge', 'shampoo', 'hair rinse', sedative treatment that produce external cooling, tonic for babies, treatment to prevent the putrefaction of corpses, treatment that pruduce a narcotic high. (1 each, in total 31)	31
Total number of preparations	182

Source: Kuby, *Folk Medicine on St. Croix: An Ethnobotanical Study*, 70–71.

A closer look at the spectrum of ailments treated by using herbs from folk medicine shows that most of the ailments are not life-threatening. Largely, they address ailments and problems the enslaved workers are known to have suffered from. For instance, the many remedies for problems in the digestive system (including intestinal parasites), respiratory diseases, and for wounds and injuries corresponds very well with the image of the diseases of the enslaved workers.

There is a certain degree of concurrence between the diseases the enslaved workers are known to have suffered from most frequently, and the 'therapeutic categories' for which the local folk medicine 150 years later prescribed the most therapies. This does not mean that the folk medicine offers an unchanged picture of illnesses and means used by the enslaved workers to treat their sick. The concurrence might be due to the fact that these illnesses are common among humans in general, and the herbal medicines used may very easily have been different, even if the local selection of plants was to a large extent the same. However, it is likely that the enslaved workers tried to treat the diseases they suffered from and that they used local plants, even though we cannot know which plants were used for which disease.

If we compare the above with the forms of therapy and remedies the Euro-Caribbean doctors disposed of there does not seem to have been much difference. Admittedly, the European pharmacopoeia at this time contained a few effective and powerful drugs (quinine, morphine etc.), yet it also still contained far more drugs of uncertain effectiveness.[197] The only field where the doctors' abilities cannot be compared to that of the enslaved healers was surgery. Here, the doctors' knowledge and abilities were far greater, and it was also in this field that they were at times capable of preventing the consequences of life-threatening injuries. Nonetheless, surgical procedures were not an everyday occurrence on the plantations and so we cannot conclude that surgery made the doctors superior in the art of healing on the plantations.

Accordingly, there seem to have been a certain similarity in the possibilities the two groups had to treat the enslaved workers. Yet, there does not seem to have been much competition between them. Apparently, they practised in two separate sectors, the 'professional' and the 'folk' sector respectively, as previously outlined in Arthur Kleinman's theory. The sectors were partly overlapping, but the different power relationships between healers (and patients) in different sectors seem to have precluded any direct competition. Normally, the doctor's position as authorised by the state and contracted by the planter was not threatened by competition from unauthorised healers, and if it was, the doctor had the law on his side.

197 See for instance: Jensen, *En verden til forskel?*

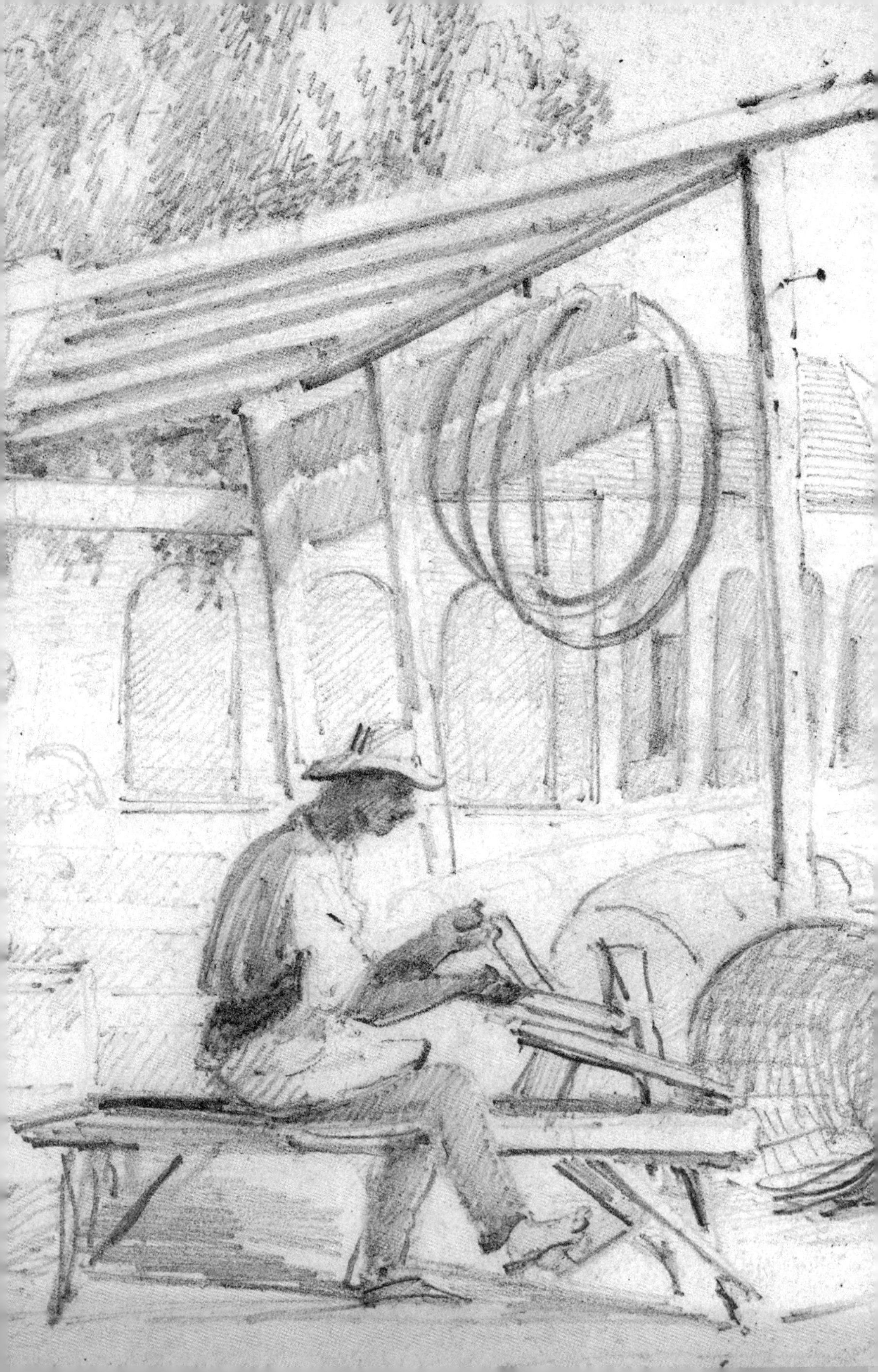

Chapter 3

Diseases, Therapies, and Causes of Death

As we have seen, the high mortality among enslaved workers in the Danish West Indies was apparently caused by a complex set of factors in the lives they lived. This raises the questions what exactly these factors were, what diseases they caused and how European and enslaved medicine tried to cope with them. In the following, I will investigate the range of diseases the enslaved suffered from, the morbidity and mortality caused by them, their possible causes, the treatments used by the Euro-Caribbean doctors to cure them, and whether the situation was similar in the British and French West Indies.

The Diseases of the Enslaved Workers and the Doctors' Therapies

The Source Material

The sources for this chapter consist primarily of two kinds of material, namely the official annual medical reports and monthly journals of plantation hospitals. The annual medical reports were produced by every doctor on St Croix and submitted via the landfysikus to the government agency of health in Copenhagen, the Royal Board of Health (*Det Kongelige Sundhedskollegium*).[198] The first report was submitted in 1803, but the next only in 1822. From then on there exist annual reports through to 1848 and beyond. The reports contain details about all the facets of a medical service that the doctors encountered in their daily work, i.e. primarily the diseases and their causes but also the treatments, the patients etc. Still, it is evident that the doctors concentrated on reporting the difficult or 'interesting' cases, and said less about diseases that were common or not life-threatening. The different disease terminology of the time can make it difficult to decipher exactly what disease they were

198 In a few cases, I shall include information from medical reports from St Thomas and St John, because they elucidate circumstances that presumably apply to all three islands but are not mentioned explicitly in the reports from St Croix.

dealing with. The quality of the reports varies from doctor to doctor but from 1822 they follow the same basic questionnaire designed by the Royal Board of Health.[199] Compared with the development in medicine during the period 1803–48, the medical reports do not show great changes. Primarily, the differences are between doctors, since some use the vocabulary and mindset of classical humoral pathology while others use a far more empirical approach in line with the new anatomic-pathologic paradigm. The therapeutic methods also seem to have remained generally the same, except in the field of surgery where the use of anaesthesia in major surgical operations from 1847 mirrors international developments.

The monthly journals originate from plantation hospitals on four royal plantations on St Croix (see Fig. 3.1). They were called 'royal' plantations because they had reverted through bankruptcy to their main creditor, the Danish Crown and state. In 1836, the Danish state owned fourteen such plantations on St Croix, which amounted to about 10 per cent of the acreage on the island.[200] Because of administrative and economic differences between these plantations and privately owned plantations in other parts of the island, these plantations are not necessarily representative of all plantations on St Croix. However, comparison with the data from the medical reports seems to show that the selected royal plantations are representative in the spectrum of diseases and the ranking of disease virulence. The hospital journals date from the years 1829–35 and they list in a schematic form the names of the patients, diseases and the dates of admission and discharge. Based on these data it has been possible to carry out a quantitative analysis of which diseases had the greatest impact on the enslaved population, i.e. which diseases respectively led to the largest number of admissions into the plantation hospital and which resulted in the longest periods of stay there. To facilitate this analysis it has been necessary to combine some of the disease categories the doctors used into larger categories comparable across the four plantations. This categorisation was not straightforward, as the doctors' terminology was based on the disease perception of humoral pathology and the miasma theory, and focused largely on what today would be called the symptoms of the disease. Furthermore, it was not the same doctor who attended to the four plantations and so the terminology varied slightly between the plan-

199 Letter from the Danish West Indian Government of 12 February 1820 and Chancellery circular of 20 December 1803. See: DNA, BH, Med.rep., 1803–1958. 1821. See also: Petersen, *Den Danske Medicinal-Lovgivning*.

200 Vibæk, 'Dansk Vestindien, 1755–1848', 325–26.

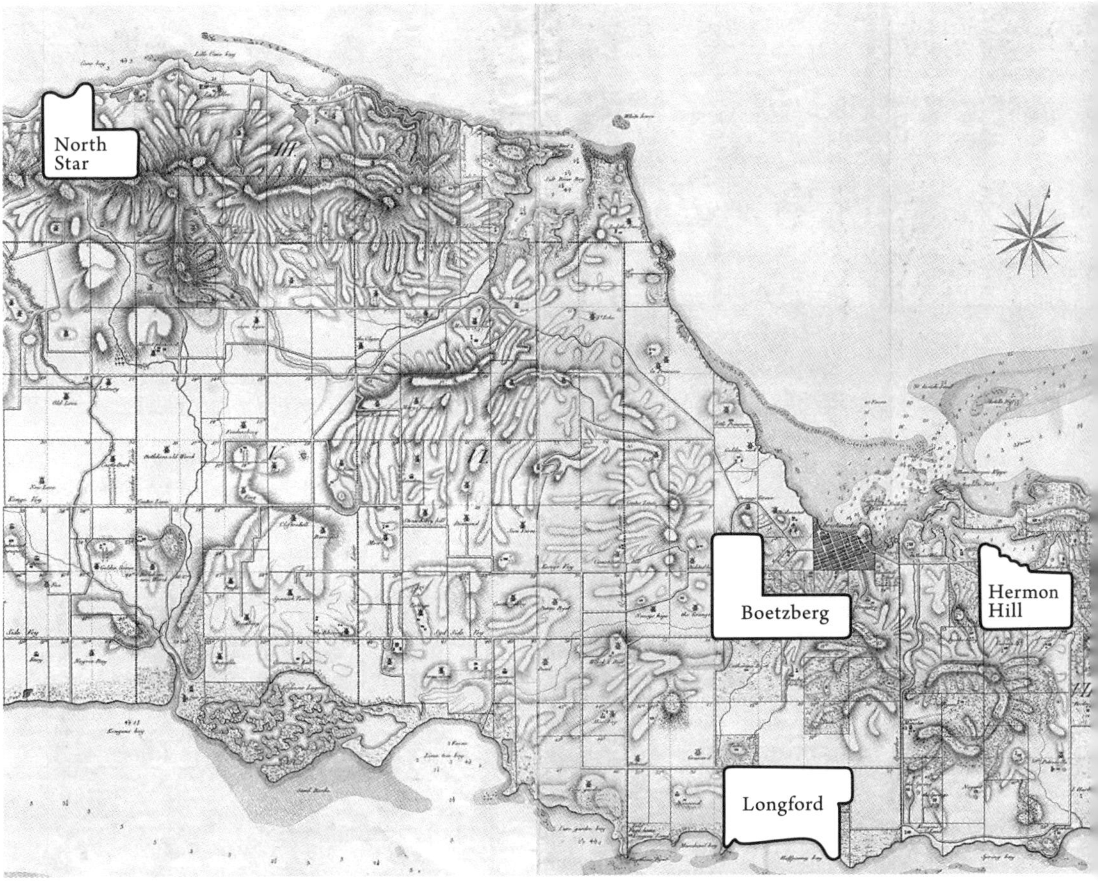

Fig. 3.1. The four royal plantations of North Star, Longford, Boetzberg and Hermon Hill. Section of Fig. 2.3.

tations.[201] Despite these circumstances, the analysis of the diseases among the enslaved workers on the four plantations shows both common features and minor variations. The four most significant disease categories were 'Fever', 'Pains and Injuries', 'Gastrointestinal diseases' and 'Boils and Sores'. These disease categories together accounted for between 60 and 95 per cent of the total

201 When lack of information has prevented the calculation of the duration of the stay in hospital, the patient in question has been excluded from the data. However, it is not possible to calculate the size of this exclusion as a percentage of all hospitalisations, because the recurrent monthly registrations of the same patient have also been removed.

number of days patients spent in the hospitals of the four plantations and they contributed by far the largest number of patients (see Table 3.1, 3.2, 3.3, 3.4). Nonetheless, the disease incidence rate of these disease categories measured in 1000 person-years-at-risk shows that the risk of an enslaved worker falling ill was not at all the same on the four plantations.

Finally, I would like to emphasise that the diseases dealt with in what follows are not necessarily the total number of diseases present on St Croix in the period 1803–48, but only the diseases mentioned in the medical reports and hospital journals.

The Doctors' Perception of the Health of the Enslaved Workers: Healthy or Fit?

The doctors on St Croix did not understand the idea of 'health' as 'a state of optimal physical, mental, and social well-being' (WHO). In fact, they only rarely used the word 'healthy' (Danish: *sund*) in the medical reports, and when they did, they seem simply to have meant the absence of visible illness. Accordingly, the word 'healthy' seems to have been an expression of an overall assessment of the physical state of the enslaved worker founded on the 'disease' perspective (see Chapter 1), and occasionally joined by the mental aspect, but always focusing on the physical ability to carry out normal work.[202] On this basis, the modern meaning of the word 'fit' seems a better match for the doctors' perception of enslaved health than the word 'healthy'. What was of primary interest to the doctors was whether the enslaved worker was capable of doing his or her job.[203] Apparently, this attitude did not only include the enslaved, but also European populations cared for by the doctors, for instance soldiers and seamen. Hence, the doctor's functional perception of the patient and the treatment both reflected the attitude of the employer or in the case of the enslaved workers the attitude of the planters. The colonial administration for its part had a more comprehensive and long-term perspective on the health of the enslaved workers, which manifested itself in a health policy with various prophylactic measures. Nevertheless, the administration also consulted the doctors concerning the preservation of the health of the enslaved, and consequently their physical perception of health was also dominant in the initiatives of the administration. In any event, the aim of both the planters and the administration was that the

202 DNA, BH, Med. rep., Danish West Indies, 1835, 1841 (Dr Stedmann), 1847 (Dr Jarvis Roebuck).

203 In the US, Euroamericans used the concept of 'soundness' to describe the enslaved in a similar way. See: Fett, *Working Cures*, 15–35.

enslaved should be able to work as much as possible without suffering permanent injury.

To what extent the enslaved perceived themselves to be in 'a state of optimal physical, mental, and social well-being' was not of interest to the doctors unless the lack of this 'well-being' affected their physical productivity. Against the enslaved workers' own perception of the disease and the cause of it, their 'illness' perspective, the doctors usually displayed scepticism and distrust, especially in relation to conditions that were not visible to the naked eye. They assumed the enslaved would lie and claim to be sick if they could get away with it in order to avoid work.

The Diseases of the Enslaved Workers and the Doctors' Treatments

FEVERS: *Intermitting and Remitting Fevers, Yellow Fever and Dengue Fever*

The annual medical reports from St Croix are generally full of references to various kinds of fever. There is not a single year without the mention of intermitting and remitting fevers as the most prominent diseases in the population as a whole. Among the enslaved, fever was also the most common disease. In 1826, Dr Hans Balthasar Hornbeck (1800–70[204]) of St John expressed this state of affairs in the following way:

> Nothing is more common among the Negroes than transitory fevers, which most often does not require anything but a purgative and a cooling drink.[205]

However, the doctors claimed in concurrence that the enslaved workers did not die from fever, not even in years when the fevers were particularly severe.[206] As we shall see later, these testimonies do not correspond at all with the causes of death registered in the church records of the island. Here, fevers had a prominent position with 19 per cent of all deaths, an average of 7.0 deaths per 1,000 enslaved (see Table 3.10).

Based on the statements concerning fever in the medical reports it is not surprising that fevers were also the most prominent category of diseases in the medical records of the hospitals of the four royal plantations. Yet, in most cases, the disease category 'Fever' was only described with that single word in the hos-

204 Kristian Carøe, *Den Danske Lægestand, 1479–1900* (Copenhagen: Gyldendal, Nordisk Forlag, 1977), III, 92 and V, 78.

205 DNA, BH, Med. rep., Danish West Indies. 1826, St John.

206 DNA, BH, Med. rep., Danish West Indies. 1825, 1838, 1841 etc.

pital records and accordingly it is difficult to make a more precise definition.[207] On the Longford and Hermon Hill plantations, fever caused the largest number of days spent in hospital among the enslaved workers, while on the Boetzberg it was only surpassed by the category 'Sores and Boils'. On these three plantations, 'Fever' caused about 30 per cent of all days spent in hospital and it was the one disease that most enslaved workers suffered from. Consequently, the average number of days spent in hospital per patient was comparably low (except on Hermon Hill). On the fourth plantation, North Star, fever ranked as only the fourth most common disease category, responsible for about 11 per cent of all days spent in hospital (see Tables 3.1, 3.2, 3.3, 3.4).

In contrast to the enslaved workers, newly arrived Europeans such as soldiers, sailors or officials succumbed in large numbers to the fevers. According to the humoral pathological disease perception of the period, the reason for this difference was to be found in the principles of constitution and acclimatisation. The perception was that the constitution of the enslaved was generally better suited for life in the tropics than that of the Europeans, because the enslaved originated in tropical Africa. Furthermore, most enslaved had lived for a long time in the West Indies, since the import of enslaved workers had been stopped in 1803, and accordingly their constitution had acclimatised to the local environment. This was also true for the Euro-Caribbeans, who were raised in the West Indies or had lived there for a long time, and were therefore also protected to a certain extent from the influences of the local environment despite their different constitution. However, newly arrived Europeans were not acclimatised and consequently they were unprotected against the harmful influences of the tropical environment, which caused the diseases.[208] This vulnerability was all too evident in the havoc caused by fevers among the newly arrived Europeans.

Modern medicine has a different explanation for the unequal distribution of the fever deaths, which is, however, not incompatible with the above explanation. First, the two most prominent types of fever, i.e. intermittent and remittent fever, usually refer to malaria.[209] Malaria is an infection caused by one or more members of a family of four parasites, *Plasmodium vivax, P. falsiparum, P.*

207 In this category I have included cases where fever is stated along with other symptoms but where fever must have been the main cause, for instance 'headache'. Furthermore, I have included single cases of 'intermitted fever' and 'Ague', i.e. fevers similar to malaria.

208 Harrison, 'The Tender Frame', 68–93.

209 Sheridan, *Doctors and Slaves*, 9.

malariae and *P. ovale*. The most deadly of them is falciparum, but the others can also be fatal. The parasites are transmitted by mosquitoes, which breed in stagnant pools and feed on both humans and animals. Today, the disease is prevalent in most tropical areas of the world, but it used to be far more common. The symptoms of malaria are periodic bouts of high fever, headache, and vomiting. The periodicity of these attacks is slightly different depending on which parasite is causing them. If the disease is not treated, it will in the long term cause serious anaemia and enlarged spleen and liver, because the parasites invade and rupture the red blood cells. This causes clogging of damaged blood cells and obstruction of blood vessels in different organs, which again can cause lethal complications.[210]

In this context, what is especially interesting about the perception of malaria in modern medicine are the types of resistance to the disease. Congenital resistance is found predominantly among people born in West Africa or of West African descent, because a large percentage of them carry a genetically determined abnormality in the red blood cells, the so-called 'sickle cell trait'. In the same population, other variants of haemoglobin occur, which are also thought to give protection against malaria. Finally, another genetic feature of the red blood cells among ethnic West Africans, namely the lack of a certain enzyme (6-phosfat dehydrogenase), also renders a certain protection against malaria. In the absence of congenital resistance, it is also possible to acquire resistance by being exposed to the disease several times. If this happens during childhood and the child survives, it will gradually acquire immunity to the local variants of malaria. The disease will only cause low numbers of parasites in the blood and accordingly the symptoms will be weak. However, the presence of the disease will weaken the defence against other diseases.[211]

The origin of these resistances against malaria explains why newly arrived Europeans, and not the enslaved workers, succumbed to the disease. The enslaved workers were largely ethnic West Africans whether they were born in West Africa or in the West Indies as children of enslaved West Africans. So, it is likely that a large percentage of them carried congenital resistances to malaria. To this were added the specific resistances to local variants of the disease, which they could acquire by growing up in an environment infected with local strands of malaria parasites. The inhabitants of European origin on

210 Kiple, *History of Human Disease*, 855–62.
211 Kiple, *History of Human Disease*, 858–59.

St Croix usually did not carry the congenital resistances, yet they could acquire the specific local resistances too if they grew up in the malarial environment of the island.[212] Accordingly, these two groups, the enslaved workers and the native Euro-Caribbeans, are likely to have had a certain resistance to malaria and did not succumb to it. In contrast, the disease wreaked havoc among the newly arrived Europeans, who rarely carried congenital or acquired resistance to the local strains of malaria, if to any at all.[213]

The other great fever disease often reported by the doctors of St Croix was yellow fever, also called climate fever (Danish: *Climatfeber*). As was the case with malaria, the victims were not enslaved workers but newly arrived Europeans. Yellow fever was such a huge problem, not just in the Danish West Indies but also in all of the West Indies and the United States that the Danish West Indian doctors partook in the lively international scholarly debate at the time concerning the causes of the disease and the possible methods of treatment.[214] According to modern medicine, yellow fever is a virus which is transmitted by infected mosquitoes. The species of mosquito responsible prefers to live near human dwellings. The symptoms are fever, headache, internal bleeding in the digestive tract and jaundice, which has given the disease its name. If the patient survives the disease, he or she will be immune for life. The disease is usually milder during childhood, which is why native populations in areas with it are usually immune. Consequently, the disease is only serious and life-threatening to newcomers, which was also the case in the Danish West Indies. For many years it has been discussed whether the enslaved workers, and by extension ethnic West Africans, had a congenital immunity to yellow fever and not just an acquired one. There are many historical examples of epidemics of yellow fever where the enslaved workers were not affected while the Europeans suffered terribly, but there is as yet no physical explanation for the difference.[215]

The last of the proper fever diseases mentioned by the doctors of St Croix was dengue fever. The first time it is identified on St Croix was in 1827, when the doctors reported that a new disease, called 'dandy fever' or 'breakbone fever', had attacked nearly everyone on the island. The doctors had heard of the disease from the other West Indian islands and read about it in the literature, but

212 Kiple, *History of Human Disease*, 500.

213 Malaria existed in many parts of Europe in the nineteenth century, even as far north as Denmark. See Carl Adam Hansen, 'Den "lollandske feber",' *Lolland-Falsters historiske Samfunds Aarbog* 1 (1913).

214 Torben Geill, 'Den gule feber i Dansk Vestindien', *Dansk medicinhistorisk årbog* (1975), 144–47.

215 Kiple, *History of Human Disease*, 1100–7.

now they recognised its typical symptoms, high fever, and swollen joints causing excruciating pain. No one died from the disease but it was noticed that the enslaved workers on the plantations did not seem to suffer as much as everyone else.[216] If this observation is true, it means that at least some of the enslaved workers had previously been exposed to dengue fever. According to modern medicine, the virus that causes the disease renders the victim immune after the first infection, yet only to that specific strand of dengue fever. In return, infection with other strands of the disease will cause severe, even lethal symptoms. Dengue fever is transmitted by mosquitoes and is rarely fatal. Today, it is endemic in most tropical and subtropical areas.[217]

The doctors' treatment of fever, regardless of its kind, was cinchona bark (quinine bark) and later the new wonder drug, quinine sulphate.[218] The alkaloid was isolated from cinchona bark the first time in 1820 and used for the first time in 1823 in the USA.[219]

OCCUPATIONAL ACCIDENTS: *Pains, Sores, Fractures, and Hernia*

According to the records for the hospitals on the four royal plantations, occupational accidents and injuries (grouped as 'Pains and Injuries') often afflicted the enslaved workers. However, the descriptions of the various ailments are too brief to determine if the problem was caused directly by hard labour or by some infection. The type of ailment occurring most frequently in this disease category is pains in the back, the side, the arms, the legs etc.[220] On the Longford, Boetzberg and Hermon Hill plantations, pains were the ailment, apart from fever, that caused the largest number of days in hospital, 17 to 25 per cent of all days in the years investigated. Still, because the number of enslaved patients with pains was high, the average number of days in hospital per patient was generally relatively low. On North Star, where the order of the disease categories was different, 'Pains and Injuries' presented the largest percentage of days in hospital; about 19 per cent (see Tables 3.1, 3.2, 3.3, 3.4).

The second most common kind of probably occupational injury was vari-

216 DNA, BH, Med. rep., Danish West Indies. 1827.
217 Kiple, *History of Human Disease*, 660–64.
218 DNA, BH, Med. rep., Danish West Indies. 1831. See also: Barclay, *Bidrag til Kundskab*, 12.
219 Philip Curtin, *Death by Migration* (Cambridge: Cambridge University Press, 1989), 63.
220 Pains in genitalia, eyes, and teeth are not included in this category unless it is obviously a work-related accident. Pains in the head are included even though they are not necessarily work-related, while pains in the stomach and intestines are not included because it seems likely that the primary cause of abdominal pain was a gastrointestinal disease and not just hard work.

ous forms of wounds (grouped as 'Boils and Sores'), generally on feet and legs, but also on fingers, hands and arms.[221] On Boetzberg, 'Sores' (and boils) caused the highest number of hospitalised days, about 32 per cent, while on Longford and North Star it ranked third with around 12 and 13 per cent respectively, and on Hermon Hill fourth with around 17 per cent. However, in contrast to both fevers and pains and injuries, boils and sores did not afflict as many patients, yet in return the time spent in hospital was markedly longer (see Tables 3.1, 3.2, 3.3, 3.4). A similar picture emerges from inventories, lease contracts and inspection reports from several royal plantations, which shows that after rose (erysipelas), different kinds of wounds ('sores', 'ulcers') on the legs were the most common and crippling ailments, especially among the older enslaved workers.[222] As the enslaved workers normally did not wear shoes it is little wonder that most of their wounds were on their feet and legs, but still it is not possible to determine if the wounds originated from occupational accidents or from infections caused by insects, parasites etc.

Other kinds of injuries were hernias, bites, cuts, sprains, and fractured limbs. A survey of inventories, lease contracts, inspection reports etc. from a number of plantations show that among these injuries hernia was the most widespread. This is also illustrated by the many hernia trusses ordered by the doctors for the enslaved workers on the plantations. Typically, hernia afflicted male enslaved workers above 30, which presumably bears testimony to the fact that they carried out the heaviest work on the plantation.[223] Among adults, hernia is a typical occupational injury caused by the lifting of heavy loads, when a loop of the intestine is pressed out through a weak spot in the abdominal wall.[224] Finally, there is one kind of injury which is notable by its absence, namely burns. The enslaved workers who laboured in the boiling house during harvest had a great risk of being scalded by the boiling sugar juice or of being burnt by the fire under the kettles, yet such cases are not mentioned anywhere. In comparison, burns

221 The category 'Boils and ulcers' (Danish: 'bylder og sår') covers skin infections excluding rose or swelling caused by oedema, since they figure in other categories.

222 See for instance: DNA, WILA, no. 46.17.54, North Star, 1838. DNA, WILA, no. 46.21, Work and Rest, 1830. NARA, RG55, Entry 1109, Box 2432, Estate Jolly Hill and Betzys Jewel, 1840. DNA, WILA, no. 46.17.6, Boetzberg, 1838.

223 DNA, WILA, no. 46.17.43, alphabetic extract of account, 1826. DNA, WILA, no. 46.58.1, Hermon Hill, 1829. NARA, RG55, Entry 1109, box 2439, report from Estate Smithfield, 1834. DNA, DSD, no. 1128, Hermon Hill, 1825 and 1836. DNA, DSD, no. 1129, Upper Love, 1843. DNA, WILA, no. 10.21, entries for J.M. Magens 1813, I.L. Müller 1812, Estate Fountain 1812, Estate Big Princess 1812.

224 Christian Blangstrup, ed., *Salmonsens Konversationsleksikon* IV (Copenhagen: Schultz Forlag, 1916 [2nd edn]), 63–64.

were very common among enslaved working in the boiling houses of the British West Indies.[225]

Returning to the annual medical reports, the doctors were concentrating on the difficult or curious ailments and the common sores and muscle pains of the enslaved workers did not belong to this category. However, there were exceptions, as when Dr Hornbeck of St John noted in 1826 that

> Old ulcers on the legs are frequent among the Negroes. Often they are so ingrown that one cannot cure them entirely without danger and often they are so deep that despite all efforts they attack the bones and kill with caries[[226]]. The leaves of physic nut (*Jatropha curcas*) is often excellent to clean up such sores, just as the fresh root of *Jatropha Manihot* (cassava); numerous wild herbs are praised as efficient home remedies, soon by one, soon by another.[227]

It is not possible to determine what caused the sores Dr Hornbeck describes, but the quotation illustrates two factors: first, the seriousness of the conditions behind the term 'Sores', and second the treatment used locally, presumably primarily among the enslaved workers. At the time and still today 'physic nut' or 'Barbados nut' (*Jatropha curcas*) grows on the US Virgin Islands, and traditionally it has been used externally to cure wounds.[228] As to the cassava (*Manihot esculenta*) it was and is a common foodstuff, and its ability to heal difficult wounds was known among doctors in the British West Indies.[229] It is interesting that Dr Hornbeck not only knew these local plants but also seems to have used them as remedies. However, the last line of the quotation also shows the scepticism of the European doctor towards the efficacy of local herb medicine.

225 Grainger, *An Essay*, 83.

226 'Caries' or osteomyelitis refers to an infection that slowly 'eats' the bone. See: Blangstrup, *Salmonsens* II, 910–11.

227 DNA, BH, Med. rep., Danish West Indies. 1826. Original Danish text: 'Gamle Ulcera paa Benene træffer man hyppigen blandt Negerne, ofte saa indgroede, at man ei uden Fare bør læge dem ganske til, og ofte saa dybt om sig ædende, at de trods alle Anstrengelser angribe Benene, og dræbe med Caries. Bladene af Physic-nut (Iatropha curcas) ere ofte fortrinlige til at gjøre saadanne Saar rene, ligesom ogsaa den friske Rod af Iatropha manihot (Cassava); mangfoldige vilde Urter roses snart af én, snart af en anden som virksomme Huusmidler.'

228 A. J. Oakes, *Poisonous and injurious plants of the US Virgin Islands* (Washington, D.C.: United States Department of Agriculture, Agricultural Research Service, 1962), 55–58. Thomas, *Traditional Medical Plants*, 85–86.

229 Collins, *Practical Rules*, 376.

GASTROINTESTINAL DISEASES

According to the records of the hospitals on the royal plantations, gastrointestinal complaints were the last of the four most common categories of ailments among the enslaved workers.[230] On the Boetzberg and Hermon Hill plantations, gastrointestinal complaints were the third most important disease category, accounting for respectively 12 and 20 per cent of the total number of days spent in hospital, on North Star it came in second with around 12 per cent, while on Longford it curiously did not figure at all (see Tables 3.1, 3.2, 3.3, 3.4). The medical reports do not attribute the same importance to gastrointestinal diseases in relation to the enslaved population in general, but mainly for the enslaved children, for whom these diseases were very serious.[231]

DISEASES AMONG INFANTS: *Tetanus neonatorum, 'Dentitio', Convulsions, Worms, and Diarrhoea*

Tetanus among newborn children, referred to by the doctors as 'Tetanus neonatorum' or 'Trismus nascentium', was a very common disease and cause of death among the newly born of the enslaved workers.[232] According to modern medicine, the disease is caused by the bacterium *Clostridium tetani* and the symptoms usually commence five to ten days after an infection caused by unhygienic dressing of the umbilical cord. The first symptom is contraction of the jaw muscles (trismus) and hence the English term 'lock jaw'. The infant's ability to suckle is impaired and a state of stiffness and cramps develops in other muscles in the body. The mortality rate is up to 90 per cent. Adults and older children infected through open wounds have a greater chance of surviving the disease, because the convulsions cease after one or two weeks.[233] On St Croix, there were also a number of these cases and the doctors stated that the disease could originate either from a wound or from the patient having exposed himself to nocturnal rain or to cold. The doctors fought for weeks to save the patients, for instance with hot sand baths and injections of opium, but they only rarely succeeded.[234] Nevertheless, in 1837 interim landfysikus Poul Elias Wintmöhl

230 The category includes unspecified problems of the gastrointestinal tract frequently referred to as 'bowels' or 'bowel complaint', 'diarrhoea' or 'dysentery'.

231 Cholera, the most deadly gastrointestinal disease of the period, did not hit St Croix when the second cholera pandemic swept the Caribbean in 1832.

232 DNA, BH, Med. rep., Danish West Indies. 1830, 1831, 1838, 1846.

233 Kiple, *History of Human Disease*, 1043–49.

234 DNA, BH, Med. rep., Danish West Indies. 1835, 1845.

Schlegel (1784–1849)[235] estimated that tetanus was not as widespread among infants as it had been previously and he ascribed this improvement to the efficient system of midwives.[236]

Another serious but very common condition among the slightly older enslaved children was the so-called 'Dentitio'. The term referred to the period when the child got its first teeth, which usually occurs about the age of four months, however the term was synonymous with at least four different 'afflictions', namely convulsions, intestinal worms, diarrhoea, and fever.[237] According to the doctors, the convulsions could be caused by the tooth eruption alone or by intestinal worms, which seem to have been very common among enslaved children and in large parts of the enslaved population in general. Several doctors expressed astonishment at the volume of worms that even healthy slaves could contain.[238] The intestinal worms were probably a result of the general lack of hygiene in the handling of foodstuffs, which is illustrated by the following quotation from 1841 by Dr William Stedman (1764–1844[239]) of Frederiksted, St Croix:

> This great prevalence of worms occurred almost solely on the estates in Northside Quarter, where great numbers of the tree, which bears the fruit named the Guava, grow wild ... It may be proper to observe that during the period when the fruit is in season the Negroes eat great quantities of them raw, often in a crude and unripe estate, and keep them for food in a variety of ways.[240]

Today, fruit is known as a frequent source of gastrointestinal infections because it is often eaten raw, and if the fruit was even stored for later use there would have been numerous possibilities for pollution with various pathogenic microorganisms, for instance worms. Judging from the descriptions in the medical reports, the types of parasitic worms that might have infected children and

235 Carøe, *Den Danske Lægestand* III, 180 and V, 92.

236 DNA, WILA, no. 10.2.1. 31 May, 1837.

237 DNA, BH, Med. rep., Danish West Indies. 1835.

238 DNA, Danske Kancelli (Danish Chancellery), Fællesafdelingen (Common department), Kommission ang. en Anordning om Medicinalpolitiet 1802–1814 (Commission regarding an ordinance on medical policy 1802–1814), Indkomne Sager, Forhandlinger og Korrespondance (Incoming cases, negotiations and correspondence), no. G125C, reports from St Croix, 1804 (Hereafter called DNA, DC, no. G125C). DNA, BH, Med. rep., Danish West Indies. 1835, 1841, 1844, 1846, 1847, 1848.

239 Carøe, *Den Danske Lægestand* III, 195–96 and V, 44.

240 DNA, BH, Med. rep., Danish West Indies. 1841.

adult enslaved are for instance pork tapeworm (*Taenia solium*), roundworm (*Ascaris lumbricoides*), whipworm (*Trichuris trichiura*) and pinworm (*Enterobius vermicularis*). Pork tapeworm, roundworm and whipworm gain access to the human organism through human excrements on raw fruit and vegetables, polluted water and dirty hands, whereas pinworm is primarily transferred in the latter way. Roundworm and whipworm can cause colic, cramps, diarrhoea etc., which corresponds very well with the descriptions, while pinworm rarely causes complications. Normally, the pork tapeworm does not cause complications either, unless during its larval state when it deposits itself in the muscle tissue of the host and causes fever, headache and muscle pains.[241] One last species of worm that is very likely to have plagued the enslaved workers is hookworm (*Necator americanus*). As a larva, it penetrates the skin on the feet of humans walking barefoot on polluted soil, after which it develops in the intestines and lives off the blood of the host organism. This can cause serious anaemia with many related symptoms such as oedema, lack of energy and indigestion.[242] Despite the different symptoms, it is common to the parasitic worms that they deprive the host organism of nutrients. According to the medical reports, intestinal worms did not cause many deaths in contrast to diarrhoea (also referred to as dysentery), which for instance in the years 1846/7 increased child mortality significantly.[243] The doctors stated that the reason for the diarrhoea was the dampness of the atmosphere caused by heavy rains.[244] The claim may have been correct in the sense that the heavy rains may have caused local flooding and so the contamination of the enslaved workers' supply of drinking water with surface water. However, the doctors did not take it too seriously if enslaved children died of diarrhoea during the 'dentition period', probably because it was so common. Apart from the children, diarrhoea also killed the old and weak enslaved workers.[245]

RESPIRATORY DISEASES: *Pneumonia, Influenza and Diphtheria/Sore throat*

In the medical reports, the respiratory diseases of pneumonia, influenza, and diphtheria (or other forms of infection in the throat) make up a complex of diseases. The diseases often appear together or in conjunction with each other and

241 Palle Johnsen, 'Snylteorme i Mennesket', *Natur og Museum* 22, no. 4 (1983).
242 Kiple, *History of Human Disease*, 784–88.
243 DNA, BH, Med. rep., Danish West Indies. 1826, 1846, 1847 etc.
244 DNA, BH, Med. rep., Danish West Indies. 1846, 1847.
245 DNA, BH, Med. rep., Danish West Indies. 1847.

can be very difficult to separate. The doctors found the cause of all three diseases in the same factor, the cool, rainy, and windy weather.[246]

Apart from the fevers, the doctors on St Croix perceived pneumonia to be the most common acute disease and, again after fever, the most dangerous for the enslaved workers.[247] However, in this respect the medical reports and the hospital records differ markedly from each other, because the records do not assign any prominent place to respiratory diseases. Pneumonia is an infection of the lungs caused by one of several agents. Many different bacteria, viruses, fungi, and parasites can cause pneumonia. Regardless of which organism causes the disease, the symptoms are always high fever and the spitting of bloody mucus. After 7 to 10 days a crisis will occur, which can be deadly. Pneumonia is more common in cold weather, because the organisms that cause the disease are more numerous in such weather.[248] Given these factors, it is no wonder that the enslaved workers contracted pneumonia, since they lived in wet and draughty houses with dry rot, a perfect breeding place for bacteria, viruses, fungi, and parasites.

Influenza is another very contagious viral disease, which especially attacks the respiratory tract and causes sore throats, coughs, runny noses, fevers, headaches, muscle pains etc. Normally, the disease is only lethal for small children, old people and people with weak immune systems, but it is also one of the most common reasons for pneumonia, where it causes many deaths.[249] In 1843 and 1847, influenza may have been the culprit behind many deaths among weak enslaved workers and enslaved children. It is impossible to ascertain if it was only influenza, because 'severe catarrhs' are also mentioned. In the instances where this condition took a serious form and became lethal, diphtheria may have been the cause.

The medical reports mention 'cynanche maligna', 'angina maligna', 'angina putrida' and 'malignant sore throat' or 'putrid sore throat', all of which refer to what modern medicine calls diphtheria.[250] The reports also mention quinsy, which is very difficult to separate from diphtheria in the text.[251] According to modern medicine, diphtheria is caused by the bacterium *Corynebacterium diphtheria*, which attacks the mucus membrane in the throat. The majority of cases

246 DNA, BH, Med. rep., Danish West Indies. 1841, 1843, 1847.
247 DNA, DC, no. G125C. W. Stedman and H. Lang, § 1. DNA, BH, Med. rep., Danish West Indies. 1828.
248 Kiple, *History of Human Disease*, 938–42.
249 Kiple, *History of Human Disease*, 807–11.
250 See for instance: Kiple, *History of Human Disease*, 265–66.
251 DNA, BH, Med. rep., Danish West Indies. 1825, 1828, 1838, 1841, 1843.

are children up to the age of 15 with a mortality rate of 30–50 per cent. Diphtheria prevails in areas where people live close together and among poor people with bad hygiene.[252]

TUBERCULOSIS (Consumption)

According to the *Oxford English Dictionary*, 'consumption' is often synonymous with 'pulmonary consumption' and 'phthisis', which are former terms for tuberculosis.[253] In the hospital records, consumption only appears on Longford plantation with one out of a total of 106 patients and even if this single patient was admitted for 183 days (9.63 percent of all days of hospitalisation on the plantation), suggesting that he suffered from chronic tuberculosis, the disease does not seem to have had the same position among the causes of disease as among the causes of death. However, it is highly likely that some of the above-mentioned respiratory diseases were in fact tuberculosis.

According to modern medicine, the bacterium *Mycobacterium tuberculosis* causes tuberculosis. The disease has killed millions since the beginning of industrialisation. It is usually a chronic disease and can linger for years, yet it also has an acute form, miliary tuberculosis, which kills swiftly by attacking almost all organs in the body simultaneously. The bacterium is transmitted by airborne droplet infection but it can survive in dry secretions (dust) if not exposed to sunlight. Consequently, the lack of indoor hygiene is an important factor in the spread of the disease. When it has entered the body, it can survive encapsulated throughout the host's entire lifespan without breaking out. The outbreak does not occur until the resistance of the host is reduced, which is often caused by specific factors depending respectively on the host and the environment. The host specific factors are age and sex. At the points during the lifetime of a human being when its resistance is at its lowest, i.e. during childhood and old age, the host is most exposed to a tuberculosis breakout. Women in their childbearing years are more vulnerable than men, apparently because their reproductive cycle increases the need for protein, and if the need cannot be fulfilled then resistance is reduced and the risk of an outbreak of tuberculosis increases. However, in the age groups above 30, men are more vulnerable than women. The environmental factors are crowding, nutrition, and working conditions. The level of crowding, i.e. how close people live to each other, is very

252 Kiple, *History of Human Disease*, 680–83.

253 See: 'Consumption' in *The Oxford English Dictionary* (OED Online, Oxford University Press, 2000), www.oed.com (accessed 30-05-2011).

important for the spread of the disease. The nutritional state of the host is also very important, because the intake of protein has a major impact on the overall resistance to diseases. For the same reason the working conditions of the host are also important, because hard physical and strenuous work weakens the resistance of the body. In contrast, climate is not an important factor, neither in bringing about nor in healing the disease, as was thought in the first half of the nineteenth century.[254]

It is no surprise to find tuberculoses among the enslaved in the Danish West Indies. The environmental factors were certainly present in the shape of a high level of crowding in the houses, bad hygiene, generally bad nutrition, and hard physical work. Source material from the period 1803–48 reports the disease being present on the islands with names such as *Lungesvindsot* (phthisis).[255] However, in the medical reports the term 'consumption' only appears in relation to visiting 'invalids', i.e. tuberculosis patients, from North America, who started to visit St Croix in 1830s to enjoy the mild climate.[256] Apart from the term 'consumption', the reports contain terms like 'pleuritis' (pleurisy), 'pulmonary disorder', and 'pneumonias', which could refer to tuberculosis or to many other respiratory diseases.

'CHRONIC DISEASES': *Elephantiasis, West Indian Rose, and Oedema*

A complex of so-called 'chronic diseases' often mentioned in the medical reports consists of elephantiasis, West Indian rose and hydrocele. It was primarily the enslaved workers and the free coloureds who suffered from the diseases in this complex, yet occasionally also poor Euro-Caribbeans.[257] The terms 'elephantiasis' and 'West Indian rose' were used almost synonymously and referred to a state of extremely swollen legs among the enslaved workers and also swollen genitals among the male enslaved.[258] In the latter instance, an enlarged scrotum could be caused by hydrocele, an abnormally large accumulation of fluid (oedema) in the membranes surrounding the testicles.[259] The swollen leg and/or genitals could attain grotesque proportions, which made it impossible for the afflicted enslaved to work in the field, if at all.

254 Kiple, *History of Human Disease*, 1059–65.
255 Barclay, *Bidrag til Kundskab*, 115–22.
256 DNA, BH, Med. rep., Danish West Indies. 1831, 1832, 1835, 1837, 1838 og 1839. Dr Stedman's reports.
257 DNA, BH, Med. rep., Danish West Indies. 1827.
258 DNA, BH, Med. rep., Danish West Indies. 1828, 1834 (landfysikus Hornbeck on St Thomas), 1845.
259 Bengt I. Lindskog, *Medicinsk Ordbog* (Copenhagen: Gyldendalske Boghandel, Nordisk Forlag A/S, 2004), 'Hydrocele'.

Today elephantiasis is called filariasis and is widespread in most of Africa, South America and South and South East Asia. Worldwide 120 million people are infected with filariasis. The disease is caused by the parasitic worms *Wuchereria bacrofti* and *Brugia malayi*, which are transmitted by bloodsucking mosquitoes. The worms live in the lymphatic system and cause accumulations of lymph in the infected tissue, as well as free access for other infections of the skin. Normally, the symptoms of the disease are only visible in adults, and in societies where the disease is endemic, 10 to 50 per cent of all men suffer from damage to the genitalia, particularly hydrocele.[260] Until 1937, when a medical programme eradicated the disease from St Croix, it was discovered that about 60 per cent of the inhabitants were infected with the parasites, Afro-Caribbean as well as Euro-Caribbean.[261]

The disease called rose, or erysipelas, is understood by modern medicine to be an acute infection of the skin, usually caused by the streptococcus bacteria. It appears when the normal immune defence of the skin is damaged by degradation, malnutrition, or other infections, for instance filariasis.[262] To the doctors on St Croix, 'rose' referred to a swelling of the skin and the lymphatic nodes caused by oedema, which to them made it look similar to elephantiasis. Some doctors assumed rose to be a preliminary stage in the development of elephantiasis, but they were generally at a loss as to the cause of the two diseases. They suggested that the cause could be sudden cold and moisture or dry weather, that the diseases were hereditary, that they were contagious, or that it was the uncleanliness of the enslaved, especially the fact that they walked barefoot in the field, that caused the disease.[263] However, whatever the reason for elephantiasis, rose, and oedema, the doctors throughout the period generally agreed that these diseases were steadily increasing.[264] Curiously, in 1803, two doctors even claimed that rose had not existed on the island twenty years earlier.[265]

According to the records of the hospitals on the four royal plantations, rose and/or 'swellings' (oedema) did not attack many enslaved workers. The two ailments only accounted for between 1 and 8 per cent of all days spent in hospital,

260 *Lymphatic filariasis*. Fact sheet no. 102. WHO Media Centre, September 2000. www.who.int/mediacentre/factsheets/fs102/en/ (accessed 30-05-2011).

261 Erik J. Lawaetz, *St Croix 500 years: Pre-Columbus to 1990* (Copenhagen: Poul Kristensens Forlag, 1990), 120.

262 Lindskog, *Medicinsk Ordbog*, 'Rosen', 'Erysipelas'.

263 DNA, DC, no. G125C. DNA, BH, Med. rep., Danish West Indies. 1825, 1828, 1834 (Landfysikus Hornbeck on St Thomas), 1836.

264 DNA, BH, Med. rep., Danish West Indies. 1826, 1827, 1828, 1829, 1830, 1832, 1833, 1834, 1841, 1845.

265 DNA, DC, no. G125C. W. Stedman and H. Lang, § 1.

but they caused long and repeated admissions. Apparently, the patients were often older enslaved workers. A survey of inventories, lease contracts, and inspection reports from a number of royal plantations shows that rose in the feet and legs was the most common crippling illness among enslaved workers above the age of 40. However, the disease is not seen in enslaved workers below the age of 25, which must be related to the fact that the disease only becomes serious (and so visible) when the immune system is no longer able to suppress it. Elephantiasis did not occur as often.[266] The doctors perceived elephantiasis and rose to be chronic, incurable diseases, but in some cases their development could be stopped, for instance by using mercurial ointments. However, the only effective remedy against elephantiasis in the leg was amputation below the knee before the disease spread further up into the body. This procedure may have been the main reason for the presence of enslaved workers with wooden legs on the plantations. The doctors claimed to be able to prolong the life of the enslaved patient through amputation, even though these diseases did not normally kill the enslaved workers, but only made them unfit for fieldwork.[267] However, these enslaved workers could perform other kinds of work that did not require full mobility. The treatment of hydrocele was also referred to as surgical, presumably because it consisted in simply draining off the accumulated fluid.[268] Another treatment was the injection of zinc sulphate, which causes the membranes to contract.[269]

In the medical reports the term 'dropsy' (Danish: *vattersot*) generally referred to other kinds of oedema than the ones mentioned above. In most cases, it was ascites (accumulation of fluid in the abdomen), but there was also anasarca (accumulation of fluid in the body generally), hydrothorax (accumulation of fluid in the chest cavity) and hydrocephalus (accumulation of fluid in the cranium).[270] However, these kinds of dropsy were quite rare. The hospital records of the royal plantations only show a few instances of dropsy.[271] In this respect, the pattern of diseases among the enslaved workers on St Croix is different from both the modern and the historic international literature on

266 DNA, WILA, no. 46.17.6, 46.17.32, 46.17.33, 46.17.44, 46.17.45, 46.17.54, 46.21. NARA, RG55, Entry 1109, Box 2432, Estate Jolly Hill.
267 DNA, BH, Med. rep., Danish West Indies. 1825, 1843, 1845, 1847 (amputations during anaesthesia with ether).
268 DNA, BH, Med. rep., Danish West Indies. 1833, 1841.
269 DNA, BH, Med. rep., Danish West Indies. 1829, 1830.
270 DNA, BH, Med. rep., Danish West Indies. 1825, 1826, 1827, 1834, 1842. See also: Barclay, *Bidrag til Kundskab*, 125–26.
271 Estates Hermon Hill, Jolly Hill, Longford med stutteri, Cotton Grove and Boetzberg.

the diseases of the enslaved, which claims that dropsy was a prominent disease.[272] According to modern medicine, oedema can be caused by a variety of problems like conditions of the heart, the liver, the urinary system or malnutrition.[273]

'SKIN DISEASES': *Leprosy, Yaws, and Scabies*

When the doctors of St Croix described elephantiasis and rose in their annual medical reports, the descriptions were often followed by comments on another group of diseases related to the skin, namely leprosy and yaws.

Previous research has claimed that the doctors in the Danish West Indies did not mention leprosy until 1849, but as will be evident from the following this is not correct.[274] The Moravian missionary C. G. A. Oldendorp mentions leprosy in his account of his visit to the island in the years 1768/9,[275] and during the period 1803–48 leprosy among the enslaved workers was a topic of great attention among planters and colonial administrators. In 1810, 'The Agricultural Society',[276] backed by the influential Council of Citizens (*Borgerrådet*), encouraged the English governor to investigate how many enslaved workers on the island were afflicted with leprosy. The aim of the society and the council was the construction of a special building to house and isolate the leprous enslaved workers to prevent them from infecting other enslaved.[277] The governor seems to have reacted promptly to the request, because in the following month lists arrived from the captains of the East End Quarter and Queens Quarter (districts) containing the number of leprous enslaved workers.[278] The lists show the number of leprous enslaved workers to have been low, a total of twenty-eight individuals in the two quarters. This was probably the reason why nothing further happened. However, leprosy was apparently so important to the members of The Agricultural Society that they revived the matter again a couple of months after the return of the Danish authorities to St Croix in 1815. In August

272 See for instance: Sheridan, *Doctors and Slaves*, 210–11; Higman, *Slave Populations*, 341–47; Kiple, *The Caribbean Slave*, 97–100; Collins, *Practical Rules*, 300–9.

273 Kiple, *History of Human Disease*, 689–96.

274 Torben Geill, 'Spedalskheden i Dansk Vestindien', *Dansk medicinhistorisk årbog* (1977), 147.

275 Christian Georg Andreas Oldendorp, *Historie der caribischen Inseln Sanct Thomas, Sanct Crux und Sanct Jan, insbesondere der dasigen Neger und der Mission der evangelischen Brüder unter denselben* I (Berlin: VWB, Verlag für Wissenschaft und Bildung, 2000– [first published Barby 1777]), 627–28.

276 The Agricultural Society seems to have been an association of planters on St Croix, existing 1808 to 1816 and possibly longer. See for instance: *The St Croix Gazette*, 1 December 1808, and *Dansk Vestindisk Regierings Avis*, 6 May 1816.

277 DNA, WILA, no. 3.56.2. 24 September 1810.

278 DNA, WILA, no. 3.56.2. 31 October 1810.

to October 1816, the colonial government requested reports on how many leprous enslaved workers existed on the island.[279] Again, lists of enslaved leprosy patients came in from the island's districts, but unfortunately they seem to have been lost. Still, they did not lead to any intervention by the administration.[280] In 1822 and 1829, the story repeated itself, yet the spread of the disease still does not seem to have been serious enough for any intervention.[281]

In the medical reports, it is evident that the doctors knew leprosy very well, with its hideous appearance of ears, nose, fingers, and toes rotting and falling off.[282] However, doctors did not know the cause of the disease, though they knew it was not very contagious and so assumed it to be hereditary.[283] There were lepers among the enslaved workers, the free coloured and poor Euro-Caribbeans,[284] but the doctors did not agree whether leprosy was an expanding disease or whether the numbers suffering from it were relatively stable.[285] A survey of inventories, lease contracts, and inspection reports from a number of royal plantations shows that leprosy was present on most plantations, but usually only with one patient on each plantation. In return, the disease afflicted all age groups.[286] In the hospital records from the four royal plantations, leprosy occurs only in one instance on North Star plantation. As one would expect, the disease was chronic; the patient was registered as being sick throughout the entire period investigated (1830–33).[287] The patient lived in isolation in a guardhouse somewhere on the plantation's land.

Apparently, no treatment existed for leprosy, except the somewhat bizarre therapy recommended for early stages of the disease by Dr William Stephen Jacobs (1779–1843)[288] in 1835.[289] The remedy was to eat raw lizards, a therapy known in the British West Indies too.[290] Curiously, the same recipe had been described in detail 50 years earlier by the Cruzian surgeon Johan Christian

279 DNA, WILA, no. 2.2.2. Case no.: 279 and 280.
280 DNA, WILA, no. 2.16.7. Case no.: 259, 296 and 298.
281 DNA, WILA, no. 10.2.3. Letter for landfysikus Block of 8 October 1822 and letter for interim landfysikus Jacobs of 16 September 1829.
282 DNA, BH, Med. rep., Danish West Indies. 1826, 1827, 1830, 1832, 1834, 1835.
283 DNA, BH, Med. rep., Danish West Indies. 1834 (landfysikus Hornbeck, St Thomas).
284 DNA, BH, Med. rep., Danish West Indies. 1827, 1835.
285 DNA, BH, Med. rep., Danish West Indies. 1827, 1830, 1832, 1835.
286 DNA, WILA, no. 46.17.6, 46.17.32, 46.17.33, 46.17.44, 46.17.45, 46.17.54, 46.21. NARA, RG55, Entry 1109, Box 2432, Estate Jolly Hill.
287 This single instance of leprosy is not included in the charts of diseases on North Star because it would be confusing.
288 Carøe, *Den Danske Lægestand* III, and V, 79.
289 DNA, BH, Med. rep., Danish West Indies. 1835.
290 Collins, *Practical Rules*, 332.

Schmidt. However, whereas Dr Jacobs prescribed lizards against leprosy, Schmidt used them against venereal disease.[291] Still, as mentioned earlier, these diseases were perceived as closely related at the time.

According to modern medicine, leprosy (Lepra) is a bacterial infection with a very long duration. It is not very contagious and rarely fatal, but causes damages to the skin and nervous system, which can be disfiguring and crippling. Today, the disease is limited to developing countries and there are around 15 million leprosy patients worldwide.[292]

Unlike the case of leprosy, the doctors on St Croix agreed that yaws was declining.[293] The doctors only mentioned yaws in connection with the enslaved workers and the plantations, which leads to the assumption that the disease normally only occurred in this population. A survey of inventories, lease contracts, and inspection reports from a number of royal plantations show that yaws was rarer than leprosy.[294] In the hospital records of the four royal plantations, yaws only occurs on Longford and Hermon Hill and only with one patient in each place. In his medical report of 1827, the interim landfysikus Schlegel linked the decline in the number of yaws cases with the ban on the import of enslaved workers from Africa.[295] Presumably, this conclusion was correct, because the climate of St Croix is warm but relatively dry, which may be one of the reasons why yaws is not endemic on the island (see below). The treatment of yaws was very similar to the treatment of syphilis, including the use of sudorific and absorbing remedies, as well as 'Plummer's Pills' containing mercury.[296]

Today, yaws or framboesia is regarded as a very contagious disease native to tropical areas with bad hygiene. The disease is caused by a bacterium, a spirochete, by the name *Treponema pallidum pertenue*. It is so closely related to the spirochete that causes syphilis, *Treponema pallidum*, that there is no morphological difference. Unlike syphilis, yaws is transmitted through skin contact, which is easier in warm, humid areas, where people wear few clothes. The disease develops in childhood and the symptoms of the early stages are suppurating boils that form crusts the same colour of a raspberry, hence the name

291 Schmidt, *Various Remarks*, viii, 26–28.

292 Kiple, *History of Human Disease*, 834–39.

293 DNA, BH, Med. rep., Danish West Indies. 1827, 1830, 1847.

294 DNA, WILA, no. 46.17.6, 46.17.32, 46.17.33, 46.17.44, 46.17.45, 46.17.54, 46.21. NARA, RG55, Entry 1109, Box 2432, Estate Jolly Hill.

295 DNA, BH, Med. rep., Danish West Indies. 1827.

296 DNA, BH, Med. rep., Danish West Indies. 1834. Concerning Plummer's Pills see: J. Edward Hutson, ed., *On the Treatment and Management of the More Common West-India Diseases, 1750–1802* (Jamaica: University of the West Indies Press, 2005), 44–45, 141.

framboesia (French: *framboise*, raspberry). After eight months, the patient often experiences a spontaneous recovery, but some of the consequences are hardly distinguishable from those of syphilis and accordingly the two diseases were often mistaken for each other until the beginning of the twentieth century.[297]

The last in this group of diseases visible on the skin was 'the itch' (scabies, Danish: *Fnat*). The doctors on St Croix often reported scabies among the enslaved children and thought it was caused by the unhygienic conditions under which the children, and their parents, lived.[298] Yet, what annoyed the doctors most was that the enslaved workers were apparently reluctant to follow the doctors' advice on the treatment of the disease.[299] As to the connection between scabies and bad hygiene the doctors were probably right, since modern medicine regards the disease as caused by poor hygiene which allows the itch mite (*Sarcoptes scabiei*) to penetrate the skin on fingers, wrists, armpits, the skin around the navel and on the nipples of women. The mite spreads rapidly, especially among people in close physical contact and the result is a strong itch in the infected places, but with no serious consequences.[300]

THE VENEREAL DISEASES: *Syphilis and Gonorrhoea*

In the medical reports, the doctors usually linked leprosy and yaws with the so-called venereal diseases, i.e. syphilis and gonorrhoea. At the time, many Euro-Caribbeans were of the opinion that the decline in the enslaved population was brought about by low fertility caused by the promiscuity and resulting venereal diseases of the enslaved themselves.[301] Therefore, it is interesting that the doctors reported the highest number of cases not among the enslaved workers but among the soldiers in the garrisons of Christiansted and Frederiksted, and among the free coloured workers in docks and plantations.[302] In the hospital records of the four royal plantations, venereal diseases also made up a very modest part of the total number of admissions, only 2 or 3 per cent. A further survey of inventories, lease contracts, and inspection reports from other royal plantations also suggests that venereal diseases were rarer than even leprosy.[303] How-

297 Kiple, *History of Human Disease*, 1096–1100.
298 DNA, BH, Med. rep., Danish West Indies. 1825 etc.
299 DNA, BH, Med. rep., Danish West Indies. 1845.
300 Lindskog, *Medicinsk Ordbog*, 'Fnat'.
301 Highfield, *Observations*, 22 (original: Brady, 1829).
302 DNA, BH, Med. rep., Danish West Indies. 1827, 1834, 1835, 1842.
303 DNA, WILA, no. 46.17.6, 46.17.32, 46.17.33, 46.17.44, 46.17.45, 46.17.54, 46.21. NARA, RG55, Entry 1109, Box 2432, Estate Jolly Hill.

ever, this result does not correspond with other information from the period after emancipation, which suggests that venereal diseases were very widespread among the Afro-Caribbean agricultural workers in St Croix.[304] Consequently, it is possible that neither doctors nor managers recorded the actual number of cases of venereal diseases. The following remarks in the first of the annual medical reports from 1803 point in that direction:[305]

> common among Negroes [are] likewise venereal complaints, which they sometimes conceal until the disease is very difficult to cure.[306]

> Venereal sickness we have much of, particularly amongst the Negroes on the estates.[307]

> Because there are old Negro women who employ themselves with the cure of this disease [syphilis/gonorrhoea] and who also avoid the most meticulous investigation by the police, it is likely that the practitioners [doctors] have not seen the majority of the venereal [patients].[308]

Based on this information, it is possible that the enslaved workers preferred their own healers in case of venereal diseases, and tried to avoid involving the manager and the doctor, if possible. Only if no enslaved healer was able to cure the disease, and it was so far advanced that the enslaved could not work, then the manager and the doctor became involved. However, it does not seem as if the doctors were overly concerned about the venereal diseases. The surgeon Vilhelm Ferdinand Feilberg (1808–71) on St John reported in 1834:

> This year I have not observed as many cases of venereal disease as last year, because I regularly overhaul all the Negroes of the entire plantation when I suspect the disease among them. In this way, I prevent it from spreading.[309]

304 Hoxcer Jensen, *From Serfdom*, 207.
305 DNA, DC, no. G125C.
306 Dr Charles Smith and Dr James Walker.
307 Dr Andrew Kenny.
308 Landfysikus Johan Mathias Frederik Keutsch. Original Danish text: 'Da der ere gamle Negerinder som beskiæftige sig med denne Sygdoms [Syfilis/Gonore] cur, og som undgaaer ogsaa den nøjeste eftersøgning af Politiet, saa er det sandsynligt at Praktikerne [lægerne] haver de fleste veneriske [patienter] slet ikke at see.'
309 DNA, BH, Med. rep., Danish West Indies. 1834. Original Danish text: 'Af veneriske Sygdomme har jeg ikke observeret saa mange i dette Aar, som forrige, da jeg af og til overhaler den hele Plantages Negere,

Presumably, the word 'overhaul' (Danish: *overhale*) is to be understood in this context as a thorough examination of all enslaved workers on the plantation to discover sores on the genitalia. Given this treatment, it is little wonder that the enslaved preferred to keep their ailment secret from the planter and the doctor for as long as possible.

According to modern medicine the symptoms of syphilis's first phase is a sore on the spot where the spirochete penetrated the body, usually the genitalia. The first phase usually ends with a spontaneous recovery after 2–6 weeks, but after another six to eight weeks the second phase sets in, characterised by rashes and sores on the skin, fever, pain in the bones, and enlarged lymphatic nodes. The third phase of the disease only occurs in a third of the cases and only after another latent period of up to twenty years. It is characterised by destruction of the skin, mucus membranes, bones, and internal organs, including a special form of mental disease.[310] Since syphilis and gonorrhoea were understood as two phases of the same disease until the middle of the nineteenth century, the characteristics of gonorrhoea, i.e. the chancre and the discharge from the urethra, was viewed as certain signs of the presence of venereal diseases. The therapy of the Cruzian doctors was similar to the one used for yaws, i.e. sudorific and absorbent drugs and mercurial pills, which is no surprise because both the first and second phases of syphilis do cause sores on the skin.[311]

Apart from the sexual transmission of syphilis, the disease can also be transmitted from the mother to the unborn child. The possible consequences of this are the child's death during birth, stillbirth or premature birth.[312] Because the above information raises doubts whether syphilis was widespread or not, it is impossible to estimate if congenital syphilis had an influence on the demographic development.

EPIDEMIC DISEASES: *Measles, Whooping Cough, and Chickenpox*

Many of the diseases described by the doctors of St Croix in their medical reports could assume an epidemic character. However, the diseases grouped together here always occurred epidemically and never endemically.

Today measles is seen as a childhood disease, but in the period in question

naar jeg har Mistanke om at Sygdommen er iblandt dem og paa den maade forhindre jeg den fra at udbrede sig.'

310 Kiple, *History of Human Disease*, 756–57, 1028–31.

311 DNA, BH, Med. rep., Danish West Indies. 1833, 1834.

312 Kiple, *History of Human Disease*, 1028–31.

here, the disease was perceived differently on St Croix. Measles seems to have been such a rare occurrence that it was not viewed as a childhood disease. When a measles epidemic broke out on the island in 1842, it resulted in more than a thousand patients and many dead among the enslaved workers, and the sick and the dead were not only children but also adults.[313] Given that an infection with measles renders the survivor immune to the disease, the fact that adult enslaved contracted the disease in 1842 means that it must have been about twenty years since the previous great outbreak of the disease. The measles epidemic in 1842 was a catastrophe for the plantations, partly because many enslaved workers died from the disease and partly because many of the enslaved were hospitalised for at least three weeks in the middle of the sugar harvest.[314] According to modern medicine, measles is caused by a highly contagious virus (*Morbilli*) and has two phases. The first phase occurs after an incubation period of fourteen days and lasts three to seven days with fever and cough. Then the second phase commences with the characteristic red rashes, which lasts four to seven days. On this basis, the three weeks of hospitalisation in the plantation hospitals seems reasonable. Other complications can occur in conjunction with measles causing secondary infections such as inflammation of the middle ear, pneumonia, or diarrhoea. The secondary infections are often the cause of the mortality connected to measles.[315]

Whooping cough occurred more often than measles on St Croix in the period 1803–48. There were reports of outbreaks in 1803, 1825, 1830, 1838, and 1843, and as one might expect the afflicted were children. An infection with whooping cough does not afford lifelong immunity and accordingly adults can contract the disease, yet in such cases, it is difficult to distinguish it from other respiratory diseases. Deaths from whooping cough were rare on St Croix, except in 1843. Today, whooping cough is described as an acute infectious disease caused by the bacterium *Bordetella pertussis*, which attacks the respiratory tract and causes persistent convulsive cough. The patient coughs up thick phlegm and the attack is often followed by vomiting, which can be dangerous to small children.[316]

Chickenpox was only reported in 1838. The outbreak did not cover the entire island and does not seem to have been very serious. Today, chickenpox is

313 DNA, BH, Med. rep., Danish West Indies. 1842.
314 DNA, BH, Med. rep., Danish West Indies. 1842, 1843.
315 Kiple, *History of Human Disease*, 871–75.
316 Kiple, *History of Human Disease*, 1094–96.

described as a viral infection caused by the *Varicella-Zoster* virus. The incubation period is ten to twenty days, after which the chickenpox emerge followed by fever and headache. Deaths are rare.[317]

INTENTIONAL or INCIDENTAL ACCIDENTS? *Poisoning, Drowning, Suicide, Injury, and Battering*

As mentioned above, the Cruzian doctors were interested in but also sceptical about the local herbal medicine of the enslaved. Presumably, the scepticism originated from the cases of poisoning caused by toxic plants, which appear in the medical reports, and from the deep concern felt by all Euro-Caribbeans towards the Afro-Caribbean knowledge about these plants. So, the interim garrison surgeon and landfysikus in Christiansted, Andreas Jacobi Crucau Aagaard (1803–76),[318] remarked in 1843:

> When poisoning occurs out here, it is almost always caused by vegetable poisons, of which there is a large number in this climate. Unfortunately, they are all too well known by the Negroes.[319]

However, the doctors' scepticism towards the medicine of the enslaved workers was also mixed with a clear respect for the positive, indeed at times almost miraculous results, which the therapies of the enslaved could bring about. As an example, landfysikus Aagaard wrote in 1844:

> In the countryside, one occasionally finds that old African Negroes know herbs, with which they can cure sores that the doctor has tried all his art in vain to cure.[320]

It was difficult for the doctors to separate the intentional poisonings from the incidental – not to mention the inexplicable sudden deaths, for which they could find no cause. A simple example of incidental poisoning could be when

317 Kiple, *History of Human Disease*, 1092–94.

318 Carøe, *Den Danske Lægestand* III, 1.

319 DNA, BH, Med. rep., Danish West Indies. 1843. Original Danish text: 'Naar Forgiftning finder sted herude, skeer det næsten altid ved Plantegifter, hvoraf der i dette Klima findes en stor Mængde, der desværre ere Negerne saare vel bekjendte.'

320 DNA, BH, Med. rep., Danish West Indies. 1844. Original Danish text: 'Paa Landet seer man undertiden at gamle afrikanske Negere kjende Urter, hvormed de kan helbrede Saar, hvorpaa Lægen forgjæves har forsøgt al sin Kunst'.

the enslaved worker named 'Doctor' on Tuesday 1 October 1833 was admitted to the hospital of the royal plantation Boetzberg because he had got the juice of the manchineel fruit in his eyes.[321] He was hospitalised for three days after the accident, which cannot be said to be a long time, since the juice of the manchineel tree (*Hippomane mancinella L.*) and its fruit is famous for its toxicity and can cause blindness.[322] A similar example is that of an enslaved woman who died after having rubbed herself with an alcohol infusion of the tobacco plant, a house remedy against lice.[323] Tobacco contains the alkaloid nicotine, which acts as an insecticide, but can also penetrate the skin and cause lethal poisoning.[324]

Regarding the intentional poisonings, they were sometimes easy to detect. For instance when an enslaved worker on Mount Stewart plantation in 1843 killed another enslaved worker by pouring the juice of the plant Kittie-McWanie (*Asclepias curassavica L.*) in his food.[325] However, just as often the detection of the crime was more incidental, as when manager Clark on Rattan plantation suddenly died under suspicious circumstances. The autopsy did not give any clue but a thorough interrogation revealed that an Afro-Caribbean woman had mixed a toxic seed in his food.[326] This is not the place to develop the details of this case, but only to conclude that intentional poisonings or murder by poisoning did occur on St Croix in the period in question, albeit rarely. So, there was an immediate reality behind the Euro-Caribbean inhabitants' fear of poisoning, even though the doctors admitted that they were probably too inclined to interpret inexplicable deaths as poisoning.[327] However, compared to other West Indian societies the fear of poisoning does not seem to have been particularly prominent in the Danish West Indies. In the French West Indies the fear of poisoning among the Euro-Caribbeans almost reached the level of a mass hysteria in this period.[328]

To the group of intentional and incidental accidents also belong cases of drowning and larger injuries. Concerning cases of drowning it is difficult to decide how common they were among the enslaved workers, to say nothing of

321 DNA, WILA, no. 46.17.5.
322 Oakes, *Poisonous and Injurious Plants*, 50–51.
323 DNA, BH, Med. rep., Danish West Indies. 1843.
324 Lindskog, *Medicinsk Ordbog*, 'Nikotin'.
325 DNA, BH, Med. rep., Danish West Indies. 1843. Asclepias curassavica is toxic and a heart stimulant. See: Thomas, *Traditional Medical Plants*, 46–47.
326 DNA, BH, Med. rep., Danish West Indies. 1843.
327 DNA, BH, Med. rep., Danish West Indies. 1847.
328 Leti, *Santé et société*, 50–56.

which cases were suicides and which murder.[329] Nonetheless, the impression is that the number of drowned enslaved workers was not very high compared to the number of enslaved on the island. The percentage was far higher among the Euro-Caribbeans. Regarding larger injuries among the enslaved workers caused by accidents, the situation is somewhat clearer. Examples of classic accidents could be when an enslaved boy of Annaberg plantation on St John in 1836 had his right hand crushed between the rollers of the sugar mill, or when another enslaved boy on St Croix in 1847 toppled over with a field cart and had his right leg crushed. In both cases, the treatment was amputation.[330] The intentional self-inflicted injuries among the enslaved were also easily recognisable, because they usually followed a pattern: the enslaved worker took a sharp instrument (axe, machete, knife) and hacked himself in the opposite arm or hand. The treatment varied from amputation of finger joints to amputation of the entire arm.[331] If the enslaved worker instead cut himself in the neck or stomach, which also occurred, the action must be interpreted as attempted suicide. Occasionally these attempts succeeded, especially in the cases where the enslaved chose to hang himself or drown himself in a well. In the source material, these obvious attempted suicides are not uncommon.[332] The reasons for the suicides and the self-inflicted injuries are not directly visible from the source material, yet it is highly likely that both were expressions of the frustration and powerlessness the enslaved workers felt because of their life situations.

Finally, the injuries of the enslaved workers could also be a result of punishment and outright abuse by the planter or manager. The source material does not contain any indication that 'ordinary' punishments (i.e. flogging) caused hospitalisation. However, as flogging was still a common form of punishment, there is reason to believe that injuries caused by such procedures were treated in the plantation hospitals. Regarding outright abuse the source material only contains a couple of instances where it can be established beyond doubt that the enslaved worker was abused by the owner, manager, or another Euro-Caribbean person.[333] Nevertheless, the research literature gives reason to believe that

329 DNA, BH, Med. rep., Danish West Indies. 1825, 1828, etc. DNA, WILA, no. 10.19 and 10.21. Accounts for 'Country Treasury', 'Land Treasury' and 'Landcass'. DNA, WILA, no. 3.81.611. DNA, DC, no. G125C. Charles Smith and James Walker, § 4.

330 DNA, BH, Med. rep., Danish West Indies. 1836.

331 DNA, BH, Med. rep., Danish West Indies. 1825, 1827, 1836 (St John). DNA, WILA, no. 3.81.611.

332 DNA, WILA, no. 3.81.611. For instance 19 October 1812, 10 January 1813 and 17 January 1817. DNA, WILA, no. 10.21. Accounts for 'Country Treasury', 'Land Treasury' and 'Estate Fountain'.

333 DNA, WILA, no. 3.81.611. For instance 10 November 1814, 27 May 1815. DNA, WILA, no. 10.21. Accounts for 'Country Treasury', 'Land Treasury' and 'Estate Fountain'.

this kind of case occurred at regular intervals and that only extreme cases led to any punishment of the Euro-Caribbean.[334]

AMPUTATION: *Ether and Chloroform*

Generally, the treatment for large injuries (and elephantiasis) was amputation. Until 1847, it was carried out without any anaesthesia, as it had always been done. However, in 1847 surgery on St Croix was revolutionised by the introduction of ether (diethyl ether) to anaesthetise patients. The first operation was conducted on 5 August by Dr Smith[335] in the presence of landfysikus Aagaard, and the patient was a middle-aged enslaved woman from the Wheel of Fortune plantation. After having inhaled ether for a full 15 minutes (!), the patient was unconscious and the amputation of her leg went according to plan. In the following months, several of the other doctors on the island followed suit, and before the end of the year a total of nine operations with anaesthesia had been carried out. All the patients were enslaved workers and in most cases the reason for the operation was elephantiasis. With the revolution of anaesthesia, amputation was so quick and painless that the patients had difficulties believing the operation was over when they woke up. Furthermore, in addition to anaesthesia with ether there was also chloroform (trichlormethane or methyl trichloride).[336] Considering that the anaesthetic properties of ether were only recognised and used in operations in the USA and Europe in 1846, and that chloroform seems to have been used for anaesthesia for the first time in 1847, the doctors on St Croix were extraordinarily quick to use the new techniques.[337] In relation to this, it is worth considering whether the enslaved workers were used as guinea pigs to test the new and potentially dangerous anaesthetics. Based on the present evidence it is not possible to give a clear answer to this question, yet it is remarkable that all of the nine patients in the first months were enslaved workers.

Moreover, the enslaved workers' relationship with the new anaesthetics was not as straightforward as it may seem at first. They were so afraid of the anaesthetic that it took a long while (15–18 minutes) before they had inhaled enough of the vapours to induce unconsciousness. In some instances where the patients were enslaved children, the anaesthetic actually never got to work properly, perhaps because the children were too scared. In contrast, the doc-

334 Olsen, 'Fra ejendomsret til menneskeret', 39–47.
335 Carøe, *Den Danske Lægestand* V, 93.
336 DNA, BH, Med. rep., Danish West Indies. 1847.
337 Porter, *Ve og Vel*, 366–67.

tors reported that on Euro-Caribbean patients the anaesthetic worked in only a couple of minutes. According to landfysikus Aagaard, the reason for the enslaved worker's fear was that they perceived anaesthesia as a form of Obeah, i.e. as a kind of magic or sorcery, which the doctor tried to set upon them.[338] In the enslaved workers' magico-religious perception of the world as inhabited by ancestors and spirits, induced sleep was a sign of magic.

DENTAL DISEASES

In the medical reports diseases of the teeth only appear in the form of the enslaved children's problems during 'dentition'. On three of the four royal plantations investigated, dental problems did cause people to be hospitalised, but only for nine days in total.[339] Given that the predominant crop on St Croix was sugar and that the enslaved were normally allowed free access to the sugar juice and the by-products of sugar production during the harvest, it is peculiar that dental problems did not occupy a more prominent position in the material.[340] Contemporary sources from the British West Indies relate that dental problems were very common and that the enslaved workers treated these problems themselves.[341] On this basis, one could suspect that the enslaved workers on St Croix took care of dental problems themselves, just as with the venereal diseases, and that they only went to the doctor or the manager if they were incapacitated by the problem and could not solve it, or if they saw other benefits in being admitted to the hospital.

APOPLEXY (Stroke, Cerebral haemorrhage/Cerebral blood clot)

According to the medical reports, sudden strokes were not uncommon among the inhabitants of St Croix.[342] The same was true for sudden deaths where no cause could be found, a sizeable part of which may have been strokes. Unfortunately, it is rarely evident from the reports if the victims were enslaved or persons from other groups in the population. However, it is clear that the victims were usually older and decrepit individuals, and few were more decrepit than the enslaved. Occasionally, victims survived with partial paralysis (hemiphlegia), which shows that the cause was a cerebral haemorrhage or blood clot.[343]

338 DNA, BH, Med. rep., Danish West Indies. 1847.
339 North Star, Longford, Boetzberg.
340 Highfield, *Observations*, 15 (original: Brady, 1829).
341 Collins, *Practical Rules*, 313–16.
342 DNA, BH, Med. rep., Danish West Indies. 1825, 1831, 1832, 1847.
343 Kiple, *History of Human Disease*, 584–87.

CACHEXIA AFRICANA *(Geophagy, Pica, Dirt eating, Mal d'estomac)*
One of the phenomena that has puzzled medical science most is geophagy or dirt eating. It has existed at all times and all over the world, but the reason for it has never been clarified. Malnutrition and psychological diseases have been suggested as possible causes, but cultural habits may also be of great importance. On plantations all over the Americas dirt eating among the enslaved workers was a great concern for planters and managers. Some thought the enslaved workers would become addicted to it and that the addiction would ultimately be fatal. The dirt eating enslaved became sick with stomach aches and breathing difficulties, followed by diarrhoea and depression. After two to three months they died. Dirt eating seems to have been especially common in the British West Indies before emancipation.[344]

In the Danish West Indies, however, the situation was somewhat different in the period 1803–48. Here, dirt eating does not seem to have been very common. The medical reports from St Croix mention in passing only two dead dirt eaters. One was a 6-year-old child who died of the disease, while the other individual drowned and so cannot be said to have died as a consequence of dirt eating.[345] The protocols from the Christiansted bailiff's office show five instances of the phenomenon in the years 1820–28,[346] whereas the plantation records from the 1830s show only two instances of dirt eating.[347] However, on St John the phenomenon was subjected to a more thorough examination and the local doctor Peter Lotharius Dons (1803–39)[348] wrote a scientific article on the problem in 1833. The article seems to show that dirt eating was more common on St John than the material from St Croix gives reason to believe. Moreover, Dons offers much information on the general state of health among the enslaved workers. Still, the most interesting part is his description of a series of autopsies of enslaved workers carried out by himself as part of his scientific investigation and entirely in compliance with the new anatomic-pathologic paradigm of the time. From these descriptions, it appears that Dr Dons did not always gain unlimited access to dissecting the bodies of the enslaved.[349] It is not clear from the text

344 Kiple, *History of Human Disease*, 927–31.
345 DNA, BH, Med. rep., Danish West Indies. 1828, 1845.
346 DNA, WILA, no. 38.22.41: 21 October 1820, no. 38.22.42: 15 August 1821, no. 38.22.41: 9 January 1822, no. 38.22.43: 8 August 1823, no. 38.22.48: 2 December 1828 (the date is the first entry of the case).
347 Cases of dirt eating: DNA, WILA, no. 46.17.31, 3 April 1830, the enslaved woman Charlotte, 19 years old. DNA, WILA, no. 46.17.46, 28 October 1833, the enslaved boy Richard.
348 Carøe, *Den Danske Lægestand* III, 40 and V, 71.
349 P. L. Dons, 'Om den saakaldte africanske Kakexie (mal d'estomac, dirteating, jordæden)', *Journal for Medicin og Chirurgie* 9 (Copenhagen, 1833), 315, 319.

who refused to let him do the autopsies, but supposedly only the relatives, i.e. other enslaved workers, could have had any reason to prevent them. Accordingly, this is another example of the clash between doctors (Euro-Caribbeans) and enslaved workers concerning the control of the bodies of the enslaved – even if these bodies were dead.

Since the cause of dirt eating is unknown, it is difficult to explain why the phenomenon was not prominent on St Croix. One possible explanation is that if dirt eating was a culturally determined practice with origins in Africa, then the increasing creolization of the enslaved population in the period in question and the declining number of Africans may have meant that phenomena such as dirt eating gradually lost their importance.

MENTAL DISEASES

The medical reports from St Croix do not contain any information on enslaved workers treated for mental illnesses. Nonetheless, materials from various plantations and the public hospital Petersfarm near Christiansted shows that a few cases did exist on the island, but it does not seem to have been a great problem.[350] It is worth considering if the cases of fatal accidents points to depressions or other psychological illnesses among the enslaved workers. In any case, the number of self-inflicted injuries indicates that there were tremendous frustrations in the enslaved population – which is no wonder considering the conditions under which they lived.

If we include the medical reports from the island of St John, however, one single instance emerges that illustrates in detail the treatment of a mentally ill enslaved worker. In 1834 a 40-year-old enslaved man was suddenly seized by 'mania furibunda', i.e. a manic condition of intense excitement and rage.[351] He was furious and threatened to kill people. When he had been subdued, the therapy was applied in the form of frequent showers, purges and a huge blistering plaster from the top of his head down his back. The treatment calmed him down but also made him depressive. The melancholia continued until he began to bleed from one ear, which eased the depression, and soon allowed him to work again as usual.[352]

350 DNA, WILA, no. 46.21. Estate Upper Love, 1835, lease contract, enslaved woman Angelicke: 'a little deranged'. NARA, RG55, Box 2407, Entry 1089, record of patients, Petersfarm, 1848. Patient no. 57: enslaved woman Madlane from Estate Humbug suffered from 'Mania'.

351 Lindskog, *Medicinsk Ordbog*, 'Mania', 'Furibundus'.

352 DNA, BH, Med. rep., Danish West Indies. 1834.

OTHER DISEASES

Apart from the diseases mentioned above, two conditions must be mentioned in closing, namely smallpox and complications connected to pregnancy and birth. These ailments are dealt with in Chapter 4, and so will not be discussed here. However, it should be mentioned that while the doctors frequently refer to smallpox vaccinations on the plantations, they hardly ever mention complications connected to pregnancy and birth. As will appear from Chapter 4, the reason for this seems to be that in general it was not the doctors but enslaved midwives who dealt with these issues. Furthermore, this division of labour also shows that this was another domain within the health services where the enslaved had some level of autonomy and did not just accept the doctors' control and interference.

Conclusion

Based on the above materials of medical reports, records from plantation hospitals, accounts, reports etc., we may conclude that the enslaved workers on the plantations of St Croix in the period 1803–48 suffered from a wide spectrum of diseases. Some were common, and not necessarily long or life-threatening, while others were rare and caused long hospitalisation and permanent injuries. The four most common disease categories were 'Fever', 'Pains and Injuries', 'Gastrointestinal diseases' and 'Boils and Sores'. On four selected royal plantations, these four categories made up 60–95 per cent of all hospital admissions and the most prominent categories were 'Fever' and 'Pains and Injuries', even though the order varied between plantations. A fifth disease category was respiratory diseases and pneumonia, which possibly caused many to be sick and many to die, particularly among the enslaved workers. However, the sources do not agree on this point. Which diseases caused the highest number of deaths among the enslaved workers is investigated later in this chapter. Among the diseases that caused a few, yet very long, hospitalisations were for instance rose, oedema, and elephantiasis (filariasis).

Despite the relative similarity among the four plantations regarding the most common diseases, it must be emphasised that the very risk of falling ill differed greatly among them. The calculation of the incidence rate per 1,000 person-years-at-risk for each disease and plantation shows a range from 2,985 incidences per 1,000 person-years-at-risk at North Star, down to only 160 incidences per 1,000 at Longford (see Tables 3.1, 3.2, 3.3, 3.4). The reason for this huge difference may partly be epidemics and so incidental to some degree;

however, the age profile of the enslaved population on each plantation seems a more likely answer. As can be seen from Table 3.5, the enslaved population on North Star was significantly older than on any of the other plantations and so likely to be more susceptible to diseases. Disease incidence rates have not been calculated for any other historical population in the Caribbean and so cannot be checked comparatively.

Returning to the general picture, it is noteworthy to what extent the diseases the enslaved workers suffered from were caused by their living conditions. Pains and injuries originated largely from the hard and strenuous work in the field, while the gastrointestinal diseases were connected to the abysmal hygiene, water supply, and nutrition. The same was true for many of the other diseases, such as rose, which is related to a failing immune system. In short, the factors specific to life as an enslaved worker seem to have been decisive for the diseases of the enslaved.

Nevertheless, the enslaved workers did not just accept the diseases and they were not just passive patients in the care of the doctors. The source material shows weak but recurring signs that the enslaved perceived certain diseases and the treatment of these diseases as domains that did not concern the doctors, which of course led to clashes with the doctors and the Euro-Caribbean authorities they represented. Examples include venereal disease, births, scabies, and dental problems, which are either conspicuous by their absence in the sources or where the enslaved workers' own handling of the disease is evident. The clashes and friction concerning these diseases between the enslaved workers and the doctors show the continuous negotiation or struggle for power over health which took place between the enslaved and doctors. In relation to this, there are examples of resistance continuing after death, because some enslaved workers resisted autopsies of their diseased family and friends. Furthermore, the use of herbal medicine was connected to the enslaved workers' treatment of diseases. This practice fascinated the doctors but at the same time worried Euro-Caribbeans in general because the enslaved occasionally used plant poisons against their masters. Finally, the use of anaesthesia for surgical operations shows the clash of perceptions of health and of the world in general, which was a part of Euro-Caribbean doctors' everyday encounter with enslaved patients. Presumably, the clashes took place in many more areas of medical treatment than presented here but as the source materials used for this investigation do not allow the enslaved to present their own views directly, this cannot be determined with any certainty.

Diseases and Therapies in Comparative Perspective

A comparison of the above investigation of the diseases of the enslaved workers on St Croix with the corresponding information from the British and French West Indies shows that the differences are few. The spectrum of diseases was virtually the same everywhere, but the ranking of the diseases in relation to their prevalence and severity sometimes differed.[353] For instance, in their seminal studies both Dr Grainger and Dr Collins claimed that gastrointestinal diseases ('disorders of the bowels') made up the largest part of the diseases of the enslaved workers in the British West Indies, followed by fever, which rarely killed the enslaved.[354] As shown above, this order was reversed on St Croix because fever occurred more frequently than gastrointestinal diseases, but despite this fever was not perceived to be a life-threatening disease, while gastrointestinal disease might be lethal, especially for children. Another difference was the incidence of oedema (dropsy). In the British West Indies, this was a frequent and serious illness,[355] but on St Croix it was not prominent. Since oedema can be caused by many different conditions, it is difficult to explain the difference. Neither was the mysterious dirt eating as widespread on St Croix as it seems to have been in the British West Indies, where it caused much illness among the enslaved workers and raised concerns among doctors and planters.[356] Again, the lack of a straightforward explanation for the 'disease' makes it difficult to single out the difference, but as mentioned one possibility is that the advanced creolization on St Croix may have had an influence. Finally, there is the question of the importance of the venereal diseases. As mentioned, these diseases occupied a special position in the continuous conflict and negotiation for power over health between the enslaved workers and the doctors, yet apart from this, they may have had a negative influence on the demographic development, as many Euro-Caribbeans claimed at the time. Bio-anthropological tests conducted on skeletons of enslaved workers excavated on Barbados indicate that congenital syphilis may have been part of the reason for the negative demographic trend.[357] As mentioned, syphilis does not seem to have been a prominent disease on St Croix, yet since it appears that the enslaved workers particularly tried to con-

353 Sheridan, *Doctors and Slaves*, 188–94, 207–21; Leti, *Santé et société*, 95–140.

354 Grainger, *An Essay*, 29–33; Collins, *Practical Rules*, 200–3, 229–30, 259.

355 Sheridan, *Doctors and Slaves*, 210–11.

356 Sheridan, *Doctors and Slaves*, 216–19.

357 Keith P. Jacobi, Della Collins Cook, Robert S. Corruccini and Jerome S. Handler, 'Congenital Syphilis in the Past: Slaves at Newton Plantation, Barbados, West Indies', *American Journal of Physical Anthropology* 89 (1992).

ceal the venereal diseases, syphilis may still have played a role in the negative demographic development.

Seasonal Morbidity

Literature from the period 1803–48 about the health of the enslaved workers in the British West Indies features a theory of seasonal variations in their morbidity.[358] At the time, it was a common observation that the highest prevalence of disease among the enslaved workers occurred during the hurricane season in the autumn, called 'hungry time' or 'the sickly season'. In his demographic studies, Barry W. Higman has tried to test this theory by comparing data from plantation journals from different parts of the British West Indies. According to his results the number of sick enslaved workers peaked at the beginning of the sugar harvest in January, decreased to a minimum a couple of months after the harvest, usually in May, and then rose again to its maximum at the beginning of the next sugar harvest. Higman suggested that the reason for this pattern was not the workload, since the agricultural regime on sugar plantations demanded the hardest work during the harvest. In contrast, Higman pointed to a combination of nutritional and climatic explanations. Because while the enslaved workers worked hard during the harvest, they also had access to a sufficient diet based on the food rations handed out to them by the planter, their own produce, and the by-products of the sugar production. Contrary to this situation, the autumn was characterised both by hard work, limited access to food and by bad weather, which caused illness among the enslaved.[359] Yet, Higman's source materials were neither as geographically nor as chronologically consistent as the plantation journals from the royal plantations on St Croix and accordingly it is interesting to test the theory on this material. The idea of a seasonal variation in morbidity was also present in the Danish West Indies, but it was not seen as specific to the enslaved population.[360]

The Source Material

The source material for this investigation originates from three of the previously mentioned royal plantations on St Croix: North Star, Longford and Boetzberg (see Fig. 3.1). The state leased its plantations to private planters, but to protect

358 Sheridan, *Doctors and Slaves*, 191.
359 Higman, *Slave Populations*, 300–2.
360 Highfield, *Observations*, 4.

them from over-exploitation the plantations were subject to regulations and inspections by the colonial government. This generated information with a degree of detail rarely seen in studies of Caribbean slavery. The rules for the treatment of enslaved workers on royal plantations seem to have been developing since the administration began to manage the first plantations that reverted to the Crown at the beginning of the 1820s.[361] At the beginning of 1833, Governor General Peter Carl Frederik von Scholten (1784–1854)[362] developed a new set of rules for the leases of royal plantations, which became effective in 1834.[363] Undoubtedly, the context for the regulations was the emancipation of the enslaved workers in the British West Indies, and thus the regulation can be viewed as a product of the efforts by von Scholten and the Danish West Indian government to improve the conditions for all enslaved on the Danish islands. However, neither the rescript of 1834 nor the law of 1840 contained any regulation of the enslaved workers' workloads, food rations, free time etc. (see the section below on 'Slaves, Laws and Health Factors').[364] Accordingly, these lease regulations of 1834 were the first efficient and sanctioned regulations in the Danish West Indies covering the central issues of importance to the health of the enslaved, i.e. work, free time, food, clothes, housing and medical assistance. However, they only applied to the royal plantations and because of these administrative and possible environmental differences (soil quality, annual rainfall etc.) it is not possible to infer that the three plantations are representative of all plantations on St Croix. Nonetheless, as the quality of information from the three plantations is superior in terms of detail and geographical density to the information used by Barry W. Higman in his 1984 study, it seems acceptable to test his hypothesis on this material.

The lease regulations consisted of two parts: the general articles and a 'plan' for the treatment of the enslaved workers, for future maintenance work and for the cultivation of the land.[365] The items in the plan fixed a series of health-related standards for the treatment of the enslaved workers, which are dealt with in various parts of this book: for instance workloads, housing and clothes

361 DNA, WILA, no. 46.20. Instructions of 3 September 1822.

362 Carl Frederik Bricka, *Dansk biografisk Lexikon* XV (Copenhagen: Gyldendalske Boghandels Forlag, 1887–1905), 255–56.

363 DNA, WILA, no. 46.20.

364 Vibæk, 'Dansk Vestindien, 1755–1848', 271–74.

365 The following is based on an examination of lease contracts and 'plans' from a number of plantations: Boetzberg 1834 (DNA, WILA, no. 2.38.2), North Star 1834 (DNA, WILA, no. 46.21), North Star 1843 (DNA, WILA, no. 46.17.54), Hermon Hill 1836 (DNA, WILA, no. 46.21), Work and Rest 1834 (DNA, WILA, no. 46.21).

(later in this chapter) and nutrition (Chapter 4). In article 6 of the regulations, the leaseholder committed himself to call in the appointed plantation doctor in case of disease among the enslaved workers. Furthermore, the manager was himself obliged to treat the disease of an enslaved worker 'in the best and proper way'.[366] Article 8 gave the government the power to terminate the agreement with the leaseholder without warning and to demand compensation if he 'treats the Negroes inappropriately', i.e. violated the rules stated in the contract.[367] Article 14 obliged the leaseholder to submit to inspections by the royal plantation inspector whenever the inspector saw fit. Article 15 obliged the leaseholder to keep a journal authorised by the Governor General, in which he was required to note everything that took place on the plantation and everything pertaining to the enslaved workers, for instance their work assignments, punishments etc. Disease and hospitalisation are not mentioned explicitly but the majority of the royal plantations kept both a weekly plantation record and a monthly hospital record.

It is evident that with the lease regulations for the royal plantations the colonial administration had set a standard assuring the enslaved workers certain rights in relation to work, free time, food rations, clothes, housing and medical assistance. However, the private plantations were not bound by similar legislation (except concerning food rations stipulated in the ordinance of 1817). So, it is possible that the conditions on the private plantations were not as good as on the royal plantations, even though they were located in areas environmentally more favourable.

The source material from the three royal plantations consists of several types of documents, but essential to this investigation is the weekly 'plantation journals'. They contain information recorded on a daily basis such as the number of enslaved workers in the hospital, the provisions handed out, tasks assigned to the enslaved work gangs etc. The following table shows the years covered by the plantation journals, including information on the total number of enslaved workers, the sex distribution, the average number of sick enslaved per day and the average age in each of the enslaved populations:

366 Original Danish text: 'på bedste og forsvarlig Maade'.
367 Original Danish text: '... uhensigtsmæssigen behandle Negerne...'.

Table 3.5: Demographic data for the three royal plantations

Plantation	Years	Number of enslaved	Sex distribution (m/f)	Average number of admitted	Average per cent of admitted	Average age
North Star	1831–33	74–76	30/44 (1833)[368]	9.5[369]	12.84–12.50	32.2 (1833)[370]
Longford	1832–36	132–140	69/69 (1836)[371]	4.0	3.03–2.86	24.2 (1836)[372]
Boetzberg	1832–33	62–64	30/34 (1832)[373]	3.0	4.84–4.69	25.09 (1824)[374]

As is evident from the table, the intervals covered by the three plantations vary in length. This is important for the interpretive value of the results from each plantation. The difference in the average number of sick is also striking, which is probably related to the average age of the population.

North Star, 1831–33

The development in the number of enslaved workers admitted to the hospital at North Star plantation in the years 1831–33 seems more or less to follow Higman's theory. As is evident from Fig. 3.2, there were variations in the monthly pattern from year to year, yet an analysis of the monthly average for all three years shows that the period October to December had a significantly higher morbidity than the rest of the year (see Fig. 3.7). Accordingly, on North Star the theory of a seasonal pattern in morbidity seems correct.

Longford, 1833–36

In the years 1832–33, the development in the number of admitted patients followed the theory, but not in the years 1834–36. In July 1835, a violent epidemic seems to have raged on the plantation, since the number of sick jumped to five times the average (see Fig. 3.3). Because no hospital records have been preserved for this period it is not possible to determine what disease caused the epidemic. However, if we eliminate the epidemic from the calculation and ana-

368 DNA, WILA, no. 46.21. North Star, report of 11 November, 1833.

369 The significantly higher number of sick enslaved must be due to the large number of old enslaved. It is clear from the plantation record that the enslaved were sick because of aging, which influences the statistics.

370 DNA, WILA, no. 46.21. North Star, report of 11 November, 1833.

371 DNA, WILA, no. 46.17.45. Report of 20 May, 1836.

372 DNA, WILA, no. 46.17.45. Report of 20 May, 1836.

373 DNA, WILA, no. 46.17.5.

374 I have not been able to find data for the average age in 1832–33. DNA, WILA, no. 10.6.1. Boetzberg, 1824.

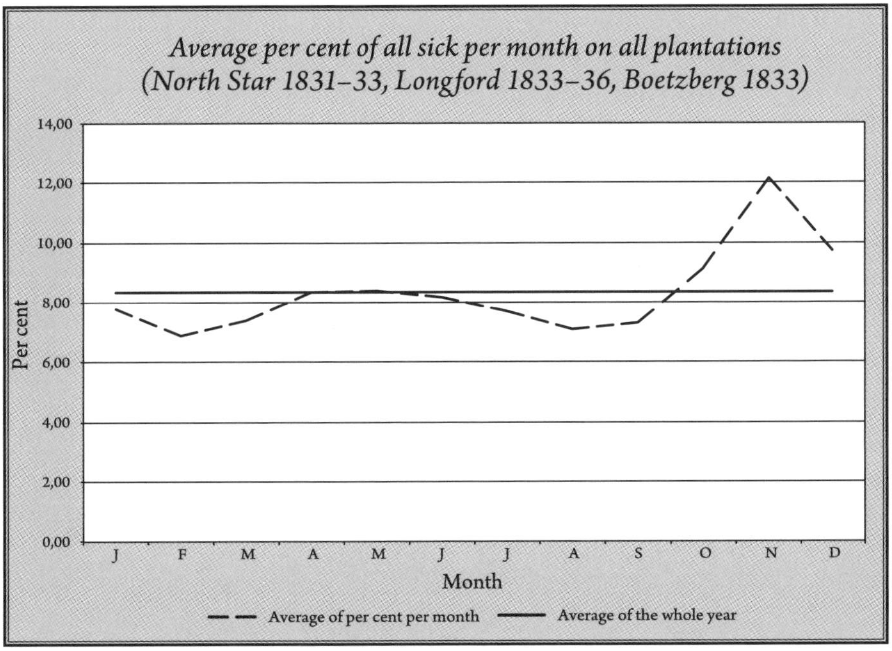

Fig. 3.10. Source: Table 3.6, 3.7 and 3.8.

lyse the monthly average for all four years, it turns out that the seasonal pattern followed the theory almost as closely as on North Star (see Fig. 3.8).

Boetzberg, 1832–33

The development in morbidity on this plantation has a weaker resemblance with the theory. An analysis of the monthly average for the year 1833 alone (data for 1832 does not cover the entire year) gives a clearer picture of the development, but still the result is that only the increase in November fits well with the theory (see Fig. 3.9).

In sum, the development in the number of enslaved workers admitted to hospital in the three plantations in question does seem to have followed the theory for about half the time covered by the years investigated. For the remaining time fluctuations occurred which go against the theory. The reason for this might be that the intervals used are too short to give a consistent result. In intervals of limited length other factors, for instance epidemics, have a relatively strong impact, which they would not have had in a larger sample. However, if we combine the monthly data from all three plantations the differences are levelled out and the main features become visible (see Fig. 3.10). The result is a more consistent picture, which clearly shows the rise in morbidity during the autumn, mentioned by Barry W. Higman. The development during the rest of the year is less clear.

Judging from this material, then, the morbidity among the enslaved workers on St Croix in the period in question does seem to have followed some kind of seasonal rhythm. However, the decisive factor for the morbidity among the enslaved does not seem to have been the workload in the quite fixed annual cycle of the sugar production (holing, harvest etc.). Instead, the decisive factors seem to have been the more unpredictable changes in the weather and the resulting ecological changes (access to food, cold, humidity etc.). Since these climatic-ecological influences were not necessarily the same throughout the island and may have been partly offset by special circumstances on the individual plantation (different standards in housing, clothes, food, drinking water, quality of the soil etc.), it is not possible to determine if the pattern of morbidity from the investigated royal plantations holds true for all of St Croix. The doctors' medical reports indicate that local variations were common, even on a relatively small island like St Croix. Still, with these reservations the investigation does confirm Higman's explanation of the fluctuations in morbidity, namely that they were caused by climatic and nutritional (ecological) factors. Accordingly, there does not seem to have been any difference between the Danish and British West Indies in this respect. Similar data is not known from the French West Indies.

Causes of Death among Enslaved Plantation Workers, 1842–47

The high mortality among enslaved workers in the Danish West Indies and the patterns of morbidity they suffered raises the question as to whether they actually died from the diseases or from something else. In the following, I will explore the causes of death among enslaved workers on St Croix, the seasonality of death, and compare these patterns with conditions in the British and French West indies.

Source Material and Calculations

The material for this quantitative analysis was collected from the records of three churches on St Croix and cover the years 1842–47,[375] the Roman Catholic St Patrick's as well as the Anglican St Paul's in Frederiksted and the Anglican St John's in Christiansted. The timeframe was decided by the fact that churches in the Danish West Indies only started to register causes of death consistently by 1842, and registration in 1848 was irregular because of emancipation. The sample consists of 1,212 diseased enslaved plantation workers above the age of 1 year. Children under that age have been excluded to make the sample comparable with the tax records, an important reference source, which does not include that age group (see below).[376]

In the period 1803–48, there were four Christian communities on St Croix, the Lutheran, the Moravian, the Roman Catholic and the Anglican. Each community had one church in each of the two towns of the island, i.e. eight churches in total.[377] The majority of the enslaved workers belonged to the latter three churches.[378] Since at this time practically all enslaved were baptised and belonged to a congregation, the majority of deaths were recorded in the church records.[379] Consequently, the population of the three churches should make up 3 out of every 8 enslaved workers on St Croix or 35–40 per cent. This estimate is clarified by the tax records, which state the total number of dead enslaved workers in 1841 to have been 563 and 542 individuals in 1847.[380] If we make a high estimate and set the average number of diseased enslaved workers to 563 annually in the years 1842–47, it amounts to 3,378 individuals in total. As the total of 1,212 dead from the three churches equal 35.9 per cent of the estimated total of 3,378 dead in the tax records, the sample amounts to at least 36 per cent of all registered deaths among enslaved workers above the age of 1 year on St Croix in the years 1842–47. Accordingly, the following data on the number of deaths per 1,000 enslaved workers for individual diseases has been calculated on the assumption that the population at risk was 36 per cent of the total enslaved population recorded in the tax records in each of the years 1842–47 (see Table 3.10, etc.). This calculation of mortality rates measured as deaths per 1,000 individuals of a known population at risk makes it possible to com-

375 This data has been collected for the St Croix African Roots Project. The church records exist in copy at the St Croix Landmarks Society Library, Estate Whim, St Croix, and the original record at the individual church offices on St Croix. I thank George Tyson for permission to use this material.

376 Asmussen, *Slavedemografi*, 33–34, appendix 2.

377 The Moravian Friedensfeld church is located mid-island.

378 Larsen, *Virgin Islands Story*, 196.

379 Hall, *Slave Society*, 209.

380 Asmussen, *Slavedemografi*, appendix 2.

pare the data with modern mortality rates. However, the existing research on causes of death among enslaved populations in the Caribbean has not used this method. Consequently, the following comparison with research on the British and French West Indies will use the less accurate measure of percentage of all deaths (see below).

Causes of Death: Comparison with the Pattern of Morbidity in the Hospital Records

The causes of death registered in the church records are many and very diverse. This was probably because it was the manager or doctors of the individual plantation who reported the cause of death and not some central coordinating authority. Another possible reason for the diversity may be that the primary purpose of the church records was not to register exactly what the parishioners died from, but who and how many had died. Consequently, the church records contain different terms for the same cause of death, just as was the case with the diseases registered in the hospital records. In the following, some of these diverse causes of death have been combined into new larger categories. This is the case with the categories 'Bowels' and 'Dysentery', and 'Old Age' and 'Infirmity'. However, the number of new combined categories is lower than in the previous section on hospital records, because the data on the causes of death are after all more precise. Accordingly, because fewer causes of death have been combined, more of the original causes of death have been retained in the analysis, which again means that many of the causes are only represented by one or two deaths. This group of causes of death, in which each cause amounts to less than 1 per cent of all deaths per 1,000 enslaved at risk, totals 10.3 per cent of all deaths per 1,000 enslaved at risk (see Fig. 3.11).

At the opposite end of the scale, four causes of death account for 56 per cent of all deaths per 1,000 enslaved at risk. These are 'Fever' (6.6 per 1,000, 17.8 %), 'Bowels and Dysentery' (5.0 per 1,000, 13.4 %), 'Consumption and Lungs' (4.6 per 1,000, 12.5 %) and 'Old Age, Debility and Infirmity' (4.6 per 1,000, 12.4 %) (see Fig. 3.11). As with the hospital records discussed previously, the categories of 'Fever' and 'Bowels and Dysentery' (gastrointestinal complaints) hold the most prominent positions. Neither is it a surprise that 'Old Age and Infirmity' holds a prominent position, since most people die of old age and the disabilities that come with aging after all. Similarly, it is no wonder that the category 'Pains and Injuries', which occupied a prominent position in the hospital records, is

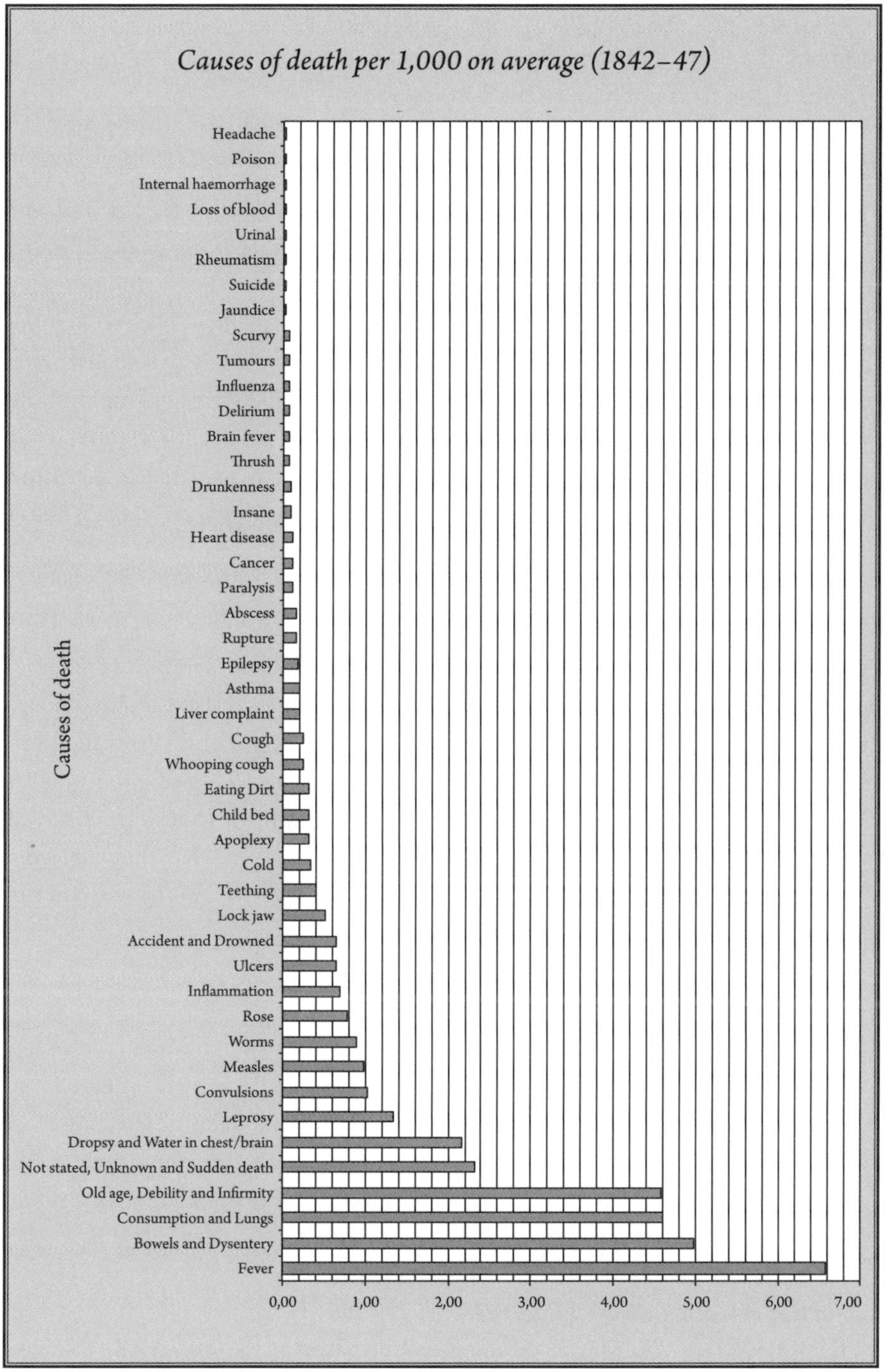

Fig. 3.11. Source: Table 3.10.

not present here, because the causes of death are more specifically stated. By contrast, the term 'Consumption' occupies a prominent position in the church records that it does not have in the hospital records.

Boils and Sores

In the hospital records, the category of 'Boils and Sores' appeared as a prominent cause of disease (12–38 % of days spent in hospital) and a cause of many extended hospitalisations. However, among the causes of death this category does not have the same importance, since only the category 'Ulcers' (1.7 per 1,000, 0.6 %) seems to have any relation to boils and sores. This suggests that even if boils and sores occurred frequently and were difficult to heal (cf. the long hospitalisations), they only rarely caused death. The reason for this is that sores need to be extremely infected before they cause shock and death. Furthermore, the doctors of the first half of the nineteenth century were generally much better at surgery than the treatment of internal diseases.

Rose, Oedema (Dropsy) and Filariasis (Elephantiasis)

In the hospital records, the disease categories of 'Rose' and 'Dropsy' (Oedema) made up 1–8 per cent of days in hospital and was characterised by long hospitalisations. Among the causes of death 'Rose' and 'Dropsy and Water in chest/brain' appear with respectively 0.8 per 1,000 (2.1 %) and 2.2 per 1,000 (5.9 %). This shows that dropsy in particular was not only a condition that some enslaved workers suffered from but a symptom of illnesses so severe that they caused a number of deaths. By contrast, 'Rose' seems to have been within the reach of the doctors' treatments, just like 'Boils and Sores'.

Yaws and Leprosy

In the hospital records, there were only two cases of yaws and one case of leprosy. Whereas the yaws patients were cured during the period investigated, the leprosy patient was chronically ill. This pattern repeats itself in the causes of death where yaws is not present at all while leprosy accounts for 1.3 per 1,000 (3.6 %). Still, the numbers are so small that leprosy did not have great importance for the overall enslaved mortality on St Croix.

'Child bed': Death during Childbirth

In the hospital records nine cases occurred, amounting to around 0.02 per cent of all days spent in hospital on the four royal plantations, in which enslaved women had been admitted to hospital or at least recorded as sick in connection with childbirth. Among the causes of death 'Child bed', i.e. death during childbirth, did have a somewhat more prominent position with 0.3 per 1,000 (0.8 %). However, the population at risk for both illness and death in connection with childbirth is obviously not the entire population, but only women of childbearing age, and accordingly the actual risk of death in this group was higher. The below discussion of causes of death per 1,000 enslaved divided by gender shows that the mortality rate per 1,000 female enslaved was 0.71 (see Table 3.11 and Fig. 3.12), yet the source material does not allow us to go any further because the precise number of enslaved women of childbearing age in 1842–47 is unknown.

'Teething'

Dental problems do not occur as a cause of death, but 'Teething' does with 0.4 per 1,000 enslaved (1.1 %). According to the doctors' medical reports, the term referred to problems occurring around the time of deciduous dentition and to a complex of the diseases 'Convulsion', 'Bowels and Dysentery' and 'Fever'. 'Teething' may also have occurred among the older children during the dentition of the permanent teeth, but did not manifest itself later in life. This is visible in the discussion below of causes of death per 1,000 enslaved divided by age, where 'teething' occurs with 1.51 per 1,000 enslaved in the age group 1–16, but only in this group (see Table 3.12 and Fig. 3.13).

Venereal Diseases

The venereal diseases were not very prominent in the hospital records and do not feature at all among the causes of death.

Age and Causes of Death

An analysis of the causes of death in the enslaved population divided into two age groups shows that both the causes of death and the mortality rate were strongly dependent on age. The two age groups are 1–16 years and 17–100+ years. These uneven age brackets are a consequence of the structure of the source materials and more specifically of the tax records. Furthermore, the tax records do not include enslaved children under the age of 1 year, which also made it necessary to exclude the 0–1-year-olds from the church records. This is very unfortunate, because the mortality among infants and children below 1 year of age is known to have been substantial and a decisive factor behind the demographic decline (see Chapter 2 on demography).

The analysis of the age groups shows that among the children and adolescents 'Fever' (12.73 per 1,000) and 'Bowels and Dysentery' (9.49 per 1,000) caused the largest number of deaths and significantly more than among the adult and old enslaved workers (see Fig. 3.13). The reason for this pattern is not immediately apparent from the available information, and besides, deaths caused by 'Bowels and Dysentery' (diarrhoea) were so common for children during 'Dentitio' that the doctors did not take much notice.

Other prominent causes of death in the age group 1–16 were 'Worms' (3.02 per 1,000), 'Measles' (2.91 per 1,000) and 'Teething' (1.51 per 1,000). As diseases/symptoms these categories would not be surprising, because they also occur among children today. Yet here, they are not just causes of illness but causes of death. What is most remarkable is the great impact of intestinal worms. Undoubtedly, the reason for this was that sometime after the first year of life breastfeeding was gradually replaced by solid food, which, apart from being of low nutritional value, may also have been infected with worms because of a lack of hygiene. At the same time, the enslaved children reached an age where children begin to move independently and so come into contact with an increasing number of sources of infection in the environment.

Regarding the age group 17–100+, adulthood and old age, other causes of death have the greatest relative importance (see Fig. 3.13). Apart from the obvious causes related to aging, 'Old Age, Debility and Infirmity' (7.01 per 1,000), the most important causes are 'Consumption and Lungs' (5.74 per 1,000), 'Dropsy and Water in brain/chest' (2.68 per 1,000), 'Leprosy' (1.83 per 1,000) and 'Rose' (1.15 per 1,000). It is interesting that 'Consumption and Lungs' is a more prominent cause of death among the adults than even 'Fever' and 'Bowels and Dysentery'. To the extent that the category is synonymous with tuberculosis the disease might have been present in the body since childhood, while the outbreak did not occur until the immune system of the enslaved worker became sufficiently weakened, for instance because of a combination of hard work and malnutrition. Another cause of death, which was also more prominent in the adult age group, is 'Leprosy'. There might have been good reasons for this similarity between 'Consumption and Lungs' and 'Leprosy', because the latter is so closely related to tuberculosis that skin tuberculosis can be mistaken for leprosy, and probably often was. Furthermore, tuberculosis is today the most common cause of death for patients with leprosy, because leprosy rarely causes death on its own but weakens the host organism so that other diseases become fatal.[381] On this basis, it is somewhat surprising that leprosy features among the causes of death at all, yet presumably the manager or doctor who stated the cause of death could not identify any other cause than the very visible leprosy. In addition, leprosy had a special status both in the European medical tradition and in the West Indies that made the fear of it greater than the number of patients actually warrants. Finally, 'Dropsy and Water in chest/brain' and 'Rose' were also conditions typically caused by a weak immune system and the increasing wearing out of the body following aging.

Gender and Causes of Death

An analysis of causes of death in relation to the gender distribution in the enslaved population at risk shows that except for births, there were only insignificant differences between male and female causes of death (see Fig. 3.12). On this basis, one can assume that the conditions that influenced the health of the two sexes, and primarily the workload and nutrition, were largely the same, or at least that their relationship to the physical capacity and needs of the sexes were about the same.

The Seasonal Mortality

An analysis of the distribution of deaths in the enslaved population during the months of the year as recorded by the church records supports the theory discussed previously about the seasonal pattern in morbidity. It turns out that in the years 1842–47 the average mortality as a percentage of all deaths (not population at risk, see below) in the months September to January was constantly above the average mortality for the whole year. The highest point was in December. In the other months (February to August) the average mortality was below the annual average (see Fig. 3.14 and Fig. 3.15). The conclusion must be that this pattern of seasonal mortality is generally concurrent with the pattern in seasonal morbidity among the enslaved workers presented by Barry W. Higman and confirmed on the royal plantations of St Croix (see above). Even though disease does not necessarily lead to death, and death is not necessarily a consequence of previous disease, the chronological coincidence of disease and death must indicate two factors. First, that the time from August to January was indeed a time of extraordinary hardship for the enslaved workers on St Croix.

381 Kiple, *History of Human Disease*, 834–37.

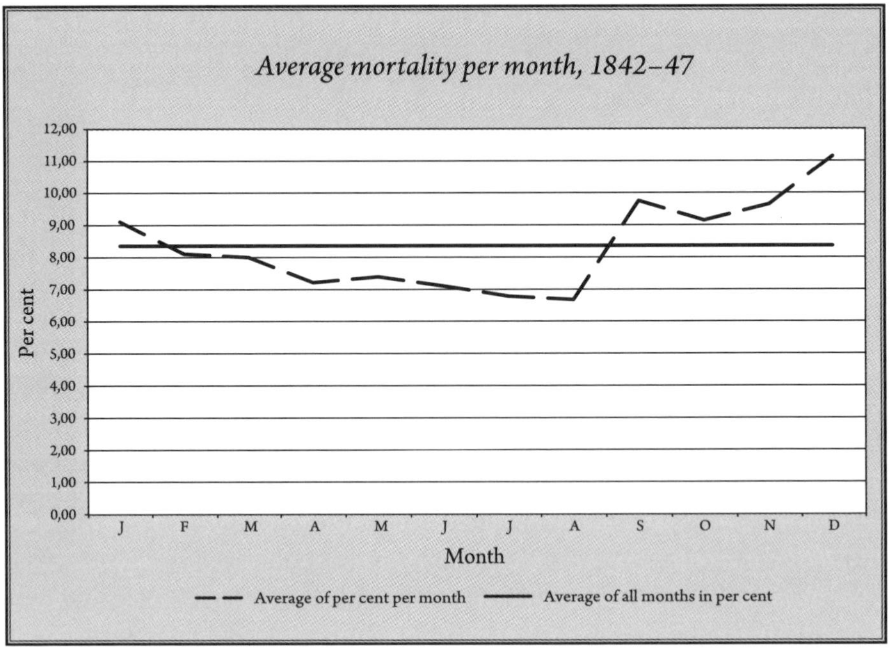

Fig. 3.15. Source: Table 3.11.

Secondly, the morbidity on the royal plantations investigated previously in this chapter followed the same pattern as the mortality on Cruzian plantations in general, and so we can also assume that their pattern of seasonal morbidity is representative of other plantations on the island. On this basis, the representativeness and credibility of both results is strengthened. Finally, it can be added that data from the period after emancipation confirm that the mortality among Afro-Caribbean workers on St Croix kept following the same seasonal pattern.[382]

Causes of Death in Comparative Perspective

If we compare the above results with the analyses by Barry W. Higman of the seasonal mortality in various British West Indian colonies, great similarities appear, but also remarkable differences. Higman's investigations have generated the most detailed data for enslaved populations in any West Indian colony

382 Hoxcer Jensen, *From Serfdom*, 209 (figure 39).

(nothing similar exists for the French West Indies). As the chronology of the data is also very close to the data from St Croix, and they originate from populations with similar demographic profiles, there is a good baseline for comparison. However, Higman did not base his calculations on the total 'population at risk' of dying but on the total number of dead in his material. This has made it necessary to use his method for the Cruzian data as well to facilitate the comparison. Unfortunately, this prevents comparison with data calculated on the 'population at risk'. Furthermore, Higman's data include the age group of 0–1 year olds, and so this group has been re-included in the sample, increasing it from 1,212 to 1,700 individuals.

According to Higman's data from Dominica, Berbice and Tobago, which correspond to data on the seasonal morbidity on Barbados, St Vincent and Jamaica, mortality among the enslaved workers was at its highest in September and lowest in March.[383] By contrast, the mortality on St Croix was above the annual average from September until and including January with the highest point in December, while it was below average and decreasing continuously from February to the lowest point in August (see Table 3.13). Higman claims that the highpoint in enslaved mortality in the British West Indies in the month of September cannot have been a direct consequence of the severe workload during the sugar harvest, because the mortality did not increase until after the end of harvest in June. Consequently, he suggests that the increased mortality was an accumulated and delayed effect of the hardship during harvest combined with a bad nutritional situation in the autumn. However, the results from St Croix suggest that there was one more reason for the fluctuations in the mortality of the enslaved workers and that the factors had a different weighting among themselves on St Croix. To begin with, the harvest on St Croix did not end in June as in Higman's material, but in August.[384] Accordingly, the harvest continued for a longer period on St Croix, since it started in January. This is important because it prolonged the enslaved workers' traditional access to the nutritious raw materials of the sugar production, i.e. the sugar cane and the sugar juice. Certainly, the harvest made the enslaved workers' working days longer, yet in return, there were nutritional benefits. Furthermore, during the harvest months the enslaved had the benefit of the crops from their own provision grounds, which had been planted in the previous autumn. Finally, the weather on St Croix from January

383 Higman, *Slave Populations*, 336–37.
384 Highfield, *Observations*, 31–32 (original: Brady, 1829).

to August is normally hot and dry, which according to the local doctors made this season healthier (i.e. with a low number of patients) than the rest of the year. To sum up, it seems that despite the long working days the better nutritional and climatic conditions in the long harvest time from January to August reduced the mortality and kept it below the annual average.

In the months September to December, the situation was completely different. In these months the main task was the holing, i.e. the preparation of the soil for the planting of new sugar cane. This was a very demanding task. The British Lieutenant Brady, who lived on a Cruzian plantation in the latter half of the 1820s, wrote:

> Holing land for canes is the hardest work that is performed by Negroes.[385]

In addition, as Higman also pointed out, the nutritional situation was worse during the autumn because the enslaved workers' supply of crops from their own provision grounds was exhausted. So, in the worst-case scenario, they only had the food rations handed out by the planter to live off, and at the same time, they had to work hard, not just with holing the sugar fields but also to prepare and plant their own provision grounds. Finally, the months from September to and including November is the time of year with the heaviest rainfall on St Croix, and the hurricane season.[386] According to the doctors' medical reports, the wet and windy weather caused increased morbidity, especially in respiratory diseases. This is also evident from the hospital records. These bad conditions is probably the reason why the planters issued extra provisions during these months in the form of 'biscuits' or 'hard bread' (hardtack), sugar water and grog for the enslaved workers, who holed the fields. The grog was intended to give warmth and to lift their spirits, while the hardtack and sugar was a welcome supplement of energy to the sparse diet (see Chapter 4).

In conclusion, it seems that it was the hard work combined with the bad nutritional and climatic situation that increased the mortality among the enslaved workers on St Croix. It is impossible to determine if the work carried out during harvest had a delayed effect as Higman suggests, but there does not seem to be any reason to believe that harvesting was harder than holing. Assuming that harvesting and holing were equally hard, it must have been changes in other

385 Highfield, *Observations*, 36 (original: Brady, 1829).

386 Sveistrup, *Bidrag*, 5–6. From 1852 to 1911 the average precipitation on St Croix in the month of October was 160 mm.

factors (i.e. the worsening nutritional and climatic situation) that caused the increased mortality during autumn. Accordingly, I will conclude that the cause of the seasonal increase in mortality among the enslaved workers on St Croix was not, as suggested by Higman, an indirect effect of the workload during harvest combined with bad nutrition, but that it was caused by hard work during holing, bad nutrition and bad weather during the months September to January.

If we take the comparison between the material from St Croix and the British West Indies to a more detailed level and focus on the importance of the various causes of death, then great similarities and remarkable differences appear. However, Higman's grouping of the causes of death is different from the one used above. This is because of the problems of interpreting the medical terminology of the period. Therefore, to permit a comparison and make it as precise as possible, the results from St Croix have been regrouped to follow Higman's grouping (see Table 3.15 and Table 3.16).

The comparison shows that the causes of death had a different weighting on St Croix than in five different British West Indian colonies: Grenada. Dominica, Tobago, Demerara-Essequibo, and Berbice (see Table 3.17). According to Higman, the most prominent causes of death in the colonies[387] he investigated were 'Diarrhoea and Dysentery', 'Dropsy', 'Fevers', 'Tuberculosis', 'Nervous system diseases' and 'Digestive system diseases'.[388] By contrast, 'Diarrhoea and Dysentery' has a very low ranking in the material from St Croix. Considering the close relation of both causes of death to the gastrointestinal system, the difference is probably due to differences in terminology among the managers and doctors who reported the causes of death in the British colonies and St Croix respectively. Nonetheless, the majority of the doctors on St Croix were trained in the English-speaking world. So, it seems that the causes of death included in 'Dysentery and Diarrhoea' and in 'Digestive system diseases' respectively have been interpreted contrarily on St Croix and in the British West Indies. 'Dysentery and Diarrhoea' on St Croix represents 3.15 per cent of all deaths and 'Digestive system diseases' 20 per cent, against respectively 18.1 and 3.5 per cent of all deaths in Demerara-Essequibo. Whatever the reason, it is clear that if the two categories are combined into one category comprising the entire digestive system, then the values become almost the same (21.25 % and 23.15 % respectively). As to the 'Tuberculosis' and 'Nervous system diseases' the values from

387 They were all new sugar producing colonies (see Chapter 2).
388 Higman, *Slave Populations*, 341.

St Croix are fairly close to Higman's. Yet, the two last causes of death, 'Dropsy' and 'Fevers', show quite different values for St Croix.

Table 3.17: Causes of death in the British West Indies, 1817–32.

Causes of death	Causes of death in per cent		
	Demerara-Essequibo, 1829–32[389]	Min.-Max., BWI[390]	St Croix, 1842–47
Diarrhea and Dysentery	18.1	16.2–25.7	3.15
Dropsy	13.9	10.7–16.0	5.31
Fevers	12.3	6.0–12.3	30.69
Tuberculosis	11.2	4.2–12.7	11.85
Nervous system diseases	11.5	7.1–11.8	6.15
Digestive system diseases	3.5	3.5–9,3	20.00
Total	70.5	47.7–87.8	77.15

Source: Table 3.14 and Table 3.16.

The difference in the number of deaths caused by 'Dropsy' is difficult to explain because there are numerous reasons for the condition. Malnutrition is one option, but 'Dropsy' might as well have been caused by cardiovascular problems, kidney problems, parasites etc. The causes behind 'Fevers' are just as numerous; however, as this cause of death was beyond comparison the most important on St Croix, and much more prominent than in the British West Indies, it is necessary to add a few more comments. As mentioned at the beginning of this chapter, the doctors on St Croix claimed unanimously in their medical reports that fever was indeed a frequent ailment among the enslaved workers but that they did not die from it. The reason why 'Fever' was nonetheless frequently stated as a cause of death may be that many of the victims of fever were children (see Fig. 3.13). With children, and particularly small children, it is difficult to get information about the disease by asking the patient. In this situation, both managers and doctors on St Croix were probably forced to rely on external symptoms, and as fever is of course a frequent symptom of disease, the managers and doctors could not report the cause of death as anything else but 'Fever'. Still, this does not explain the discrepancy between the doctors' statements concerning the mortality by fever among the enslaved in, respectively, the annual medical reports and in the church records.

389 Demerara-Essequibo is an illustrative example of the causes of death in an individual colony in the British West Indies.

390 BWI = British West Indies.

Conclusion

The above quantitative analysis has demonstrated the most important causes of death among the enslaved workers on St Croix in the 1840s (measured per 1,000 enslaved at risk) to have been 'Fever', 'Bowels and Dysentery', 'Consumption and Lungs' and 'Old Age, Debility and Infirmity'. The two first categories correspond well with the diseases most prominent among the enslaved workers, while the last category is a common cause of death among humans in general. However, for unknown reasons the category 'Consumption' occupied a much more prominent position among the causes of death than among the diseases. The mortality and the ranking of the causes of death differed greatly according to the age of the enslaved. The child mortality, age 1–16, was caused particularly by the categories 'Fever' and 'Bowels and Dysentery', whereas 'Consumption and Lungs' was a much more prominent cause of death among the adults, age 17–100+. In contrast to the age distribution, there were no significant gender differences in the causes of death.

The development of mortality throughout the year turned out to be seasonal in the same way as the morbidity was previously shown to be. The lowest number of deaths occurred in August and the highest in December. By comparison with Barry W. Higman's results from the British West Indies, it became clear that the seasonal pattern of mortality was a little different on St Croix, yet that the factors behind the pattern were the same: hard work, bad nutrition and bad weather in the months from September to January. However, Higman's hypothesis about an indirect and delayed effect of work during harvest is not confirmed by the data from St Croix.

Finally, a comparison of the importance of the various causes of death (as a percentage of all deaths) in the enslaved populations of St Croix and the British West Indies (Higman) respectively has shown that there were great similarities. Unfortunately, the differences are hard to explain, because the different terminology at the time obscures the causality behind the deaths.

Slave Laws and Health Factors

Some of the factors that influenced the health of enslaved workers in the Danish West Indies were subject to more or less consistent legislation. In the following, I will introduce the somewhat incoherent state of the slave laws in the Danish West Indies, examine five factors of particular importance to the health of the enslaved and compare with the situation in the British and French West Indies.

The Lack of a Slave Law

In the period 1803–48, the legislation governing the enslaved workers in the Danish West Indies was based on a confusing collection of older laws and local ad hoc legislation. The earliest and founding law was still Governor Phillip Gardelin's (governor of St Thomas and St John, 1733–36)[391] draconian slave law of 1733. The Gardelin slave law focused on the position of the enslaved worker as the private property of the owner and listed brutal mutilating punishments for any behaviour deviating from the wish of the master. The law did not grant the enslaved any rights, not even regarding food, clothes, and housing. Not until the takeover of the Danish West Indies by the Danish Crown in 1755 were such rights granted to the enslaved workers by King Frederik the Fifth's slave law of that year. However, even these rights could not satisfy the physical needs of the enslaved, but at least they might have prevented the worst abuses.[392] Unfortunately, the slave law of 1755 was never promulgated. The Governor General in charge at the time, Baron Christian Lebrecht von Prøck (1755–66),[393] chose to shelve the law out of consideration for the sensitive relationship between the Danish colonial administration and the planters. In 1783, the titular councillor of state Wilhelm Anton Lindemann (1739–1801)[394] submitted a proposal for a new slave law. The proposal included a number of rules, which would further improve the health conditions of the enslaved workers in comparison with the unpublished law of 1755. For instance, the planter was to build houses for the enslaved, allocate land to them for their own production of provision crops and a weekly day off to work on this land. Finally, medical treatment of sick enslaved workers was to be mandatory and all conditions concerning weekly food rations, punishment and disease were to be recorded in a special plantation journal. Sadly, Lindemann's proposal suffered the same fate as the law of 1755: it was never implemented. The same happened to a similar proposal from a royal commission set up in Copenhagen under Count Adolph Sigfried von der Osten (1726–97)[395] in 1785.[396] Not even the royal commission for the abolition of the slave trade, set up in Copenhagen in 1791, dared to encroach upon the planters' private rights of ownership. The commission was fully aware that

391 Kay Larsen, *Guvernører, Residenter, Kommandanter og Chefer samt enkelte andre fremtrædende Personer i de tidligere danske Tropekolonier* (Copenhagen: Arthur Jensens Forlag, 1940), 33, 67.
392 Hall, *Slave Society*, 56–59.
393 Bricka, *Dansk biografisk Lexikon* XIII, 302–3.
394 Bricka, *Dansk biografisk Lexikon* X, 312.
395 Bricka, *Dansk biografisk Lexikon* XII, 450.
396 Hall, *Slave Society*, 65–67.

the abolition of the slave trade was closely related to the question of the conditions of the enslaved workers on the plantations, because bad conditions there caused a negative demographic development. If these conditions did not change, the preservation of a stable enslaved work force would remain dependent on imports of new enslaved workers. However, it was also the firm conviction of the commission that the abolition of the slave trade in itself would bring about improvements in the conditions of the enslaved workers, because the planters would no longer be able to replace dead enslaved workers with new imports. This would force the planters to change the conditions of the enslaved in their own self-interest. Besides, the commission could not agree to set new rules for food rations, clothes, housing, and care for pregnant women, children, and the sick.[397]

In the period 1803–48, new proposals for a cohesive slave law were submitted in 1802 and 1817 (after each of the two British occupations), but each time they were shelved. About 1830, the question of a consistent legislation was raised again, but at this time there was great uncertainty regarding the future of slavery because of the British debate on the subject of emancipation, and so the Danish colonial administration chose to wait and see.[398] In 1834, the emancipation of the enslaved workers in the British West Indies put the Danish legislation under great pressure regarding the enslaved. The reaction was the rescript of 22 November 1834, which was however only published in the ordinance of 1 May 1840, but confirmed the enslaved workers' rights to independent property and to purchase their own freedom. With this, the full human rights of the enslaved workers had in fact been admitted and it was only a question of time before the final emancipation would become a reality. The motive for the delay of emancipation until 1848 was due to the administration needing time to sort out the many practical problems connected to emancipation.[399] In this process, the slave law of 1755 was finally published in a rescript of 18 February 1843.[400]

The absence of a cohesive legislation concerning the enslaved workers meant that in everyday life the administrators of the colonial government had to navigate a suitable course between the many different rules the legislation had come

397 Vibæk, 'Dansk Vestindien, 1755–1848', 182–83 et passim.
398 Olsen, 'Danske Lov', 309.
399 Olsen, 'Fra ejendomsret', 49.
400 Tage Algreen-Ussing, *Kongelige Reskripter og Resolutioner, Reglementer, Instruxer og Fundatser, samt Kollegialbreve, med flere Danmarks Lovgivning vedkommende offentlige Aktstykker* (Copenhagen, 1845). 'Reskript af 18. februar 1843 ang. Forbedringer i Negerslavernes Stilling' (Rescript of 18 February 1843 concerning improvements in the situation of the Negro slaves).

to consist of. Accordingly, the limits of the planter's authority over his slaves-bondsman/woman were defined by legal practice, both in the islands, and when cases were occasionally tried before the Supreme Court in Denmark.[401] Another consequence of the lack of a slave law was that the rights of the enslaved workers in relation to food, clothes, housing, work hours and medical treatment seems to have been largely guided by customs.

The Workload

It is obvious that the work of the enslaved workers had a great impact on their state of health. This impact was partly due to the work-related injuries (cuts, sprains, fractures etc.) and the general degradation caused by the work, partly due to the workload itself, i.e. how hard and how long the enslaved had to work. The latter issue was of special importance, because the enslaved workers' access to food, and so to the energy required by their work, was limited. Accordingly, the workload was a decisive factor for the health of the enslaved workers.

The daily work hours of the enslaved working in the fields does not seem to have changed much during the period in question. The special inspector on the plantations of the Schimmelmann family, Viscount Martin-Marie-Charles de Boudens de Vanderbourg (1765–1827),[402] wrote in his report of 1798 that outside harvest time the enslaved worked from sunrise at 5 or 6 in the morning to sunset at 6 or 7 in the evening; a working day of ten to eleven hours. Furthermore, the enslaved had to cut grass for the cattle twice a day. Around 8 o'clock in the morning, the enslaved workers would take a break of about one hour to eat, and from around midday to 2 p.m. there was a break for lunch. During harvest (January–August) the working hours were longer, because the sugar cane had to be cut down, pressed and the sugar juice boiled in one operation. However, outright night work does not seem to have been common as it was in other parts of the West Indies. Despite the long working hours, harvest time was the favourite time of the year for the enslaved workers, probably because of the abundance of food. By contrast, the rest of the year (September–December) was characterised by a limited food supply, which was why this season was called 'hungry time'. During this time, the enslaved had half the Saturday off and all of Sunday.[403]

401 Olsen, 'Fra ejendomsret', 47, and Olsen, 'Danske Lov', 312–14.
402 Gustave Vapereau, *Dictionnaire universel des literatures* (Paris: Hachette, 1876), 2012.
403 Tyson and Highfield, *The Kamina Folk*, 142.

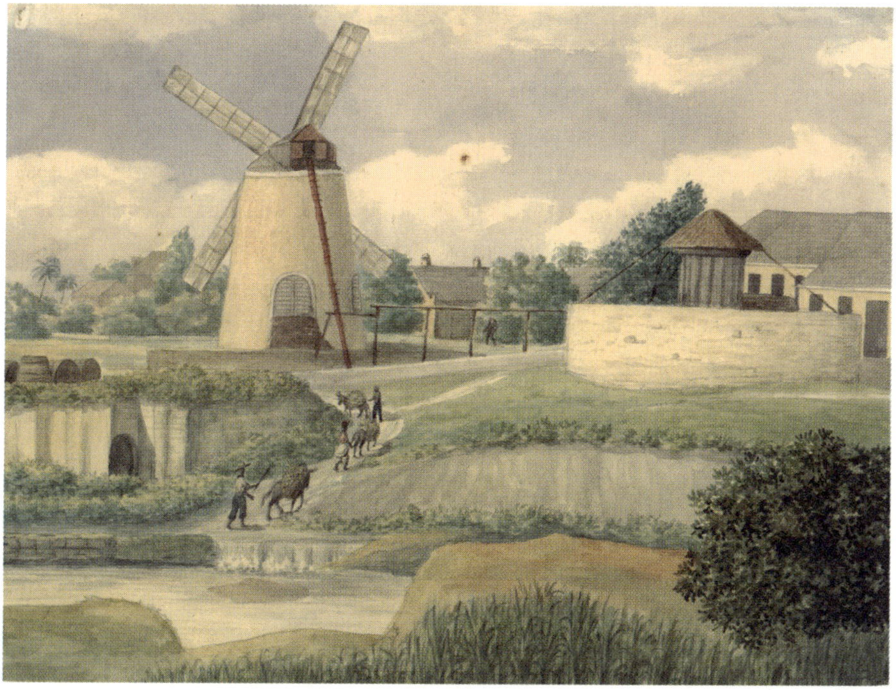

Fig. 3.16: The transport of sugar cane on mules from the fields to the mill was often the job of older enslaved children. Coloured drawing by Frederik von Scholten, the brother of Governor General Peter von Scholten, showing the plantation Castle on St Croix, August 1833. Danish Maritime Museum, Elsinore, Denmark.

Later descriptions of the working hours of the enslaved from the 1820s to the 1840s follow the same scheme with insignificant variations.[404] Nevertheless, there are signs that the effort, the energy, forced from the enslaved during the working day was rising during the period.[405] This factor cannot be measured directly or with any precision, but Lieutenant Brady remarked that on some plantations both the soil and the enslaved workers were 'forced' to the limit.[406] The reason for this was the declining price of sugar, the huge burden of paying instalments on loans in the plantations and the continuously rising demand for labour. It is evident that this growing pressure must have had an impact on the

404 Tyson and Highfield, *The Kamina Folk*, 187, 204, 207; Highfield, *Observations*, 10, 30–31 (original: Brady, 1829).
405 Vibæk, 'Dansk Vestindien, 1755–1848', 272.
406 Highfield, *Observations*, xvii, 30, 99 (original: Brady, 1829).

enslaved and increased their energy expenditure and so their wearing out and need of energy from food; a need that seems to have been difficult to fulfil (see Chapter 4).

Presumably, it is in the light of this development, as well as the emancipation in the British West Indies, that we must regard the colonial administration's attempts to set the maximum hours of work. The first attempt was on the royal plantations where the lease regulations of 1834 essentially fixed the traditional work scheme mentioned above. However, the traditional work scheme did not prevent the leaseholder increasing the pace of the work and so injuring the enslaved workers and the state as their owner. To prevent this, article 6 of the lease regulations prescribed that the leaseholder was obliged to follow a cultivation plan, prepared by a commission set up for that specific purpose.[407] The cultivation plan should ensure that the number of acres under sugar cultivation was equivalent to what the number of enslaved workers on the plantation could manage within a 'normal' work effort.[408]

The legislation did not go further than this until 1843 when a royal rescript ordered that the enslaved workers were to have the whole of Saturday off all year round. However, the enslaved could choose to rent themselves out for money on this day off.[409] Apart from this rescript, no legislation was issued pertaining to the work of the enslaved in the period in question, even though in 1834 Governor General von Scholten had discussed such legislation with a royal commission for the emancipation of the enslaved workers. In fact, through a flexible clause von Scholten had the authority to issue legislation on the work conditions of the enslaved, if it proved necessary. However, he did not use this option because as long as law and order were maintained in the colony there was no reason for drastic interventions, which would no doubt cause unrest.[410] If such legislation on work were issued, it would be a serious encroachment on the most primary concern of the planters, namely the exploitation of the labour of their enslaved workers. A reduction by law in the working hours of the enslaved could make plantations unprofitable and so destroy the economy of both the planters and the colony with a single blow. Neither the planters nor the colonial

407 DNA, WILA, no. 46.19. 'Reglement for Negernes Behandling m.m. på de Kongelige Plantager som er bortforpagtede' (Rules for the treatment of Negros etc. for the royal plantations on lease). § 1, § 6.
408 See for instance: DNA, WILA, no. 2.38.2. Lease contract for Estate Boetzberg, 1834.
409 Algreen-Ussing, *Kongelige Reskripter.* Rescript of 18 February 1843.
410 Vibæk, 'Dansk Vestindien, 1755–1848', 271–74.

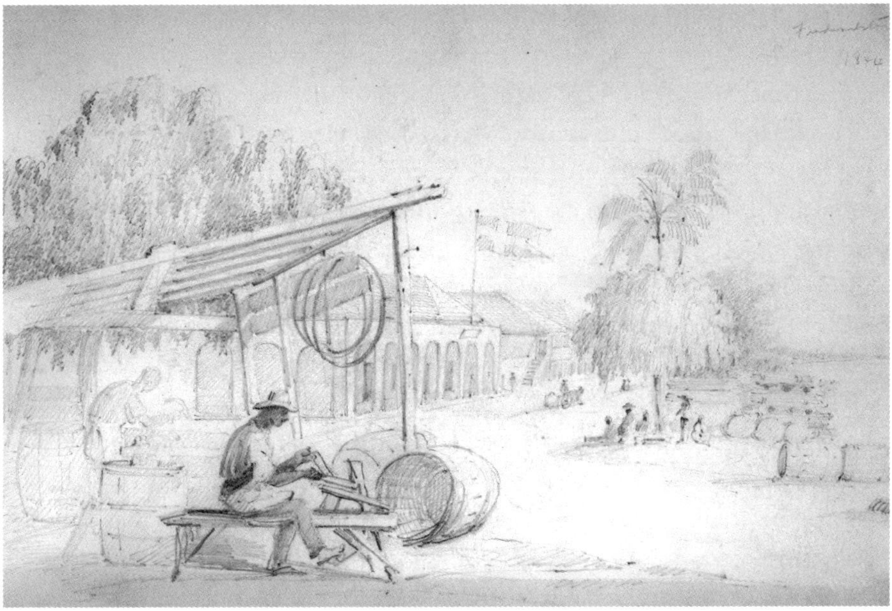

Fig. 3.17: Not all enslaved workers toiled in the sugar fields. Enslaved artisans, for instance, like the cooper on this drawing, had a less physically destructive job. Drawing by Reverend Henry Jackson Morton, Frederiksted 1843–44, titled 'Bay Street Looking South From the Fort'. St Croix Landmarks Society, St Croix.

administration had any interest in measures with such potentially devastating consequences.

Enslaved workers not working in the fields did not necessarily have such a demanding and rigorous work scheme. This was true for instance for the enslaved artisans, domestics, sick-nurses, herdsmen, watchmen etc. These functions were rarely as physically demanding as the fieldwork, yet in return the hours could be longer. Children and old people undertook various tasks in the fields and elsewhere that did not demand the same level of physical strength and endurance. For instance, many of the old people worked as watchmen, while the older children took care of the transport of sugar cane on mules from the field to the sugar mill.[411]

On sugar plantations in the British and French West Indies, the working hours were very similar to those on St Croix. In the British colonies in the east-

411 Highfield, *Observations*, 34–35 (original: Brady, 1829).

ern part of the Caribbean the working hours were about ten hours a day, except on Barbados where they were only nine hours. However, this was only outside harvest time. During harvest, night work in shifts was not unusual, but the practice was being phased out. In 1831, a royal ordinance fixed the working hours at nine hours per day in the British Crown colonies of Trinidad, Demerara-Essequibo, and Berbice. In 1823, a similar ordinance had relieved the enslaved of working on Sundays, which had however been the norm since the turn of the century. During the 1820s, it became common to give the enslaved a half day off on Saturday outside harvest time. The ordinance of 1823 was a part of the efforts of the British government to ease the conditions of the enslaved workers, and in relation to this the government encouraged the introduction of the so-called 'task-work' or piecework system on plantations. The idea was that the enslaved worker should not work for a set number of hours a day but carry out a specified task. In this way, the enslaved had an incentive to work harder, because they could finish their work faster and get more time on their own. However, the system was only introduced in the Crown colonies where the British central government had the largest virtual power.[412]

In the French West Indies (here exemplified by Martinique), the workload was similar. The legislation prescribed that work should commence by sunrise (at 5–6 a.m.) and end around 5 p.m. or at sundown. Between midday and 2 p.m. there was a lunch break. Furthermore, the enslaved had to cut grass for the cattle twice a day. However, these regulations did not apply during harvest time, when the enslaved worked in shifts through the night. The legislations prescribed Sunday as a day off for the enslaved workers and in addition it was the custom to give the enslaved part of or all of Saturday off to work on their own provision grounds.[413]

Comparing the workload among the enslaved in the Danish, British, and French West Indies there is not much difference. A somewhat larger difference is visible in the degree to which the authorities intervened in the field. As in many other instances, the intervention of the French state is clearly visible throughout the period whereas the efforts of the British authorities were less consistent because of the various forms of government in the different colonies (see Chapter 2). However, the interventions of the Danish state and local colo-

412 Higman, *Slave Populations*, 179, 181–83, 187.

413 Dale W. Tomich, 'Slavery in Martinique in the French Caribbean', in *Caribbean Slavery in the Atlantic World: A Student Reader*, ed. Verene Shepherd and Hilary McD. Beckles (Jamaica: Ian Randle Publishers, 2000), 422–25.

nial administration in this field seem to have been even weaker than those of the British. In the Danish West Indies, no general law was issued on the length of the enslaved workers' working day or the special circumstances during harvest time. Only the royal plantations got such regulation in 1834. Despite the fact that the Danish administration was very active in preserving the health of the enslaved workers in other fields, working hours was an issue of such importance to the planters, and by extension for the economy of the entire colony, that the colonial administration did not find it opportune to intervene.

The Weather

According to the medical reports from the Cruzian doctors, the weather in the period 1823–48 was characterised by recurring droughts. Eleven of the 26 years in this period are described as unusually dry and were consequently seen as healthier than average in accordance with the humoral pathological perception of the importance of the weather.[414] These conditions were expressed in a general way by Dr William Kerr (1794–1837)[415] in 1834:

> As far as my experience goes this island is becoming more healthy every year, especially among the native and those accustomed to the climate, which may be accounted for by the increased dryness of the state of the atmosphere.[416]

The doctors explained the better conditions of health among both Afro-Caribbean and Euro-Caribbean inhabitants by stating that the drought prevented the decomposition in the fallen leaves induced by humidity and warmth, which created the disease-producing miasma (see Chapter 2).[417] However, the dry weather caused problems for the crops. Not only for the sugar crop, which was of course of vital importance to the planters and the economy of the colony, but also for the crops on the enslaved workers' provision grounds. None of the sources mention a lack of food, let alone famine, but there are references to years of 'general distress' caused by drought.[418] When the enslaved workers could not supplement it with crops from their provision grounds, their diet must have become

414 DNA, BH, Med. rep., Danish West Indies. 1824, 1831, 1832, 1833, 1834, 1835, 1840, 1841, 1842, 1845, 1847.

415 Carøe, *Den Danske Lægestand* III, 107 and V, 80.

416 DNA, BH, Med. rep., Danish West Indies. 1834.

417 DNA, DC, no. G125C, 1803. DNA, BH, Med. Rep., 1803–1958, 1822 (Dr. Bloch). DNA, BH, Med. rep., Danish West Indies, 1841 (Dr. Stedman).

418 DNA, BH, Med. rep., Danish West Indies. 1835.

even more unbalanced with only the distributed food rations of corn meal and salt fish (see Chapter 4).

When the rain finally came after a long drought, other health problems emerged. The heavy showers were always followed by epidemics of dysentery and diarrhoea among the enslaved workers, and particularly the children died from gastrointestinal problems, fever and convulsions.[419] With modern knowledge about disease-causing micro-organisms, the reason for the gastrointestinal problems seems to have been that the heavy showers contaminated the drinking water with infected surface water (see below).

Other kinds of diseases perceived to be caused by the weather were influenza and respiratory diseases (whooping cough, pneumonia, and diphtheria). Low temperatures, rain and strong winds from the north heralded many cases of these diseases among the enslaved, which is no surprise considering the low standard of their houses and clothes (see below).[420]

In the British and French West Indies, the enslaved experienced the same problems with the weather and entertained the same perceptions of it.[421]

The Water

Even by the standards of the period 1803–48, the resources of drinking water accessible to the enslaved workers were inferior. As already mentioned, St Croix occasionally experienced heavy rainfall, yet very irregularly. Consequently, the island did not have any freshwater streams of importance, and those that did exist quickly dried out during droughts. Furthermore, the well water (groundwater) was saline and accordingly the inhabitants collected water from the roofs or from special brick-built catchments (in Danish: *regnbakker*) and stored it in barrels or cisterns under the houses.[422]

At the time, the water from the cisterns was praised as 'the purest water in the world',[423] but it is doubtful how clean it actually was. Accounts from a later period with knowledge of the link between the quality of water and the health of the population suggest that the conditions may occasionally have been even extraordinarily bad. From the roofs leaves, dust, and bird excrement was washed down into the cistern with the rainwater forming a layer of sludge on the bot-

419 DNA, BH, Med. rep., Danish West Indies. 1835, 1846, 1847.

420 DNA, DC, no. G125C. DNA, BH, Med. rep., Danish West Indies. 1843, 1847.

421 Sheridan, *Doctors and Slaves*, 190–91; Leti, *Santé et société*, 56–81.

422 Schmidt, *Various Remarks*, 3–4.

423 Bernhard v. Petersen, *En historisk Beretning om de dansk-vestindiske Øer, St Croix, St Thomas og St Jan* (Copenhagen, 1855), 231. Original Danish text: '... det reneste Vand i Verden...'.

tom. In times of drought, when the water level was low in the cistern, the sludge polluted the remaining water and the same happened when heavy rainfall filled up the cistern and so disturbed the sludge. Accordingly, it was quite natural that the population suffered gastrointestinal diseases after heavy rainfall.[424] A similar connection between heavy rainfall and gastrointestinal diseases can be found in the period 1803–48.[425] Furthermore, the cisterns doubled as breeding places for the mosquitoes,[426] which transmitted for instance malaria, yellow fever, and filariasis.[427]

The water in the cisterns was normally reserved for Euro-Caribbeans. Accordingly, the enslaved workers had to make do with what they could get from other sources.[428] Prior to the period dealt with here the enslaved collected water for their own consumption from the roofs of their houses and stored it in barrels.[429] This practice is not mentioned in later times but it seems reasonable to assume that such a simple and necessary practice was continued in the period in question. Besides collected rainwater, the enslaved also obtained water from the same source as the cattle, namely the brackish water from the wells and the few streams. The well water was lifted with hand wheels and buckets or by a windmill.[430]

The well water seems to have been of very low quality. This is evident from the first medical report of 1803 where landfysikus Johan Mathias Frederik Keutsch (1775–1815)[431] described how recently arrived sailors came down with life-threatening diarrhoea because the lack of cistern water had forced them to drink 'pool water' (Danish: *pytvand*), i.e. bad well water.[432] Similarly, landfysikus Johan Frederik Bloch (1780–1827)[433] reported in his medical report of 1822 that cases of diarrhoea, dysentery, and colic had been common during the months of October and November. In his opinion, this was because of the well

424 Christian Ditlevsen, 'Om sanitære og hygiejniske Forhold i Dansk Vestindien', *Atlanten: Medlemsblad for Foreningen 'De danske Atlanterhavsøer', Særskilte Artikler og Foreningsanliggender* 4 (1917), 4–5, 9–10.

425 DNA, BH, Med. rep., Danish West Indies. 1847. Dr Jarvis Roebuck Sr, Christiansted.

426 J.L. Carstens, *En almindelig Beskrivelse om alle de Danske, Americanske eller West-Jndiske Ey-Lande: Dansk Vestindien for 250 år siden* (Copenhagen: Dansk Vestindisk Forlag, 1981), 144.

427 Ditlevsen, 'Om sanitære og hygiejniske Forhold', 15–20.

428 Jensen, 'Sundhed, citroner og slaver', 6.

429 Oldendorp, *Historie der caribischen Inseln* I, 190–92.

430 Henry Morton, *St Croix, St Thomas, St John. Danish West Indian sketchbook and diary – Skitsebog og dagbog fra Dansk Vestindien, 1843–44* (Copenhagen: Dansk Vestindisk Selskab and St Croix Landmarks Society, 1975), 68, 72.

431 Carøe, *Den Danske Lægestand* III, 107 and V, 19–20, 80.

432 DNA, DC, no. G125C. 1803.

433 Carøe, *Den Danske Lægestand* III, 18 and V, 67.

water, which many people had been forced to drink because it was a dry year and they had run out of cistern water.[434] If we are to believe the doctors of a later age, the morbidity caused by the well water was not only due to its salinity, but more likely to the fact that the wells were often exposed to pollution from dunghills, waste water, washing etc.[435]

Nevertheless, the quality of the water in the streams seems to have been even worse. So, a *plakat* (a local ordinance or proclamation in the form of a public notice) of 27 July 1804 focused attention on how 'sess ponds' (sic, presumably cesspools) would often overflow during heavy rainfall and pollute streams, which were used for drinking water by both humans and animals. This situation was detrimental to public health and accordingly the Governor General emphasised that in the future cesspools had to be situated in such a way that the neighbour, his enslaved workers and animals would not come to any harm if they overflowed.[436] Besides cesspools, most plantations had dunghills for the waste from animals and humans, and under heavy rainfall runoff from them may have polluted any nearby streams or wells.[437] The same streams were used for washing, so it is not surprising if the water could be hazardous to the health.[438]

Because of the irregular rain, shortage of water was a recurring problem. For instance, in 1842 no rain fell for eight months, which made all plants wither.[439] In such situations water had to be brought to the plantations in carts to prevent the enslaved workers from dying like the cattle.[440] On this basis, it is relevant to ask if the enslaved workers normally got the amount of drinking water they needed. Obviously, there is no clear answer to that question, but assuming that the enslaved collected water from the roofs of their houses it turns out that *in theory*, at least, they did have the possibility of collecting much more drinking water than they needed. From the roof of a standard, stone-built, slave house from this period it was possible to collect about 42,480 litres of water in a year with average rainfall.[441] In comparison, an adult enslaved worker doing hard

434 DNA, BH, Med. rep., 1803–1958. 1822, case no. 292, 1824.
435 Ditlevsen, 'Om sanitære og hygiejniske Forhold', 6–10.
436 DNA, WILA, no. 2.1.6.
437 Oxholm, *De danske Vestindiske Øers Tilstand*. See Plan I, which shows two dunghills.
438 Tyson and Highfield, *The Kamina Folk*, 205.
439 DNA, BH, Med. rep., Danish West Indies. 1842.
440 See for instance the plantation record for the royal plantation North Star, months of April and May 1833 (DNA, WILA, no. 46.17.55). Furthermore, the process of boiling sugar depended on a stable supply of water.
441 Roof size of typical slave house: 16 × 26 feet = 38.65 m² (see: William Chapman, 'Slave Villages in the Danish West Indies', *Perspectives in Vernacular Architecture* 4 [1991], 112). Average annual precipitation

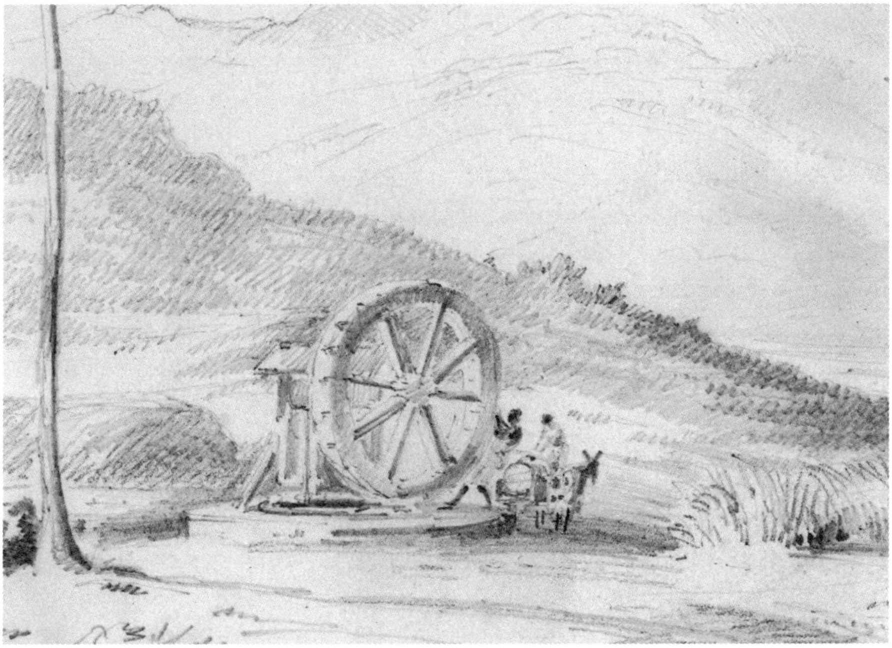

Fig. 3.18: Hand-drawn water well, St Croix, 1843–44. Section of drawing by Reverend Henry Jackson Morton, titled 'Blue Mountain from Slob'. St Croix Landmarks Society, St Croix.

physical work would need to drink up to 10 litres of water per day, i.e. around 3,650 litres per year.[442] As the standard slave houses normally accommodated two to four individuals, the water collected from the roof could easily, at least *in theory*, cover their need for drinking water.[443] However, it is important to stress that this was *only* possible in years with an average amount of rain, and that a large amount of rain would inevitably be wasted, partly because of the storage and limited keeping qualities and partly because of evaporation.

As mentioned, the enslaved workers had to resort to well water during the dry season and during water shortages.[444] Apart from the danger that the water

in Christiansted: 1,099 mm (see: Cappelen and Jensen, *Jordens Klima*, www.dmi.dk/dmi/tr01-17.pdf, 153. Accessed 30-05-2011). 38.65 m² × 1,099 m = 42.48 m³ (42.480 litres).

442 *Work-Rest and Water Consumption Tables* (Maryland: US Army Center for Health Promotion and Preventive Medicine, 2004), Table A-3, A-5. http://safety.ucanr.or g/files/2901.pdf (accessed 30-05-2011).

443 Asmussen, *Slavedemografi*, 80.

444 Highfield, *Observations*, 69 (original: Brady, 1829).

was polluted it also had a high salinity. The reason for the high content of salts in Cruzian groundwater is partly that the aquifer releases mineral salts into the water and partly that salts from seawater is washed into the groundwater with the rain. Today, the salinity of the groundwater is so high that according to modern standards it is generally useless as drinking water (often more than 1,000 milligrams of chlorides per litre).[445] It is not possible to determine if the salinity was equally high in the period 1803–48, but even if the concentrations were lower, the enormous need for drinking water among the hardworking enslaved workers would have given them a considerable intake of salts, if indeed they drank well water. This intake may have caused them problems such as hypertension, kidney problems and disorder in the gastrointestinal system.[446]

In the literature about the enslaved workers and their conditions in other West Indian colonies, the water supply is poorly documented. This is somewhat surprising since water is a fundamental necessity for the life and health of all human beings. One possible explanation is that the water supply was better in most other islands, which had either better groundwater or mountains of higher altitude that could secure a more stable rainfall. However, it does seem as if the situation on Barbados was in many ways similar to St Croix, as people there were also forced to collect rainwater and use dams and ponds.[447]

The House

The houses of the enslaved workers on St Croix seem to have been significantly improved in the period 1803–48. According to archaeologist William R. Chapman, the period 1790–1830 saw a replacement of the former huts made of wattle and daub with roofs of grass or leaves. They were replaced by houses of stone with shingled roofs. The new houses could be single-family houses or built together in row houses with two, three, or more units in each. Each single-family house consisted of two rooms, which also offered the possibility of two single enslaved workers occupying the house. These single-family houses measured about 16 × 26 Danish feet (5.0 × 8.2 metres)[448] and usually they had doors, windows with

445 Perry G. Olcott, *Ground Water Atlas of the United States. Alaska, Hawaii, Puerto Rico and the U. S. Virgin Islands* (Virginia: U.S. Geological Survey, Cartography and Publishing Program, 1985), HA 730-N. http://capp.water.usgs.gov/gwa/ch_n/N-PR_VItext5.html (accessed 30-05-2011).

446 WHO *Public Health Initiatives – Investigation of Gastrointestinal Diseases and Water Supply Structures in Central Asian Republics*. Seminar report: Health Impact of Highly Saline Waters (Denmark: WHO regional office Europe, 2003), 12–15.

447 Jerome S. Handler, 'An Archaeological Investigation of the Domestic Life of Plantation Slaves in Barbados', *Journal of the Barbados Museum and Historical Society* 34 (1972).

448 1 Danish foot = 0,3141 metre. See: Birkeland, *Mål & Vægt*.

shutters and raised wooden floors. The houses were located along the entrance-way to the plantation, in terraces on a hill or in a special area with walls around it. Often the houses were laid out according to an architectural plan with equal space between them. The inspiration for this architecture probably came from contemporary British industrial architecture (houses for workers) where ideas of economy, health, and order were given the pride of place.[449]

Chapman's description of the houses of the enslaved workers corresponds fairly well with contemporary accounts, even if the replacement of the wattle and daub huts seems to have been a somewhat slow process, continuing until emancipation.[450] According to Chapman, it was not until 1840 the Danish colonial administration implemented a building code for slave houses, prescribing the dimensions of the houses and the distances between them.[451] However, this is not entirely correct as the first set of rules on St Croix concerning slave houses is found in the 1834 lease regulations and so only applied to the royal plantations. The lease regulations prescribed that all slave houses had to be constructed of masonry and that the inside dimensions should be 12 × 18 Danish feet (3.7 × 5.5 metres). The distance between houses should be about 30 feet (9.2 metres).[452]

Archival material from the royal plantations shows clearly that the lease regulations brought about an increased focus on the houses of the enslaved workers, yet also that most slave houses at this time were still made of wattle and daub or wood. Furthermore, many of the slave houses on the royal plantations were in dire need of repair, regardless of whether they were made of wattle and daub, wood, half-timbered or entirely of stone. Leaky roofs, cracked walls, and rotting floors were general problems, not least for the preservation of the health of the enslaved workers.[453] This focus on health becomes visible through the investigations carried out by the royal plantation inspector, for instance when water penetrated the floors and walls of the slave houses.[454] It is likely that the humidity in the houses created optimal conditions for the growth of fungi, mould and bacteria, which may have injured the health of the enslaved workers. In other

449 Chapman, 'Slave Villages', 108–20.

450 Tyson and Highfield, *The Kamina Folk*, 186, 210.

451 Chapman, 'Slave Villages', 119.

452 DNA, WILA, no. 46.19. 'Reglement for Negernes Behandling m.m. paa de Kongelige Plantager som er bortforpagtede'. DNA, WILA, no. 2.38.2.

453 DNA, WILA, no. 46.21. Inventory for Estate Longford, 1837. Inventory for Estate Cotton Grove, 1833. Report from Estate Grange, 1835. Report from Estate Upper Love, 1835. Report from Estate Springgarden, 1833. Report from Estate Rust up Twist, 1838.

454 DNA, WILA, no. 46.21. Report from Estate Rust up Twist, 1838. DNA, WILA, no. 46.17.32. Pro Memoria, 1838 and inspection report, 1846.

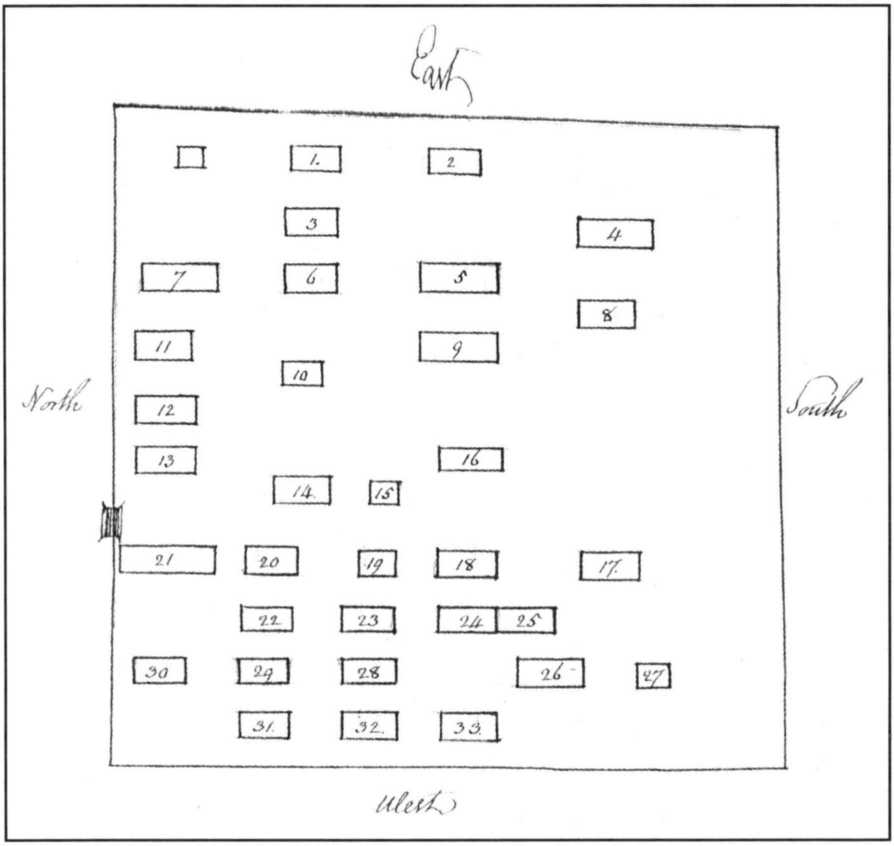

Fig. 3.19: This is a simple sketch from 1838 of the village of the enslaved on the royal plantation Rust up Twist (North Side B Quarter). The alignment of the houses is far from perfect but the symmetric design is clearly visible. DNA, WILA, no. 46.21. Report from estate Rust up Twist, 1838. Courtesy of the Danish National Archives.

words, many of the slave houses on the royal plantations, and probably on some private plantations too, were not in a good state in the 1830s. This must have had an impact on the health of the inhabitants of the houses, yet it is not possible to give more precise information on the hygienic conditions inside the houses.

A similar development from wattle and daub huts via wooden houses to buildings of stone seems to have taken place in the British and French West Indian colonies, though with great variations. These variations make it impossible to compare the housing conditions on St Croix with the other colonies and so determine if they were worse or better. However, in this field, it seems that government interventions in the British and French West Indies were either completely absent or later respectively than in the Danish West Indies.[455]

Clothes and Shoes

There is no doubt that clothing and footwear were important for the preservation of the health of the enslaved workers. Clothes protected against both injuries during work and against the weather, be it sun, rain or wind. The first precise description of the amount of cloth handed out to each enslaved worker as a part of his or her allowance originates from Lieutenant Brady on St Croix in the 1820s. According to Brady, the statutory annual allowance per male enslaved worker was 7 yards (6.4 metres)[456] of 'Osnaburg', a coarse type of linen, and 3.5 yards (3.2 metres) of 'Bamboo', a coarse woollen cloth. Female enslaved workers received one more yard of Osnaburg and the enslaved children in proportion according to their age. In addition, each enslaved person received one blanket every other year. On the plantation where Brady lived, Mannings Bay, every male enslaved worker also received one hat every year and the women two scarves. Brady maintained that this allowance of cloth was only just enough to cover the needs of the enslaved workers and that the Osnaburg would make one shirt and one pair of trousers for the men and the Bamboo a coat or cape.[457]

Whether the amounts of cloth referred to by Brady were in fact statutory is unclear, because in the 1820s the only regulations in the field were the unissued slave code of 1755, which was not published until 1843. According to this code, every enslaved worker was entitled to an annual allowance of either two suits of linen or eight Danish 'alen' (about 5 metres)[458] of linen and had to sew the clothes themselves.[459] In other words, there does not seem to be any connection between Brady's account and the undisclosed legislation.

As in many other fields pertaining to the health of the enslaved workers, the lease regulations of 1834 also had an impact on the amount of cloth handed out on the royal plantations. The regulation prescribed that every enslaved person above the age of 15 was to receive annually six yards of Bamboo (5.5 metres) and 12 yards 'Brown' (11 metres), a brown linen cloth, plus one hat or one scarf.[460] The cloth was to be handed out in two half-yearly rations, and every third year

455 Higman, *Slave Populations*, 218–23; Leti, *Santé et société*, 241–43.
456 1 yard = 0,914 metre. Birkeland, *Mål & Vægt*.
457 Highfield, *Observations*, 17 (original: Brady, 1829).
458 Birkeland, *Mål & Vægt*.
459 Algreen-Ussing, *Kongelige Reskripter*. Rescript of 18 February 1843.
460 Tyson and Highfield, *The Kamina Folk*, 207 (note 4).

every enslaved person was to receive one blanket. Enslaved children under 15 years of age were to receive cloth in proportion to their age.[461] It is possible that the orders of the lease regulations were later extended to include enslaved workers on the private plantations. In any case, Victor Schoelcher reported from his visit in the 1840s that all enslaved workers in the Danish West Indies received 12 yards of Bamboo, 24 yards Brown and two hats annually.[462] The consistent doubling of the quantities mentioned above indicates that Schoelcher misunderstood the clause that the handout was to happen twice annually, yet only as half rations. If this assumption is correct, and if Schoelcher's statement in fact included all enslaved workers and not just those on the royal plantations, it means that the lease regulations had also increased the size of the allowance of the enslaved workers in relation to clothes.

Regarding footwear, it was not something that the enslaved workers on St Croix received or wore. This is slightly puzzling if one considers the many wounds on feet and legs that the enslaved received during their work, which caused many admissions to the plantation hospitals. These admissions might have been prevented if the enslaved had worn some kind of footwear. However, some enslaved workers did receive shoes or boots. For instance, the accounts of the private Upper Bethlehem plantation from 1829 shows the purchase of '4 pairs [of] shoes for [the] invalids' and in 1831 '1 pair [of] shoes for [the] Driver', plus '[a] pair [of] shoes for [a] sick Negro'.[463] Similar instances occurred on the royal plantations.[464] The footwear was given to two groups of enslaved: firstly, the sick and the invalid, who most likely had a special need to protect their feet. Secondly, the driver and the mason, who were the highest ranking enslaved workers.

The conditions in other West Indian colonies seem generally to have been very similar to those in St Croix. There, too, were several rules for the amount of cloth to be handed out, but the role of the authorities in relation to the clothing of the enslaved does not seem to have been either more or less prominent than in the Danish West Indies. Shoes were a rarity among the enslaved everywhere.

461 DNA, WILA, no. 2.38.2. Lease contract for Estate Boetzberg, 1834.

462 Tyson and Highfield, *The Kamina Folk*, 207.

463 DNA, WILA, no. 41.6.6. Upper Bethlehem, 1829.

464 NARA, RG55, Entry 1109, Box 2438, Mount Victory. Accounts, 2 March 1828: 'Paid for a pair of boots for Driver on Doctor's request'. Accounts, 25 March 1831: 'One pair of shoes for mason as ordered by Doctor'.

Conclusion

The initial examination of the Danish West Indian slave laws, or the lack of them, reveals some general structures in the relationship between the colonial administration, the planters, and the enslaved workers. Firstly, the administration's weakness in the face of the economic arguments of the planters is evident. Secondly, however, it is also evident that the administration continually tried to improve the conditions of the enslaved. Finally, it appears likely that the conditions of the enslaved did improve, at least after 1834, because the unissued code of 1755 was published in 1843 without protest.

A closer look at a number of circumstances influencing the health of the enslaved and at the efforts of the administration towards these circumstances reveals an ambiguous situation. Obviously, the administration did not control the weather, and accordingly the water supply of the enslaved workers was not something the administration tried to control. The situation was the same in the British and French West Indies. Regarding the houses, clothes, and footwear of the enslaved the initiatives of the Danish colonial administration do not stand out compared to the British or French, even though its efforts regarding slave houses may have been slightly greater. In terms of the last remaining factor, the workload, the situation was however quite different. This was the single most important adjustable factor in the economy of the planters as well as in the health of the enslaved workers. Here, the interventions of the Danish colonial administration were generally weaker than in both the British and French West Indies, which probably illustrates the immense importance of the work of the enslaved for the planters, for the sugar production, and for the colony's economy and very existence. It appears that the administration did not have the necessary strength to intervene in this field. On this basis, it may seem inconsistent that the administration intervened relatively more forcefully in a number of other fields (see Chapter 4), yet in my opinion this only illustrates the power relations that existed between the administration and the planters, and which health policy the administration was capable of implementing given this power relation.

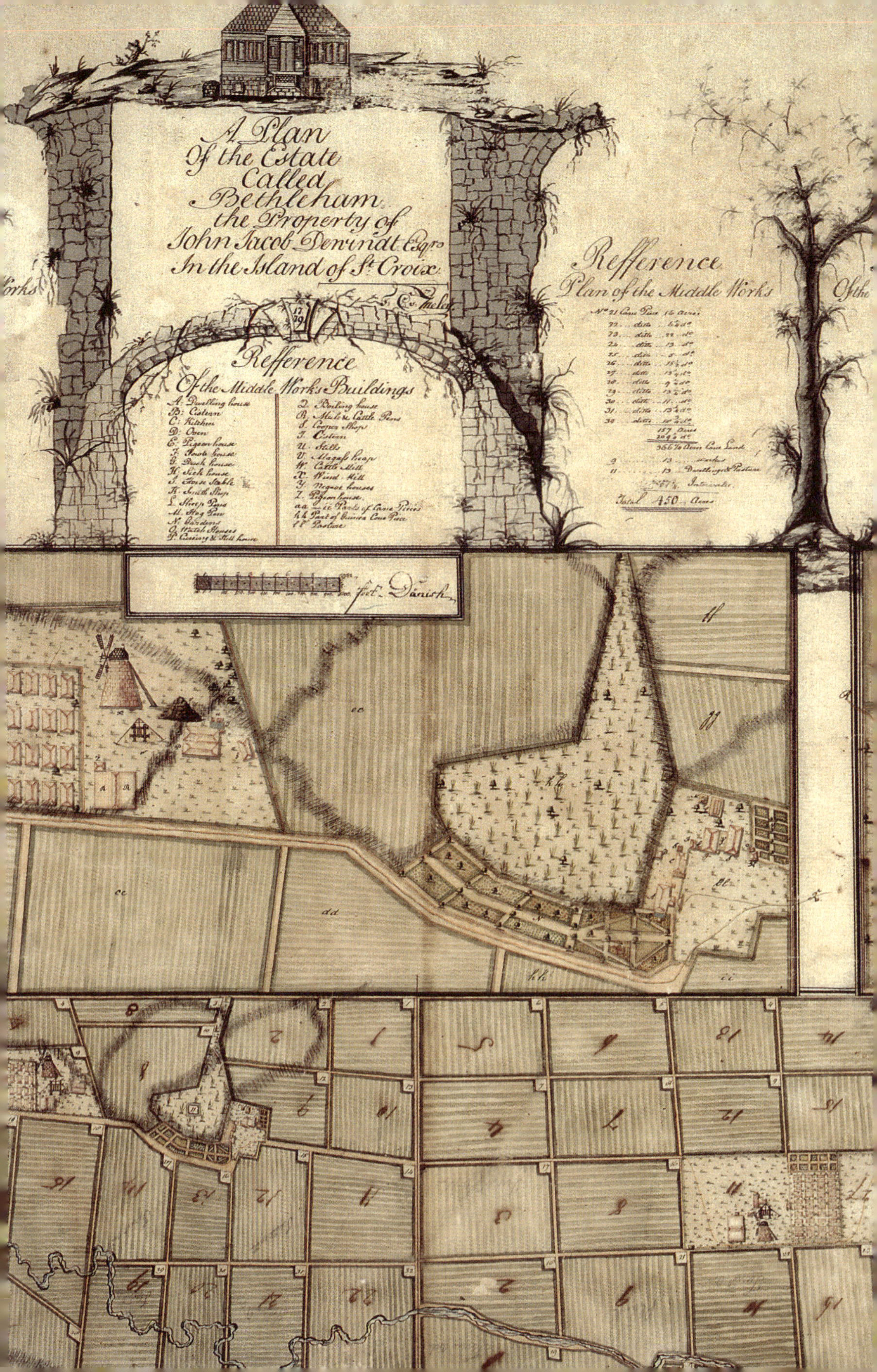
A Plan
Of the Estate
Called
Bethleham
the Property of
John Jacob Dewindt Esq.re
In the Island of St. Croix
C. v. Theler
1779
Refference
Of the Middle Work's Buildings
A: Dwelling house
B: Cistern
C: Kitchen
D: Oven
E: Pigeon house
F: Fowle House
G: Duck house
H: Sick house
I: Horse Stable
K: Smith Shop
L: Sheep Pens
M: Hog Pen
N: Gardens
O: Watch Houses
P: Curing & Still house
Q. Boiling house
R. Mule & Cattle Pens
S. Cooper Shops
T. Cistern
U. Stills
V. Magass heap
W. Cattle Mill
X. Wind Mill
Y. Negroe houses
Z. Pigeon house
aa ii Parts of Cane Pieces
hh Part of Guinea Cane Piece
ee Pasture
feet Danish
Refference
Plan of the Middle Works
No. 21 Cane Piece 16 Acres
Total 450 Acres

Chapter 4

Three Case Studies of the Health Policy of the Danish Colonial Administration

The previous chapters have dealt with the first level of this book investigating a range of contextual questions concerning the structure of health services in the Danish West Indies, morbidity and mortality among the enslaved workers, the factors causing disease and death etc. We now move to the second level to explore the two central questions of what health policy initiatives the Danish administration instigated to deal with the excess mortality in the enslaved population, and what these initiatives reveal about the power relations between the administration, the planters and the enslaved workers concerning the health of the enslaved. To answer the questions, I will present three case studies of the most important initiatives in the administration's health policy, namely nutrition, vaccination, and midwifery.

The Puzzle of Nutrition: Requirements, Rations, Crops and Natural Resources

Nutrition is one of the most important and broadest subjects related to the health of enslaved workers. In the following, I will investigate its multiple aspects with the aim to establish a more comprehensive picture of the nutritional state of the enslaved on St Croix and to analyse the role of the Danish colonial administration in relation to the food supply and nutrition of the enslaved. Furthermore, the conditions on St Croix will be compared to the conditions in the British and French West Indies.

In historical research, two different groups of investigations have previously dealt with the broad field of nutrition and food production among enslaved populations in the Caribbean. First, there is a rather large group of investigations concerning the individual food production of the enslaved.[465] This is a well-established field where the focus on work and land of anthropologist Sidney Mintz and the Marxist perception of history has been prevalent.[466] Second, there is a much smaller group of investigations focusing on the nutritional value of food and the health of the enslaved workers who consumed the food. This subject is much more debated and its best known and most controversial book is *The Caribbean Slave: A Biological History* by Kenneth Kiple (1984). Because Kiple's book has been the inspiration for this case study, and since the problems and limitations of his approach are important for the structure of the following, it is necessary to discuss his main arguments.

In his investigation, Kiple tries to establish a connection between malnutrition among the enslaved in the Caribbean and the fact that the enslaved rarely managed to sustain their numbers through reproduction. In general, he successfully demonstrates the importance of nutrition, but there are clear problems. The presentation of nutrition as the explanation for the decline in the enslaved population is unbalanced, because Kiple's conclusions do not take account of temporal changes in the diet and because his sources originate in only three very different geographical areas.[467] Furthermore, Kiple does not take account of contributing factors like workload, hygiene, living conditions, clothes, accidents, and punishments.[468] Neither does he deal with the differences in ration size between different groups of enslaved workers nor with the contribution of the surrounding environment to the diet.[469] Finally, Kiple seeks to argue from certain dietary problems to certain nutritional diseases, which is extremely difficult based on historical sources that are inaccurate with regard to quantities and symptoms.[470]

With this in mind, the following investigation is located within a narrow geographical and temporal frame. The analysis emphasises the differences between food resources available to different groups in the enslaved popula-

465 See for instance: Ira Berlin and Philip D. Morgan, *Cultivation and Culture: Labor and the Shaping of Slave Life in the Americas* (London: University Press of Virginia, 1993).

466 See for instance: Sidney W. Mintz and Douglas Hall, *The Origins of the Jamaican Internal Marketing System* (New Haven: Yale University Press, 1960).

467 K. David Patterson, 'The Caribbean Slave: A Biological History', *Isis* 77, no. 2 (1986), 365.

468 Richard Sheridan, 'The Caribbean Slave: A Biological History', *The Hispanic American Historical Review* 66, no. 3 (1986), 585.

469 Rebecca Huss-Ashmore, 'The Caribbean Slave: A Biological History', *The American Anthropologist* 88 (1986), 998; E.L. Jones, 'The Caribbean Slave: A Biological History', *The Economic History Review* 39, no. 2 (1986), 324.

470 Lydia A. D'Alois, 'A Response to "Slave Mortality",' *Journal of Social History* 11, no. 2 (1977), 292–94.

tion and especially the importance of the environment for both the cultivated and collected parts of the diet.[471] Most investigations of the food resources of the enslaved neglect the latter aspect, perhaps because it is very geographically specific. However, this is exactly why it is important to attempt to include it.[472] In recognition of the great uncertainties related to the detailed analysis of the nutrients in food described in historical records, the following analysis will focus on the macronutrients, i.e. carbohydrate, protein and fat, especially the first two. Micronutrients like vitamins and minerals will also be dealt with but not in detail. The above-mentioned contributing factors neglected by Kiple are not included in this case study, but they are dealt with elsewhere in the book.

The Supply System: Imported Foods and Local Food Production

The task of establishing a clear picture of how, what and how much food the enslaved workers on Cruzian plantations received at various times in the period 1803–48 involves great difficulties. Obviously, food for the enslaved workers was a central resource for all West Indian plantations and planters. This was partly because food was often imported and therefore expensive and partly because the work performed by the enslaved depended to a large degree on the amount of food they received. From the planters' point of view the enslaved had to be fed exactly enough food to do their job but to give them more would be unprofitable. Consequently, the planters tried to adjust the supply of food precisely to the immediate and local conditions in terms of economy, ecology, and social relations.

Generally, there were three ways of dealing with food supplies in the West Indies. First, to import all supplies and distribute them to the enslaved in weekly rations. After the British abolition of the slave trade and the outbreak of the Napoleonic War in 1807, planters rarely used this system on its own, because it was vulnerable to changes and interruptions of trade, which might lead to famine. The second method meant the production of provisions on the plantations in the same way as the main crop, i.e. with enslaved workers working in gangs. The planter distributed these provision crops to the enslaved as weekly rations. The third method was to assign a plot of land and a certain amount of free time to each enslaved worker and so give them the possibility of producing their own

471 This is an approach that can also be found in Higman, *Slave Populations*, 205.
472 Tyson Gibbs, Kathleen Cargill, Leslie Sue Lieberman, and Elizabeth Reitz, 'Nutrition in a Slave Population: An Anthropological Examination', *Medical Anthropology* 4 (1980), 175–76.

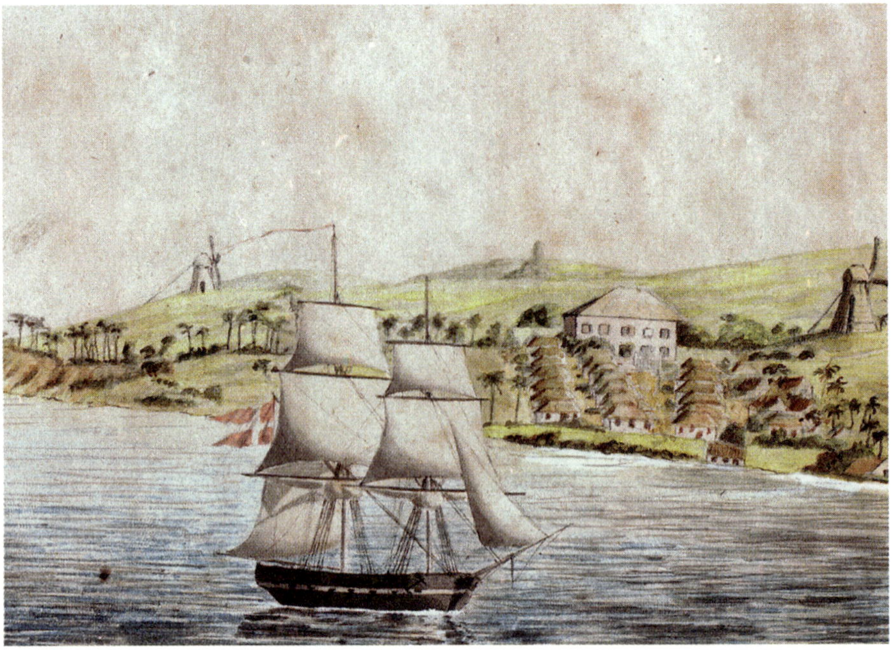

Fig. 4.1: View of the private plantation Sprat Hall on the western end of St Croix (North Side A Quarter) around 1840. Notice the houses of the enslaved workers arranged in rows below the great house. Usually the enslaved had small gardens between their houses as well as larger garden plots located elsewhere on the estate. Coloured drawing attributed to Frederik von Scholten, Danish Maritime Museum, Elsinore, Denmark.

provisions. Under the last two methods, the remaining part of the provisions, i.e. meat and/or fish, were imported and handed out by the planter.[473]

Because the food supply was always closely adjusted to the local economic, ecologic, and social conditions, the three supply systems are rarely seen in their pure forms. Accordingly, the food supply system on St Croix in the period in question seems to have been a combination of all three systems. The planter handed out the largest part of the food as rations consisting of imported foods and/or of foodstuffs produced as part of the plantation's crop. The enslaved produced the remaining part of the food individually in their provision grounds.

473 Higman, *Slave Populations*, 204.

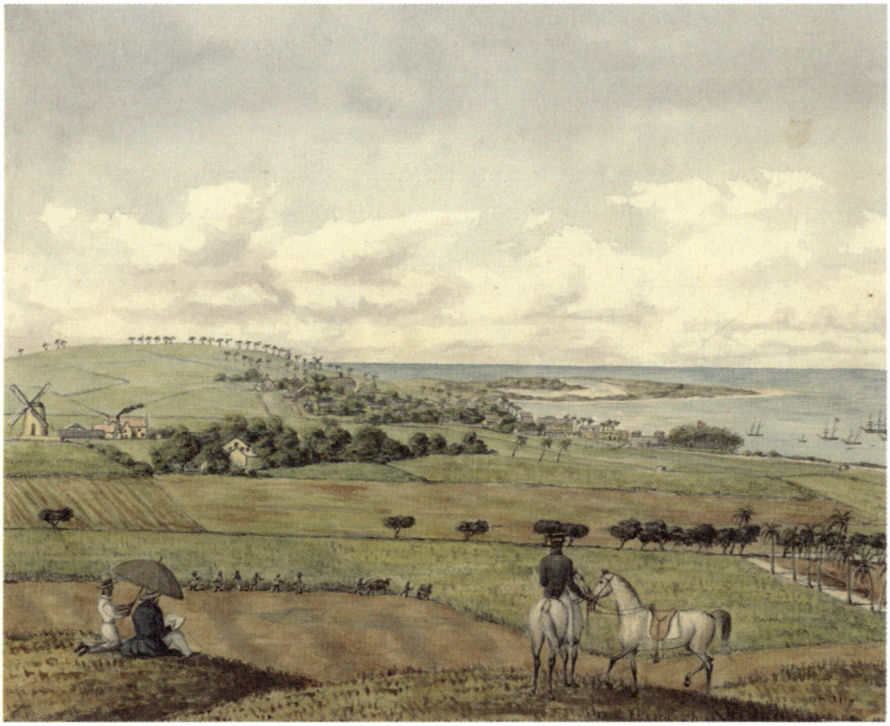

Fig. 4.2: View of the town of Frederiksted and the private plantation La Grange on the western end of St Croix. Notice the enslaved workers harvesting sugar cane in the lower left side of the picture. Coloured drawing by Frederik von Scholten, March 1837. Danish Maritime Museum, Elsinore, Denmark.

Finally, the enslaved also obtained foodstuffs from the natural world surrounding the plantations: the sea, the mangroves, and the bush.

Food Rations: Practices, Standards, and Legislation

As previously mentioned, the Danish West Indian legislation governing the conditions of the enslaved workers was incoherent at best. As regards food rations and the size of them, there existed no legislation at the beginning of the period in question, apart from the unpublished slave law of 1755. However, sources from around 1800 indicate the existence of a customary 'standard ration'. In 1798, inspector de Vanderbourgh of the Schimmelmann plantations wrote in his above-mentioned report that during harvest time, i.e. four months of the year, 25 pounds of yams were issued per week to each enslaved worker, which amounted to food for five days. The rest of the year only five pounds of corn meal were issued per enslaved worker per week, which would only feed the individual for two and a half days. The distribution of salt fish or meat, the other staple in the rations of the enslaved workers, is not mentioned. Vanderbourgh added that the enslaved were themselves responsible for obtaining the rest of their food from small plots of land given to them by the planter, from raising pigs, goats, or chicken or from trading forage grass, firewood, or other items in the towns. However, the inspector also emphasised that the 'standard ration', i.e. the 5 pounds of corn meal, was too small, especially during the 'hungry season' when the enslaved workers' possibilities of obtaining other foods were few, even in good years. Accordingly, Vanderbourgh advised Count Schimmelmann to follow other, to use his term, 'humane' planters on the island and increase the ration by 50 per cent, i.e. to 7.5 pounds of corn meal per enslaved per week. To go further than that and hand out a double ration, i.e. 10 pounds of corn meal, would furnish the enslaved workers with all the food they needed. Yet, that was not an expedient approach, Vanderbourgh explained, partly because it would deprive the enslaved of the incentive for private industry (gardening, rearing of livestock etc.) and partly because it would create discontent among other planters, who handed out smaller rations to their enslaved workers.[474]

It is not known if the ration on the Schimmelmann plantations was in fact increased to 7.5 pounds (3.75 kg)[475] of corn meal per week, but it seems likely that in the years around 1800 there existed a lower 'standard ration' on St Croix of 5 pounds (around 2.5 kg) of corn meal per adult enslaved worker per week outside harvest time. During harvest, experience had shown that the size of the issued ration was less important, because the supply of foodstuffs in nature was more abundant both in terms of the enslaved workers' own crops and in terms of sugar cane and sugar juice, which the enslaved were allowed to consume. As is evident, the Cruzian standard ration was not a legally sanctioned quantum but a local practice, which may have been influenced by practices in the neighbouring British islands. So, in the British Leeward Islands[476] the statutory weekly ration for adult enslaved workers was in 1798 8 pints (ca. 2.5 kg)[477] of corn meal and 1.25 pounds of salted fish.[478] The same ration size of corn meal appears to

474 Tyson and Highfield, *The Kamina Folk*, 153–57.

475 1 Danish pound weighed (pre-1839) 0.50045 kg. 7.5 × 0.50045 = 3.75 kg.

476 The islands of St Kitts, Nevis and Antigua.

477 1 British pint = 0.568 litre. 8 × 0.568 = 4.544 litres. 1 litre corn meal = 550 g. 4.544 litres × 550 g = 2.4992 kg corn meal.

478 Sheridan, *Doctors and Slaves*, 170.

have been common on Barbados until the 1820s.[479] Finally, this collective evidence for a 'standard ration' of about 2.5 kg of corn meal per week casts doubts on a famous Danish account of the size of rations on St Croix, namely headmaster Hans West's *Description of St Croix* from 1793. Here, the anti-abolitionist West claimed that each enslaved worker received ten to twelve pots of corn meal twice a week plus an unspecified amount of salt meat or fish.[480] As this would amount to a total of more than 10.5 kg corn meal per adult enslaved worker per week, which is about twice as much as the double ration mentioned by Vanderbourgh, West's claims are not plausible.[481]

The function of the standard ration as an actual norm in the plantation society of St Croix is supported by the fact that the size could indeed be exceeded, yet only to a certain degree unless unrest were to develop among the enslaved workers on other plantations and cause discontent among the planters. It is not possible to discern whether some planters issued smaller rations than the standard, but it is highly likely. Still, there is no doubt that rations much smaller than the standard would also inevitably generate a fermenting discontent among the enslaved workers, which again *could* set off a rebellion. Accordingly, because of considerations of security, rationing below the standard must have been frowned upon among the planters, unless it was offset by, for instance, larger provision grounds for the enslaved workers. Having said that, it was of course an advantage for the planters that the standard ration was only a custom and not fixed by law, because this gave them a wider scope for action and prevented the colonial administration from intervening on behalf of the enslaved workers – except in the very gravest of cases.[482]

Governor General Bentzon's Minimum Ration, 1817

In the years after the second British occupation, the standard ration for the enslaved workers changed again, but this time due to the active intervention of the Danish colonial administration. On 13 June 1817, Governor General

479 Higman, *Slave Populations*, 207.

480 1 pot = 0.9661 litre. 0.9661 litre × 20 = 19.322 litres. 1 litre corn meal = 550 grams. According to Vanderbourg, 1 gallon of corn meal weighed about 5 pounds. Because 1 British gallon contained 4.546 litres and 1 Danish pound (pre-1839) weighed 0.50045 kg, 5 pounds of corn meal equalled 2.50225 kg. 2.50225 kg / 4.546 litres = 0.550 kg corn meal per litre. Accordingly, in the late years of the 1790s 1 litre of corn meal weighed ca. 550 g. 19.322 litres × 550 g = 10.63 kg corn meal per enslaved worker per week.

481 West, *Beskrivelse over St Croix*, 72–73.

482 In several instances planters withheld rations to punish the enslaved. See for instance: DNA, WILA, no. 2.16.5, case no. 168, 11 December 1807. DNA, WILA, no. 2.16.7, case no. 393, 2 November 1816.

Adrian Benjamin Benoni Bentzon (1777–1827)[483] issued a public proclamation condemning planters who instead of handing out provisions gave their enslaved workers Saturday off to work in their provision grounds. The reason for this behaviour among the planters was allegedly the current drought, which had destroyed the provision crops for the enslaved. The Governor General regarded the planters' behaviour as extremely illegal and irresponsible, both towards the enslaved workers, who according to him should be treated as fellow human beings, and towards the security and property of other planters. The security problem probably stemmed from the danger of a rebellion among the enslaved workers. To Bentzon not even a bad economy sufficed as an excuse 'because he who cannot feed his Negroes must not posses any plantation'.[484] Finally, the Governor General stipulated that 6 quarts (around 3.75 kg)[485] of corn meal, or the equivalent in other vegetable provisions, was the minimum ration per adult enslaved worker per week. Unfortunately, he did not mention the size of rations in salt fish or meat. The Danish anthropologist Karen Fog Olwig has claimed that Bentzon's proclamation only published the rules regarding food rations from the shelved slave law of 1755, but this is not correct.[486] The 1755 law stipulated that any enslaved worker above 10 years of age was to receive a weekly ration of 2.5 pots of cassava or corn meal (around 1.3 kg)[487] or the equivalent in other vegetables, and 2 pounds of salted beef or 3 pounds of salted fish.[488] Hence, a much smaller quantity of vegetable food than the roughly 3.75 kg stipulated by Bentzon, but with the addition of some animal foods.

The idea of ensuring a minimum allowance for the enslaved workers was not new to Bentzon,[489] but from where did he get the inspiration for a minimum ration of this particular size? A legally sanctioned ration of exactly this size does not appear to have existed anywhere else in the West Indies. However, we find a better basis for comparison in the customary ration sizes of the time. According to inspector Vanderbourg a customary ration of exactly the same size (7.5

483 Bricka, *Dansk biografisk Lexikon* II, 66.

484 DNA, WILA, no. 2.1.5. Original Danish text: '... thi den som ei kan føde sine Negere maa ingen Plantage besidde...'.

485 Probably British quarts, 1 quart = 1.136 litres (US quarts for dried goods = 1.1012 litre). 6 × 1.136 = 6.816 litres. Corn meal weighed ca. 550 g per litre. 6.816 litres × 0.550 kg = 3.75 kg corn meal per week.

486 Olwig, *Cultural Adaptation and Resistance*, 30.

487 1 pot = 0.9661 litres. 0.9661 × 2.5 = 2.41525 litres. Unless otherwise indicated, all of the following measures are taken from Birkeland, *Mål & Vægt*, 25, 29, 38–39, 79.

488 Algreen-Ussing, *Kongelige Reskripter*. Rescript of 18 February 1843.

489 Susanne Ahlmann Svensson and Signe Thylstrup, *Slaveriet i Dansk Vestindien – Ideal eller virkelighed? Den komplekse legitimering af slaveriet i Dansk Vestindien* (unpublished MA thesis, Department of History and Society, Roskilde University, 1997), 83–84.

pound or 3.75 kg) had existed on St Croix since the beginning of the century. It is possible that this 'humane' ration size had been used on St Croix since the days of Vanderbourg and that it was now just elevated to law by Bentzon's proclamation. Another possible source of inspiration – mentioned in the book *Practical Rules for the Management and Medical Treatment of Negro Slaves in the Sugar Colonies* (1811), written by the British doctor and planter David Collins of St Vincent – was a ration size used in the British West Indies, that was regarded as more humane and rational, even if it was not sanctioned by law.[490] Collins described two different rationing systems, which were both supplemented by the enslaved workers' own production on their provision grounds. The first system was an existing, yet outdated system with rations of six to 7 pints of corn meal and the same number of salted herring per enslaved worker per week. In the second system rations amounted to 10–12 pints of corn meal per enslaved worker per week.[491] Seven pints of corn meal equals around 2.2 kg, which is a little less than the old 5 pound standard ration on St Croix, whereas 12 pints is the equivalent of 6 quarts and so exactly the same as the 'humane' ration of 3.75 kg of corn meal. Accordingly, it would appear that the minimum ration stipulated by Governor General Bentzon was not only regarded as humane and progressive in the West Indies at the time, but it also seems to have existed for some time among 'humane' planters on St Croix.

The proclamation of 1817 seems to have had an impact on the colonial administration's ability to intervene against the planters in cases where the enslaved workers complained of undersized rations. If we look at the period 1800–17, which is difficult, however, because of poor recordkeeping during the British occupations, there occur very few cases about the size of rations and they do not seem to have had any consequences for the planters involved.[492] After the proclamation of 1817, the news of which apparently spread quickly among the enslaved workers, the situation looks very different. In the months following the proclamation, several complaints came in from enslaved plantation workers concerning ration sizes. It turned out that the complaints were justified and the planters were severely reprimanded or fined for not following the proclamation.[493]

490 Sheridan, *Doctors and Slaves*, 32.

491 Collins, *Practical Rules*, 75, 80.

492 For instance: DNA, WILA, no. 38.9.11, case no. 1802–06. 5 March 1802. DNA, WILA, no. 2.16.5, vol. 155, case no. 66, 3 August, 1807.

493 DNA, WILA, no. 2.16.8. Case no. 1151, 1340, 1351.

When assessing the vigour of the colonial administration in utilising the new rules it is, however, important to be aware of the context. The proclamation of 1817 was occasioned by an emergency, i.e. the drought that had apparently damaged the provision crops. Accordingly, it became necessary for the planters to buy and distribute expensive imported foodstuffs to the enslaved workers, and the less food they handed out to the enslaved, the more money they saved. It was in this situation the Governor General felt compelled to act, even though there were probably also purely ethical considerations of human dignity behind his actions. However, the problem of supplying the enslaved workers with the necessary food was far from new and it did not disappear with the proclamation of 1817.

The Years 1817–48

In the years from 1817 to 1848, the legally sanctioned ration of 6 quarts of corn meal seems to have been observed on St Croix. Around 1828, the previously mentioned Lieutenant Brady wrote in his detailed account of the conditions of the enslaved workers on the island that the planters were at liberty to either hand out provisions to the enslaved or to assign them an extra piece of land and an extra day off to work it, besides Sunday. Nonetheless, Brady explained, the latter method was rarely used and the statutory weekly ration for adult enslaved workers was 6 quarts of corn meal or 24 pounds of yams or other root crops plus six salted herring or other salt fish. To the last item, Brady added that in practice, the number of fish handed out was higher, but as the universal principle behind the volume of provisions in all of the West Indies was that the enslaved should provide for their own food on the seventh day of the week, the number of herring was customarily 6 per week.[494] Besides these regular rations, Brady also listed a special Christmas ration and extra rations during the holing in the autumn. The latter consisted of one hardtack and a dram of rum when work began in the morning, 2 pints of sugar water in the morning and one hardtack and a grog in the afternoon. In case of rain, the enslaved would receive another dram of rum. Later we shall see that these extra rations were in fact a significant contribution to the diet of the enslaved. Finally, Brady observed that the general conditions of the enslaved, and so also their food supply, were heavily dependent on the economic situation of the planter.[495] Brady's account seems to show

494 Highfield, *Observations*, xxi–xxiii, 12–13 (original: Brady, 1829).
495 Highfield, *Observations*, 6, 13 (original: Brady, 1829).

that the proclamation of 1817 was in fact followed in the later years of the period. However, the alleged freedom of the planters to let the enslaved produce all the food for their own consumption does not seem to agree with the proclamation of 1817. Another very useful piece of information is the indication of the size of the ration of salted fish, the other important article in the rations of the enslaved workers.

We can only assume that the conditions Brady describes pertain primarily to the prosperous plantation he himself lived on (Mannings Bay) and so his descriptions are not necessarily representative of all the plantations on St Croix. However, a number of later accounts by visitors to the island during the 1830s and 1840s (Hovey, Tuckerman, Schoelcher, Weed) also describe the rations issued to enslaved workers on Cruzian plantations. They all agree on 6 quarts of corn meal as a fixed unit, yet are less clear regarding the volume of other rations.[496] On this basis, it appears that the legally sanctioned amount of corn meal was in fact followed, while the equally common but unfixed ration of salted fish varied in size.

The above illustrates what were the general standards and customs on privately owned plantations on St Croix. However, the royal plantations had a firmer set of rules. The previously mentioned lease regulations of 1834 prescribed, in accordance with the proclamation of 1817, that all enslaved workers above 15 years of age were to receive a weekly allowance of 6 quarts of corn meal plus 'the agreed quantity of herring'.[497] According to the regulations, younger enslaved workers were to receive proportionally smaller rations according to their age, but it appears from reports from some royal plantations that this age group occasionally received larger rations than prescribed.[498] Similarly, other special groups in the enslaved population seem to have received a larger allowance then was formally due to them. This was for instance the case with the driver (the gang boss), the carpenter, the sick-nurse, and those who herded the cattle.[499] The reason for the larger ration for the driver was probably his responsibility as the leader of fieldwork, while the other groups received larger rations because they did not have Sunday off. Finally, the lease regulations in their original form did not prescribe the handing out of hardtack, rum, and sugar water

496 Tyson and Highfield, *The Kamina Folk*, 185–86, 201, 207, 211; Tuckerman, *Letter Respecting Santa Cruz*, 4, 24.

497 DNA, WILA, no. 46.20. Original Danish text: '...det vedtagne Kvantum Sild...'

498 DNA, WILA, no. 46.17.54. Report, 1834.

499 DNA, WILA, no. 46.17.43. Pro Memoria, 1830. NARA, RG 55, Entry 82, Box 342. Some plantation inventories. Dr Johnson and S. Abott's status.

during holing. Yet, from the regulations and records of some plantations, it is clear that hardtack was handed out.[500]

In addition to the above, both the private and royal enslaved workers had time-honoured rights of another kind of seasonal ration during the sugar harvest. They were allowed to eat the ripe sugar cane and to drink as much as they liked of the fresh sugar juice from the mill or the cooked juice from the boiling house. The enslaved workers seem to have been very fond of this food and allegedly they lived almost entirely from it during harvest, which gave them the opportunity to save and sell their weekly rations.[501] At the time sugar juice was universally regarded as very nutritious and healthy, which is not altogether wrong, since the raw sugar juice contains not only large amounts of carbohydrates but also far more minerals than refined sugar.[502]

We can conclude that in the period 1803–17 there seems to have existed an unsanctioned weekly standard ration for adult enslaved workers of about 5 pounds (around 2.5 kg) of corn meal or equivalent vegetable foods. With Governor General Bentzon's proclamation of 1817 this standard was increased to 6 quarts (around 3.75 kg) of corn meal and legally sanctioned, a standard that was maintained until 1848. However, the ration of protein in the form of salted fish (or meat) was never legally sanctioned and consequently it varied throughout the period. The most common size of this ration seems to have been six herring per week, yet the following investigations will show that larger rations were by no means unusual. In other words, from 1817 to 1848 the Danish colonial administration utilised legislation and the courts to maintain a minimum standard for the amount of food the enslaved workers were entitled to receive on both private and royal plantations. There are several reasons for the administration behaving this way. At the time, there was a general wish for a more humane treatment of the enslaved workers, yet it was just as important to avoid rebellion among the enslaved and the economic disaster that would follow. Furthermore, it is clear that through the legislation concerning the allowance of the enslaved the colonial administration assumed a power over the enslaved workers that had previously belonged to the planters.

Government Protection of Food Imports

As previously mentioned, the food supply for the enslaved workers on St Croix

500 DNA, WILA, no. 46.20.
501 North Star, 1843 (DNA, WILA, no. 46.17.54). Hermon Hill, 1842 (DNA, WILA, no. 46.17.33).
502 Highfield, *Observations*, 15 (original: Brady, 1829). Smith, *Winter of 1840 in St Croix*, 109.

was vulnerable. Consequently, the local colonial administration felt compelled to intervene to safeguard the health of the enslaved, and by extension the enslaved worker's ability to work, and the economy of the island. There were several reasons for the vulnerability of the food supply. Firstly, the largest part of the foodstuffs was imported. This made the food supply sensitive to the consequences of the international wars that raged in the Caribbean during the first two decades of the nineteenth century and to problems in the economic system, which could also block the shipments. Secondly, the local food production was always vulnerable to drought, one of the main ecological problems on St Croix. Regardless of the cause, breakdown in the food supply could cause an imminent famine among the enslaved workers, which in turn could incite a rebellion.

The problem of the dependence on imported foodstuffs occurred for the first time in the period in question in 1807, just prior to the second British occupation. At this time, Denmark and its colonies were no longer neutral as they had been during the international wars of the eighteenth century,[503] during which time the supply problem does not seem to have been as disastrous as in other colonies.[504] During the second British occupation of the islands, the problem continued and in 1813 it became so grave that the British Governor, Major General George William Ramsay (1770–1838), established a commission of local planters to be in charge of the purchase of the necessary provisions for the entire island of St Croix.[505] Each planter reported to the commission what provisions he needed and how much.[506] Furthermore, the British Governor issued a *plakat* ordering every planter to plant an extra 1.5 acres of land in provision crops for each ten enslaved workers he owned, in addition to the provision grounds of the enslaved.[507] However, the crisis seems to have continued in 1814 with scarcity of provisions and famine on some plantations.[508]

When the Danish administration returned to the islands in 1816, the *plakat*

503 Ole Feldbæk, 'Den lange fred, 1700-1800', in *Gyldendal og Politikens Danmarkshistorie* IX, ed. Olaf Olsen (Copenhagen: Gyldendals Boghandel, Nordisk Forlag and Politikens Forlag, 1990), 301–2, 344–50.

504 Vibæk, 'Dansk Vestindien, 1755–1848', 77–78, 139–40; Sheridan, *Doctors and Slaves*, 154–62.

505 DNA, WILA, no. 45.1.3.

506 NARA, RG 55, Entry 56 (box 122).

507 DNA, WILA, no. 2.1.5. Plakat of 16 October 1813.

508 DNA, WILA, no. 3.56.7. 6 January and 2 February 1814. Ben Kessler, *Priceless Heritage: History and Lore of Estate St George, Home of the St George Village Botanical Garden of St Croix, U.S. Virgin Islands* (Frederiksted, 1980), 35.

of 1813 was abolished.[509] This turned out to be unfortunate, because the problem of maintaining an adequate food supply returned in 1817, though this time not because of blocked supply lines, but because of drought. As mentioned above, Governor General Bentzon reacted by issuing his proclamation of 1817.[510] However, a few years later, in 1822/3, the problem reappeared, but this time for a very different reason. At this time, the planters of St Croix were financially distressed because of the postwar business conditions with falling prices on sugar combined with heavy mortgage debts. The planters were practically incapable of paying for the shipments of foodstuffs. Accordingly, the North American merchants and captains who supplied St Croix with most of its food, including the vital slave provisions, refused to extend their credit. This made the danger of famine and an ensuing rebellion imminent and in December 1822 the Danish West Indian government was forced to issue a state guarantee to the merchants for the planters' outstanding debts.[511] By order of 9 March 1823, the Danish West Indian government followed the example of General Ramsay and established a special commission consisting of officials and representatives of the planters to carry out the purchase of provisions for the Cruzian planters with state funds.[512] To supervise this public credit facility the government established a special office, which was effective until 1898.[513] In relation to these government interventions to secure the food supply, Governor General Johan Frederik von Bardenfleth (1772–1833) restored the English legislation ordering the planters to grow extra provisions on the plantations.[514]

In the years 1823–48, the food supply does not appear to have caused problems, despite the fact that drought was a recurring problem and the economic situation continued to be poor. A contributing factor must have been the colonial administration's tight control of the food supply via the credit commission.

We can conclude that after 1817, the Danish colonial administration used legislation and intervention against violations of the same to ensure that the enslaved workers on St Croix received a standardised minimum amount of food. Likewise, the administration followed the example of the previous British occupying power in ensuring that the supply of food remained stable, which

509 DNA, WILA, no. 2.1.5. Plakat of 4 January 1816.
510 DNA, WILA, no. 2.2.2. Case no. 659.
511 Vibæk, 'Dansk Vestindien, 1755–1848', 312–18.
512 DNA, WILA, no. 2.1.5.
513 Vibæk, 'Dansk Vestindien, 1755–1848', 318. DNA, WILA, no. 58.1–8.
514 DNA, WILA, no. 2.1.5.

was of the utmost importance in these years of economic decline. Accordingly, the administration encroached on the planters' rights over their enslaved workers to an extent not seen before. The reason for this approach was undoubtedly a wish for a more humane treatment of the enslaved workers; however, it was just as important to avoid rebellion among the enslaved and the economic disaster that would follow. The instability of the food supply in the period enhanced the need for government intervention, not least because the state owned several plantations, which were among the most vulnerable in terms of food supplies. Consequently, the colonial administration had to maintain a delicate balance between humane, economic and safety-related priorities considering the ongoing negotiation of power over the food resources between the administration, the enslaved workers and the planters.

Actual Ration Sizes, Nutritional Content and Dietary Needs

Having established which laws and practices existed on St Croix in the period 1803–48 concerning the size of the allowance of the enslaved workers, it is interesting to examine two questions. First, whether rations issued on the plantations actually followed the legislation and, second, if the estimated nutritional content of the rations would meet the estimated dietary needs of hardworking enslaved workers. I shall try to answer these questions through an analysis of three selected plantations on St Croix: the royal North Star plantation (Northside B Quarter) and the private plantations of Upper Bethlehem and Fredensborg (King's Quarter). It is important to be aware of the geographical position of the plantations as they are all located around the centre of the island. This is an area with fertile soil and good access to fresh water, which gives reason to assume that the life of the enslaved on these plantations may have been relatively better than on plantations with inferior soils.

It is equally important to be aware that the following calculations are subject to a number of uncertainties. This is because the historical measures of volume used in the source material are often difficult to convert into current measures. Similarly, it has been necessary to estimate the nutritional value of historical foodstuffs. Finally, it has been necessary to estimate how much energy a grown enslaved worker needed on average to carry out his or her work and other obligations. Every single one of these estimates is debatable but I believe them to be sufficiently reliable at the general level to which interpretations like these based on samples from single plantations will always belong. Accordingly, it is not the aim of this investigation to make a thorough examination of all the nutrients in the diet of the enslaved because the basic estimates do not allow for such a detailed analysis. Instead, the aim is to reveal the general macronutritional problems, i.e. problems with carbohydrate, protein, and fat, inherent in the diet of the enslaved workers on the plantations of St Croix. Micronutrients like vitamins and minerals will only be touched upon.

Estate North Star (1832–33)

The records of the royal plantations are generally very detailed and the records of North Star exceptionally so. This has allowed a summation of all the provisions handed out each week to the enslaved workers on the plantation during the years 1832 and 1833. As can be seen in Table 4.1, corn meal and salted herring were the two recurrent and most important foodstuffs in the ration of the enslaved. However, during 1832 substantial quantities of peas and barley flour partly replaced both of these items. This temporary change had a very beneficial influence on the amount of energy (mostly from carbohydrate) and protein in the ration. According to the above discussion of laws and practices, it was not unusual to replace corn meal with other imported or locally grown stables and this of course makes it difficult to generalise about the nutritional content in the food issued to the enslaved workers.[515] Besides the mentioned foodstuffs, the seventy-four enslaved workers on North Star also received extra rations during holing. The energy in this supplement was substantial if measured on the total amount of energy in the ration.

The amount of energy in the ration per enslaved worker per day shows a marked difference between the years 1832 (10.46 megajoule) and 1833 (8.91 megajoule). This was not only due to the use of peas and barley flour instead of corn meal but also due to other variations in the amounts of food issued. Again, this is a warning that the variations make it difficult to say anything precise about the nutrition of the enslaved even if investigated at plantation level. Of course, the variations were even greater between plantations and especially between colonies.

A comparison of the standard ration of corn meal stipulated by the colonial administration in 1817 and 1834 with the actual rations handed out on North Star in 1832/3 shows that the ration of corn meal issued was too small. In 1832, this was not a problem because other staples were issued instead which made up for the deficit, yet in 1833 the corn meal was not supplemented by anything but

515 NARA, RG 55, Entry 1109, Box 2435, letter concerning Estate Belvedere, 1822.

herring and extra rations during holing. Accordingly, the amount of corn meal issued in 1833 was about 8 per cent smaller than stipulated.[516] This of course had an impact on the amount of energy per enslaved worker per day. The reason for this variation in ration size, even on the fairly regular and controlled royal plantations, is unknown.

In addition, the ration of herring also differed from the expected. Judging by the above-mentioned norm of six herring per enslaved worker per week the ration of herring handed out on North Star was 67 per cent larger in 1832 and 90 per cent larger in 1833.[517] This equals about ten herring a week in 1832[518] and about eleven herring a week in 1833.[519] This larger ration size is interesting because it is supported by the contemporaries Lieutenant Brady in the 1820s and Joseph Tuckerman in 1836/37.[520] On this basis, we may hypothesise that the 'agreed quantity of herring' referred to in the lease regulations were in fact not a ration of six herring per week but of ten to twelve herring per week.

Nevertheless, the most important question in relation to the rations is whether they were sufficient to meet the energy requirement of the hardworking enslaved plantation workers. Based on current estimates from United Nation's Food and Agriculture Organisation (FAO), World Health Organisation (WHO) and United Nations University (UNU), I have made the following estimate of the daily total energy expenditure of the enslaved fieldworkers:

Table 4.2: Estimated daily total energy expenditure of enslaved fieldworkers[521]

Age	Men (ca. 1.64 m, BMI 18.5, ca. 50 kg):	Women (ca. 1.56 m, BMI 18.5, ca. 45 kg):
18–30 years	13.3 MJ/day	10.6 MJ/day
30–60 years	13.3 MJ/day	11.1 MJ/day

Total Energy Expenditure at PAL 2.20, i.e. high level of physical activity.

516 12,445.24 kg/year / (13,515.67 kg/year / 100) = 92.08 %.

517 1,811.35 kg/year / (1,080.14 kg/year / 100) = 167.70 %. 2,053.68 kg/year / (1,080.14 kg/year / 100) = 190.13 %.

518 (36,227 herring/year/52 weeks) / 69.24 enslaved = 10.06 herring per enslaved per week.

519 41,073.5 herring/year/52 weeks) / 69.24 enslaved = 11.41 herring per enslaved per week. The weight of one herring is estimated at around 50 g. 6 herring × 50 g/herring = 300 g.

520 Tuckerman, *Letter Respecting Santa Cruz*, 4, 24.

521 *Human energy requirements* (Rome: FAO, 2004), Chapter 5: 'Energy requirements of adults'. The figures are taken from Table 5.4, 5.5, 5.7 and 5.8. www.fao.org/docrep/007/y5686e/y5686e00.htm#Contents (accessed 30-05-2011).

The estimate is based on several assumptions: First, Barry W. Higman's calculations of the height of enslaved adult male and female individuals in the British Virgin Islands in the years 1819–25, which is the closest we can get geographically and temporally to the height of the enslaved in the Danish West Indies.[522] Second, I have assumed that the Body Mass Index (BMI) of the enslaved, which indicates the relationship between height and weight, was generally very low because they probably had problems getting sufficient nutrition to make up for their high energy expenditure. Today a BMI value of 18.5 and below is considered low. It is possible that the BMI of the enslaved was even lower, yet there are no archival or other sources to confirm such a hypothesis. Third, I have assumed the daily workload of the enslaved to be equivalent to the high level of physical activity experienced among agricultural workers in present-day developing countries. The Physical Activity Level (PAL) is indicated by a value of 2.20, which is possibly a low estimate, but a PAL value of more than 2.40 is known to be difficult to sustain for a longer period. The stated total energy expenditure and energy requirement for enslaved men of 13.3 MJ/day is an average of all days throughout the year. During harvest and holing the activity levels were higher than average. Recent research has shown that energy expenditure among South African and Colombian agricultural workers harvesting sugar cane can be as high as 14 MJ/day.[523] Overall, my assumptions add up to a conservative estimate of the total energy expenditure and energy requirements of an adult enslaved individual working in the cane fields.[524] It is important to note that the energy requirement of enslaved women was higher than it appears in Table 4.2. Pregnant women have an additional energy requirement of 1.18 MJ/day on average (first trimester 0.35 MJ/day, second trimester 1.2 MJ/day and third trimester 2.0 MJ/day),[525] whereas lactating malnourished women require an extra ca. 2.8 MJ/day (well nourished women only about 2.1 MJ/day).[526] Regardless of whether the women were malnourished or not, it is highly likely that they were pregnant or lactating during large parts of their adult lives in the same way as many

522 Higman, *Slave Populations*, 283, Table 8.2.

523 M.I. Lambert, E.J. Cheevers and Y. Coopoo, 'Relationship between Energy Expenditure and Productivity of Sugar Cane Cutters and Stackers', *Occupational Medicine* 44 (1994), 190–94; K.J. Collins and D.F. Roberts, *Capacity for Work in the Tropics* (Cambridge: Cambridge University Press, 1988), 17.

524 Kenneth Kiple estimated the energy requirement to be 3,000 kcal on average, i.e. 12.5 MJ, which is too low. Kiple, *The Caribbean Slave*, 78.

525 *Human energy requirements*, Chapter 5 and 6.3.

526 *Human energy requirements*, Chapter 5 and 7.2.

women in the developing countries of today.[527] Accordingly, the daily energy requirements of the enslaved women were in fact just about as high as that of the men even if the women seem to have had a smaller workload during and after pregnancy.[528]

Apart from the enslaved fieldworkers there were other groups of enslaved on the plantations that for various reasons had different energy requirements. For instance the skilled tradesmen, i.e. carpenters, coopers, masons, sugar boilers etc., did not necessarily have the same soaring energy requirement as the fieldworkers. Their work was generally less strenuous. The same applies to the enslaved working as domestics and the old and invalid enslaved who often worked as watchmen. Finally, sick enslaved workers and enslaved children constituted two groups with special needs. As to the sick, a diet sufficient for a healthy individual can be insufficient when special dietary needs arise, for instance because of infection. An individual's nutritional state is decided not just by the intake of food but also by the digestion of it, the absorption and the use made of the energy and nutrients during a period of time. Disease can influence each of these biological processes as well as an individual's dietary needs, and accordingly the type and amount of food are two critical nutritional variables during illness.[529] The sick enslaved workers in the plantation hospital received a special individual diet as part of their treatment. This consisted for instance of salep (flour of the roots of various kinds of orchids), tapioca (flour of cassava or manioc), barley, rice, wine and fresh meat from sheep and chicken.[530] Something similar seems to have been the case with the small children,[531] but as can be seem from the lease regulations of 1834 the size of children's rations was decided by the child's size, i.e. the amount of work he or she could carry out, and did not necessarily correspond to their needs for growth. Bio-anthropological investigations of skeletons from burial grounds of enslaved people in other Caribbean colonies suggest that malnutrition caused growth crises among the

527 Michael C. Latham, *Human nutrition in the developing world* (Rome: FAO, 1997), Chapter 5, www.fao.org/DOCREP/W0073e/w0073e00.htm#TopOfPage (accessed 30-05-2011).

528 Tyson and Highfield, *The Kamina Folk*, 205.

529 Gibbs, Cargill, Lieberman, and Reitz, 'Nutrition in a Slave Population', 200–1.

530 See for instance the accounts of the private plantations Upper Bethlehem and Fredensborg mentioned below. DNA, WILA, no. 46.17.43, Estate Longford, alphabetical register of items, 1828. DNA, WILA, no. 46.17.33, Estate Hermon Hill, letter of 7 January 1843.

531 DNA, WILA, no. 46.17.43, Estate Longford, alphabetical extract of accounts, 1826.

children. Such crises might have been the result of a rationing policy similar to the one in the Danish West Indies.[532]

Returning to Table 4.1 it is evident that the estimated amount of energy in the food issued on North Star in 1832 and 1833 was respectively 10.46 MJ and 8.91 MJ per enslaved individual per day. In comparison, Table 4.2 shows an estimate of the daily energy requirement of the enslaved to be around 13.3 MJ per adult enslaved individual per day. In other words, the rations handed out by the planter left every adult enslaved individual 3–4 MJ short every day and so with only between three quarters and two thirds of the energy they needed to sustain their daily lives.

Besides the lack of energy, the amount of protein in the ration was another great problem. Today the recommended daily intake of protein for healthy individuals is a minimum of 15 per cent of the total energy in the diet.[533] In comparison, the protein content in the ration issued at North Star was only respectively around 10.5 per cent and 7.5 per cent of the total energy requirement of the enslaved workers.[534] In other words, the enslaved not only had to supplement the ration with energy from carbohydrates, which they could grow in their provision grounds, but they also had to secure important proteins that were far more difficult to obtain.

The problem of protein was, however, more far-reaching than is evident at first glance. Proteins are crucial components in a large number of functions in the human body, for instance in cell formation, the reconstruction of damaged skin and muscle tissue, in the immune system, the energy conversion, the production of hormones, enzymes, blood etc.[535] Proteins consist of amino acids of which some are essential for the production of proteins. Yet, the human body is not capable of producing all essential amino acids and therefore these acids have to be present in the proteins we ingest. Animal foodstuffs like meat, eggs, and milk contain all the necessary amino acids while proteins in vegetable foodstuffs are

532 Jerome S. Handler and Robert S. Corruccini, 'Plantation Slave Life in Barbados: A Physical Anthropological Analysis', *Journal of Interdisciplinary History* 14, no. 1 (1983); Mohamed Rakieb Khoudabux, *Effects of Life Conditions on the Health of a Negro Slave Community in Suriname* (doctoral thesis, University of Leiden, 1991), 48–49; Jacobi, Cook, Corruccini and Handler, 'Congenital Syphilis in the Past', 145–58; David R. Watters, 'Mortuary Patterns at the Harney Site Slave Cemetery, Montserrat, in Caribbean Perspective', *Historical Archaeology* 28, no. 3 (1994), 56–73.

533 Sick and malnourished individuals have greater needs.

534 1.34 MJ / (13.3 MJ/day / 100) = 10.08 %. 1.42 MJ / (13.3 MJ/day / 100) = 10.68 %.
1.0 MJ / (13.3 MJ/day / 100) = 7.52 %. 0.99 MJ / (13.3 MJ/day / 100) = 7.44 %.

535 Arne Astrup et al., *Menneskets ernæring: Fra molekylærbiologi til sociologi* (Copenhagen: Munksgaard Danmark, 1997), 101–3.

less complete in their combination of amino acids and so vegetable foods have to be combined in certain ways to fulfil the nutritional needs. Because of this special problem with protein it is less important what percentage of energy in the diet of the enslaved came from protein if the combination of amino acids in these proteins did not cover the nutritional needs.[536] The protein present in the ration issued to the enslaved workers on North Star was predominantly vegetable protein because it originated for the most part from corn meal and peas. Corn meal specifically has a low content of the amino acids tryptophan and lysine whereas peas have a high content of lysine and so could alleviate the shortage in the corn meal.[537] However, it is evident from the above-mentioned provisioning laws and practices that corn meal was the standard foodstuff while peas were only one of several vegetable substitutes for corn meal. Accordingly, the combination of protein in the issued vegetable foodstuffs must often have been insufficient. This deficit may have been alleviated partly by the salted herring, which added much needed complete animal proteins to the diet. However, it is questionable what condition the herring and their protein were in after several months of pickling during the voyage across the Atlantic and storage in the tropical heat.[538] On this basis, it is likely that the protein content in the ration issued at North Star was not only too small but also too incomplete in terms of amino acids to cover the nutritional needs of the enslaved workers.

In addition to the incomplete combination of proteins the ration issued was probably also lacking some important vitamins, minerals and fat. For instance the content of vitamin A, B1 (thiamine), B2 (riboflavin) and B3 (niacin), and the minerals iron and calcium seem to have been too low compared to current recommendations.[539] The low content of fat in the diet was also critical for several reasons. First, because fat has the highest energy content of all nutrients. Second, because certain essential fatty acids are not produced by the human body and must be obtained through the diet. Third, because some important vitamins are only soluble in fat and so can only be absorbed in the body with fat. Children have a special need for a constant intake of fat to sustain normal growth. From the time they stop breastfeeding till about two years of age a child needs to receive 30–40 per cent of its energy from fat.[540]

536 Latham, 'Human Nutrition', Chapter 9.

537 Kiple, *The Caribbean Slave*, 80–81, 87.

538 Kiple, *The Caribbean Slave*, 80.

539 For a discussion see Kiple, *The Caribbean Slave*, 82–86.

540 J.R. Lupien et al., 'Edible Fats and Oils', *Food, Nutrition and Agriculture* 11 (1994), www.fao.org/docrep/T4660T/T4660T00.htm (30-05-2011).

Based on this analysis of the foodstuffs issued as rations on the royal plantation North Star in the years 1832/3 it is evident that the amount of food was larger than stipulated in the proclamation of 1817 and the lease regulations of 1834. Nevertheless, the nutritional content could not meet the needs of an adult worker – or a child for that matter. To make up for the lack of food the enslaved had to grow their own crops on special provision grounds assigned to them by the planter or they could try to obtain the food in other ways (see below).

Estates Upper Bethlehem and Fredensborg (1829–31)

As the conditions on royal plantations like North Star are not necessarily representative of the private plantations on St Croix, the following analysis will concentrate on the ration issued on the two private plantations, Upper Bethlehem and Fredensborg (King's Quarter). These plantations had the same owner and were managed as one plantation with one record of the food supply.[541] The analysis is based on this collective record for the year 1831 combined with similar records for the years 1830 and 1829. Because the source materials consist of accounts and not a journal with precise weekly entries as was the case on North Star, it is not possible to determine with the same level of certainty whether the enslaved workers received all the food bought for the two plantations. Some of the foodstuffs could have been consumed by the manager or other Euro-Caribbeans living on the plantations, but the absence of typical European foods like wheat flour and pork indicates that there was no substantial Euro-Caribbean household on these plantations. Similarly, certain heavy goods like unground oats and corn may just as well have been given to horses as to enslaved workers and so these goods have been excluded from the analysis.

In the years 1829–31, the supplies purchased for the 121 and 161 enslaved individuals of Upper Bethlehem and Fredensborg respectively consisted almost exclusively of corn meal and salted fish (see Table 4.3).[542] In 1831, the volume of the supplies were a little smaller than in 1829 and 1830 which gives reason to believe that calculations based on the year 1831 will give a conservative estimate. Compared to the ration of corn meal stipulated in the proclamation of 1817 the amount purchased in 1831 was a little larger. However, as the difference was only 2–3 per cent,[543] the reason for the increase cannot be that the ration sizes used were larger than the 6 quarts per adult enslaved worker per week specified

541 DNA, WILA, no. 41.6.6, 1840.
542 This total figure of 282 enslaved workers dates from 1832.
543 51,672.08 kg/year / (50,293.90 kg/year / 100) = 102.74 %.

in the proclamation of 1817. The ration of salted fish was also larger than prescribed by the norm of six herring per adult enslaved worker per week, yet here the difference was a significant 83 per cent.[544] This would amount to around 11 herring per adult enslaved worker per week.[545] As in the example from North Star this amount is remarkably similar to the ration of ten to twelve herring per adult enslaved worker per week mentioned in Joseph Tuckerman's narrative from 1836/7. So, the evidence seems to indicate that the rations of herring or other salt fish on both the royal and private plantations were often considerably larger than the above-mentioned 6 herring per adult enslaved worker per week.

Because of the larger amount of corn meal and herring in the ration that *could* have been issued on Upper Bethlehem and Fredensborg, the energy content is estimated to around 8.96 MJ per adult enslaved worker per day. This is of course higher than stipulated by the proclamation of 1817 (7.91 MJ) plus the norm of 6 herring per week (0.47 MJ). However, as I have estimated the total daily energy requirement of an adult enslaved worker to be 13.3 MJ, the enslaved on these private plantations also lacked about one third of the energy they needed to carry out their work and daily routines. In addition, the foodstuffs on Upper Bethlehem and Fredensborg had the same insufficiencies in the amount and combination of protein as was the case on North Star.

Based on the above analyses of the two samples from a royal and two private plantations on St Croix, and bearing the necessary estimates in mind, it seems probable that the enslaved workers on the Cruzian plantations were given rations of corn meal that corresponded to the laws and regulations of the day. The ration of salted fish, however, seems to have been significantly larger than the norm known from contemporary sources, yet nonetheless in accordance with some accounts from the period. Despite this, the energy content of the ration was too low to meet the estimated requirements of an adult enslaved fieldworker. First of all, the ration lacked between a quarter and a third of the required energy. Enslaved individuals with lower requirements, for instance old people, invalids, domestic workers and trades people with lighter workloads, could possibly acquire the necessary energy from the ration but even they must have had problems with the low content of protein and the insufficient mixture of amino acids, not to mention the lack of certain vitamins, minerals, and fatty acids. The poor nutritional content of the ration could occasionally be

544 7,382.50 kg/year / (4,024.80 kg/year / 100) = 183.43 %.

545 (147,650 herring/year / 52 weeks/year) / 258 enslaved individuals = 11.00 herrings per enslaved per week.

improved by substitution of corn meal with alternative foodstuffs like beans, but everything points to the fact that corn meal and herring were the standard foodstuffs throughout most of the year. Accordingly, there can be no doubt that the enslaved workers had to supplement their food on their own accord in order to survive, which also seems to have been an intention deeply ingrained in the rationing system.

The Supplementary Food Resources of the Enslaved

The enslaved workers could supplement their insufficient rations with foodstuffs of many different kinds and from many different sources. Several of these food resources were dependent on local ecological and geographical circumstances and the season. Because of these diverse and ever-changing conditions, it is neither possible to determine exactly how the remainder of the diet of the enslaved was composed nor if it was nutritionally sufficient. Nonetheless, an analysis of the available food resources can establish the basis for a closer evaluation of which of these resources the enslaved had access to and to what extent they were in fact capable of getting a diet sufficient for their needs from these sources.

Provision Grounds, 'Negro Grounds', and Gardens

The food supply for the enslaved workers on St Croix in the period 1817–48 seems to have been based on a combination of the three known supply systems. The imported foodstuffs have been dealt with above, but in the following the focus will be on the locally produced food crops. These crops can be divided in two types: food crops grown for the planter as part of the collective fieldwork of the enslaved and used to replace or supplement imported provisions, and food crops grown by the enslaved individually during their free time and for their own use. However, it is difficult to discern how much land was cultivated under these two systems because the sources rarely distinguish clearly between them. This is a problem because crops grown for the planter were used for rations and accordingly are not relevant for an analysis of the food resources cultivated by the enslaved individually to supplement their rations. In the following, I shall try to distinguish between the two systems of cultivation and estimate how much land the enslaved might have had individually for their own use, as well as how they used this land and the size of the crop the land may have yielded them.

In the years prior to the period dealt with here, it was the custom to give the enslaved their own plots of land for the cultivation of extra rations and to raise pigs, goats, chickens etc.[546] From an island-wide survey of 1805, it is possible to estimate that an average of around 403 square metres were allocated to each enslaved individual, regardless of age.[547] This figure is of course too general for a calculation of the quantity of crops from the provision grounds per enslaved worker. However, from the second half of the period it is possible to get a more precise estimate of the size of these grounds. In 1828, Lieutenant Brady wrote that the enslaved had two kinds of plots at their disposal. Firstly, a small piece of land next to their houses in the village of the enslaved on the plantation, which was occasionally used as a garden. Secondly, a larger piece of land which was issued anew each year and meant for the cultivation of vegetables. This piece of land varied in size according to the whim of the planter and the quality of the soil, yet on Estate Mannings Bay (Prince's Quarter) where Brady lived, the size of these plots were usually 35 feet square (113.9 square metres).[548] Every adult enslaved worker had one of these plots, half-grown teenagers had one plot to share between two, and small children were assigned one third of a plot. Finally, Brady added that the enslaved had the right to keep goats, pigs and chickens of which the two former had to be kept in pens in the village.[549] Sylvester Hovey, visiting St Croix in the middle of the 1830s, described a similar system. He did not mention the small 'gardens' next to the houses of the enslaved but he estimated the separate plots for cultivation of vegetables to be 20–30 feet square (37.2–83.7 square metres). He also mentioned pigs and chickens.[550] Joseph Tuckerman told a similar story when he visited the island in the 1830s,[551] and travellers Victor Schoelcher and Thurlow Weed who visited the island in the 1840s mentioned larger garden plots cultivated by the enslaved but not the size of them.[552]

Another indication of the size and use of the enslaved workers' provision

546 Arnold R. Highfield, ed., *Hans West's Accounts of St Croix in the West Indies* (US Virgin Islands: Virgin Islands Humanities Council, 2004). Tyson and Highfield, *The Kamina Folk*, 142.

547 Peter Lotharius Oxholm, *Nogle Anmærkninger over en Afhandling om Negerhandelens Ophævelse udi Maanedskriftet Minerva af Febr. 1805* (Copenhagen, 1806), 12, 29. 2,257 'St Croix-acres' (7.15 % of the land) were laid out for provision grounds for 22,076 enslaved individuals on the plantations of St Croix, which equals around 403 m² pr. enslaved regardless of age. One 'St Croix-acre' = 3,940 m² according to Daniel Hopkins, 'The Eighteenth-Century Invention of a Measure in the Caribbean: The Danish Acre of St Croix', *Journal of Historical Geography* 18, no. 2, (1992), 168.

548 I assume that Brady, being a British subject, measures in British feet. 1 British foot equals 30.5 cm. 35 feet square = (30.5 cm × 35 feet) × (30.5 cm × 35 feet) = 113.95 m².

549 Highfield, *Observations*, 10–11, 15.

550 Tyson and Highfield, *The Kamina Folk*, 186.

551 Tuckerman, *Letter Respecting Santa Cruz*, 22.

552 Tyson and Highfield, *The Kamina Folk*, 208, 211.

grounds in the last two decades before emancipation comes from the regulations of 1834 concerning the lease of royal plantations and the records generated because of this regulation. The 1834 regulation stipulated that:

> Every one of these [the enslaved] who are more than 10 years old shall always be granted a piece of land for their own cultivation, which should preferably be located close to the Negro houses.[553]

As is evident from this, the regulation did not specify the exact size of the plot, but this information can be found in the reports from the official inspectors on the royal plantations. For instance, a report from Estate Work and Rest (Queen's Quarter) states that the area surrounding the houses of the enslaved was so large that it would be easy to parcel out a plot 60 feet square (334.9 square metres) as 'permanent gardens' for each enslaved individual in accordance with wishes of the colonial administration.[554] Reports from the Estates Retreat and Hermon Hill (Company Quarter) stated that in both places 4 acres of land had been parcelled out as 'Negro Grounds',[555] which would give each enslaved individual respectively 202 and 181 square metres regardless of age. Furthermore, the report from Retreat states that in addition to 'a constant Negro Ground', which is most likely referring to the 4 acres mentioned, some leftover pieces of land were also given to the enslaved to cultivate on a temporary basis. On Estate Jolly Hill (West End Quarter), 5 acres had been parcelled out to the enslaved as 'constant provision grounds' located close to the great house.[556] This area would give each enslaved individual on the estate around 205 square metres. In the reports from the estates Rust up Twist and Longford it only says that there is plenty of land for 'Negro Grounds', yet at the same time the reports emphasise the words of the lease regulations that the situation of the plot is important. On estate Rust up Twist the provision grounds of the enslaved workers were situated in the mountains, and despite the slope the enslaved preferred this land to any other.[557] On estate Longford, the available land was situated close to the village of the enslaved workers and so the conditions here were in

553 See for instance DNA, WILA, no. 46.21. Estate Hermon Hill, 1836.
554 DNA, WILA, no. 46.21. Lease contracts concerning royal plantations, Report, Estate Work and Rest, 1833.
555 DNA, WILA, no. 46.21. Estate Retreat, 1839 (78 enslaved). DNA, WILA, no. 46.17.45 (87 enslaved).
556 NARA, RG 55, Entry 1109, Box 2432, Estate Jolly Hill, 1840 (96 enslaved).
557 Rust up Twist was situated on the North shore in North Side B Quarter.

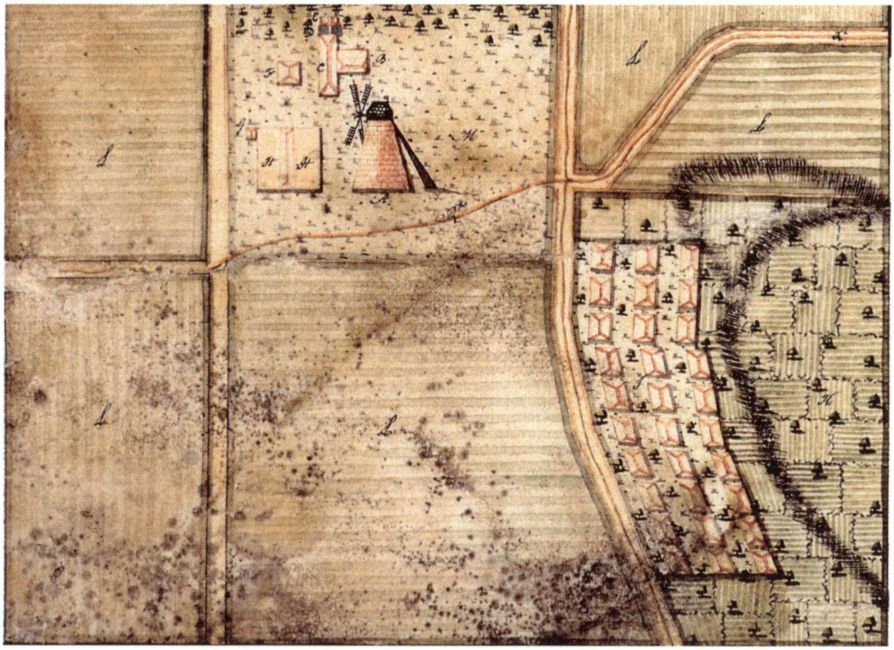

Fig. 4.3: Section of a map of the private Estate Bethlehem around 1779 showing the Bay Works, i.e. the southernmost of the three factory complexes making up the plantation. Notice the houses of the enslaved arranged in rows on the hillside and behind them the small garden plots with trees. Coloured drawing by Frederik Christian Meley, Danish National Museum, Copenhagen, Denmark.

better accord with the lease regulations.[558] On estate Springfield, the manager considered relocating the plots of the enslaved to a location closer to their village to follow the regulations better. However, the enslaved workers seem to have been in favour of keeping the plots they had because they were situated in a large fallow area within which they could choose the place to cultivate as they pleased.[559] Similarly, on estates Cotton Grove and North Star the enslaved workers wanted to decide the location of their plots themselves.[560] Finally, some royal plantations did not comply with the regulations because of their geographical location, for instance Estate Upper Love located in Prince's Quarter

558 DNA, WILA, no. 46.21. Rust up Twist, 1838. DNA, WILA, no. 46.17.45. 1836.
559 DNA, WILA, no. 46.21. Springgarden, 1833.
560 DNA, WILA, no. 46.21. Cotton Grove, 1839 and North Star, 1833.

in the fertile central plain on the island. Here the government inspector found it unprofitable to use the high quality land for provisions and instead he recommended that the enslaved use all their time on sugar production. Presumably the enslaved were compensated by means of larger rations.

So, based on the above information from narratives and the reports from royal plantations from the period 1817–48 we have estimates of the size of the enslaved workers' provision grounds ranging from 0 to 60 feet square (334.9 square metres). That the most usual plot size lay somewhere in between these extremes is indicated by the fact that after emancipation in 1848 each of the former enslaved workers retained a plot of land measuring 30–50 feet square (83.7–232.6 square metres) as part of their wages for working on the plantations.[561] The obvious reason why these provision grounds had no standard size is that the quality of the soil varied greatly according to local conditions on each plantation (access to water, exposure to sun, elevation etc.). This was probably also the reason why the lease regulations of 1834 did not specify the size of the plots although it did specify the amounts of other items to which every enslaved worker was entitled. This scattered image makes it difficult to estimate how much food the enslaved might have been able to cultivate on their provision grounds. Nevertheless, in the following I shall try to arrive at a useful estimate.

Crops and Yields

The crop mentioned most frequently in relation to provision grounds on St Croix was yams (*Dioscorea spp.*).[562] However, it has not been possible to find any source mentioning the average annual yield of yams on St Croix during the period in question and consequently it has been necessary to use a modern estimate. The FAO has estimated that the average annual yield of yams in present-day developing countries is approximately 9 tons per hectare.[563] The reason for the relatively low yield is problems with lack of water and fertilisation (no artificial fertiliser) which seems very similar to the situation in St Croix. There is no reason to assume that the average yield of yams was any higher on St Croix – quite the opposite in fact. Firstly, the quality of the soil (fertilisation, location, exposure

561 Adolph Frederik Bergsøe, *Den danske Stats Statistik* (Copenhagen, 1853), 618.

562 See for instance: Eva Lawaetz, *A Report from Governor General P. L. Oxholm to The Royal Westindian Chamber in Copenhagen Dated May 4, 1816. St Croix*, trans. and ed. Eva Lawaetz (Christiansted, 1977), 8.

563 *Roots, tubers, plantains and bananas in human nutrition* (Rome: FAO, 1990), table 9.2, www.fao.org/docrep/T0207E/T0207E00.htm (accessed 30-05-2011). *Realizing the Promise and Potential of African Agriculture* (Amsterdam: InterAcademy Council, 2004), 80, www.interacademycouncil.net/CMS/Reports/AfricanAgriculture.aspx (accessed 30-05-2011).

to sun) and the lack of water (rain, streams) seem to have been general problems on the provision grounds of the enslaved. As mentioned above the plots were often located in places unsuited to other kinds of agriculture because of topography (hillsides). In addition, the lack of water was a recurring problem on St Croix.[564] Finally, yams need attention on a regular basis. If the enslaved or the individual's family/friends could not take care of the plants because of the sugar harvest, disease etc. the yield would inevitably decrease.

The FAOs estimate of 9 tons of yams per hectare equals 0.9 kilograms per square metre which on an average plot size of around 200 square metres would amount to 180 kilograms of yams annually. However, the entire harvest could not be converted into food. Today, yam farmers save about 30 per cent of the harvest to plant next year's crop and this was probably also the case on St Croix.[565] Finally, there is a considerable amount of waste during storage and the preparation of yams for food. Consequently, perhaps only 60 per cent of the yam harvest could be used as food by the enslaved workers, i.e. around 108 kilograms annually. Compared to the above estimate of an additional need of 3–4 MJ a day per adult enslaved worker this amount would not be sufficient. Boiled yams contain approximately 0.487 MJ per 100 gram, which means that 600–800 grams a day could cover the need for 3–4 MJ.[566] On an annual basis, this would amount to 219–292 kilograms of yams, more than twice as much as the effective yield of 108 kilograms from a 200 square metre plot.

Based on these estimates and calculations it seems that not even the largest provision grounds of 60 feet square (334.9 square metres) mentioned in the sources above would have been sufficient to compensate the enslaved for the lack of energy in the rations issued by the planter. Even if we include the few square metres in the 'gardens' surrounding the houses of the enslaved, it would still not be enough. Regarding the need for protein mentioned above, a crop of yams this size would have been even more insufficient because yams are a very poor source of protein. However, some enslaved workers may have had access to provision grounds larger than 60 feet square and so they may have been capable

564 Sveistrup, *Bidrag*, 3–6.

565 R. Asiedu, H. Mignouna, B. Odu, and J.d'A. Hughes, 'Yam Breeding', in *Plant Virology in Sub-Saharan Africa: Proceedings of a Conference Organized by IITA*, ed. Jacqueline d'A Hughes and Babajide O. Odu (Ibadan: International Institute of Tropical Agriculture, 2001), 467. http://old.iita.org/cms/details/virology/pdf_files/466-475.pdf (accessed 30-05-2011).

566 USDA National Nutrient Database, www.nal.usda.gov/fnic/foodcomp/search/, 'Yam, cooked, boiled, drained, or baked, without salt' (accessed 30-05-2011).

of growing enough crops on their land to sustain their energy needs. Yet, this is not the common picture.

In the above analysis, the crop of the enslaved was assumed to consist entirely of yams. This was a way of simplifying the estimates and calculations, but it has nothing to do with the actual conditions on St Croix. According to the annual medical report from the doctors on the island and the previously mentioned authors Brady, Smith and Weed, the enslaved workers produced a whole range of tubers, vegetables and fruits on their plots. For instance tubers like cassava, sweet potatoes and tannia, vegetables like okra, red pepper, beets, cabbage, onions and pigeon peas, and fruits like banana (sweet and/or plantains), oranges, tomatoes, lemon, lime, pineapple, avocado, mango, coconut, peanuts, passion fruit etc.[567] Many of these vegetables and fruits are mentioned in relation to the markets and they were probably cultivated for sale rather than for the enslaved themselves.

Some of these fruits, however, seem to have come from wild trees and bushes. From this source, the enslaved also got firewood both for their own use and for sale. This was an increasing problem because there was very little wood left on the island in the period.[568] In addition, the recurrent hurricanes destroyed the trees of the island, which reduced the availability of fruit significantly.[569] On this basis, there is no reason to believe that St Croix had an abundance of fruit trees and consequently there cannot have been as much fruit available for the enslaved workers as one might expect in a tropical climate.[570] Hence, it is likely that the enslaved did eat some of the fruit they gathered from their own fruit trees and from nature, but that a large part of this harvest went to the market.

Regardless of the volume of this possible harvest of vegetables and fruits it is important to point out that neither its energy content nor the yield per square metre could exceed that of yams. Accordingly, the enslaved would not have been able to cover their need for energy any better by choosing crops other than yams. Still, many of these vegetables and fruits contain far more vitamins and minerals then yams, which is why they would have been an indispensable supplement to the nutritionally insufficient ration issued by the planter. Even so,

567 DNA, BH, Med. rep., Danish West Indies. 1841. Highfield, *Observations*, 14. Tyson and Highfield, *The Kamina Folk*, 186, 204, 216–17.

568 Highfield, *Observations*, 95.

569 Tuckerman, *Letter Respecting Santa Cruz*, 10.

570 The situation was the same a hundred years later: Trandailer Jones, *Impressions of Nutrition Habits in the Virgin Islands* (US Virgin Islands: Virgin Islands Department of Health, Nutrition Division, 1952), Bulletin 2, 17.

vegetables and fruit do not contain a sufficient quantity and quality of protein and fat to satisfy the needs of the enslaved and accordingly the enslaved workers had to find other sources for these macronutrients.

Fishing, Hunting, and Gathering

In the period 1817–48, almost the entire island of St Croix was laid out for agriculture, grazing or other kinds of use. Still, there were food resources to be found on the edges of or outside the plantation system, i.e. in the island's natural environment. To begin with, it is obvious that the inhabitants of an island would try to get part of their food from the sea. In contrast, freshwater fish was a resource reserved for the fortunate few because the island had no streams or lakes of any significance.[571] However, for the enslaved both fishing and hunting was restricted by legislation. Since the middle of the eighteenth century, laws had prohibited the use of boats and canoes by enslaved individuals unless with written permission from their owner. The intention was to prevent the enslaved from escaping by sea.[572] Nonetheless, some plantations had a 'fisher slave' whose job it was to provide fish for the planter and possibly for purposes of sale.[573] Furthermore, the enslaved were neither allowed to fish in Great Pond, a large salt pond on the south coast of the island, nor to hunt without written permission from their owner. In the nineteenth century hunting was further restricted to individuals carrying a special hunting permit issued by the government.[574]

Despite all these limitations, there is no doubt that the enslaved fished and hunted for their own consumption and not only to satisfy the planter. Lieutenant Brady describes how the enslaved caught fish, land crabs, turtles, iguanas, and terrestrial animals like cats and rats, and that they fished from rafts.[575] Archaeological investigations of kitchen middens on St Croix have shown that the inhabitants of the eighteenth and nineteenth centuries, Afro-Caribbeans as well as Euro-Caribbeans, ate both local fish and various shellfish. Among the shellfish were various kinds of mussels and sea snails living in the water surrounding the island or in the mangroves (Krause Lagoon, Salt River, Altona Lagoon etc.). Among these, the most significant was the large conch (*Strombus*

571 Smith, *Winter of 1840 in St Croix*, 69.

572 DNA, WILA, no. 2.1.4. Proclamations prohibiting hunting and fishing dated 13 February 1742, 17 May 1756, 30 April 1771, and 31 March 1786.

573 For instance DNA, WILA, no. 46.21. Report, Estate Cotton Grove, 1839. Samuel, 36 years old, fisherman.

574 DNA, WILA, no. 2.1.6. Proclamation of 15 August 1836, p. 267.

575 Highfield, *Observations*, 14–15.

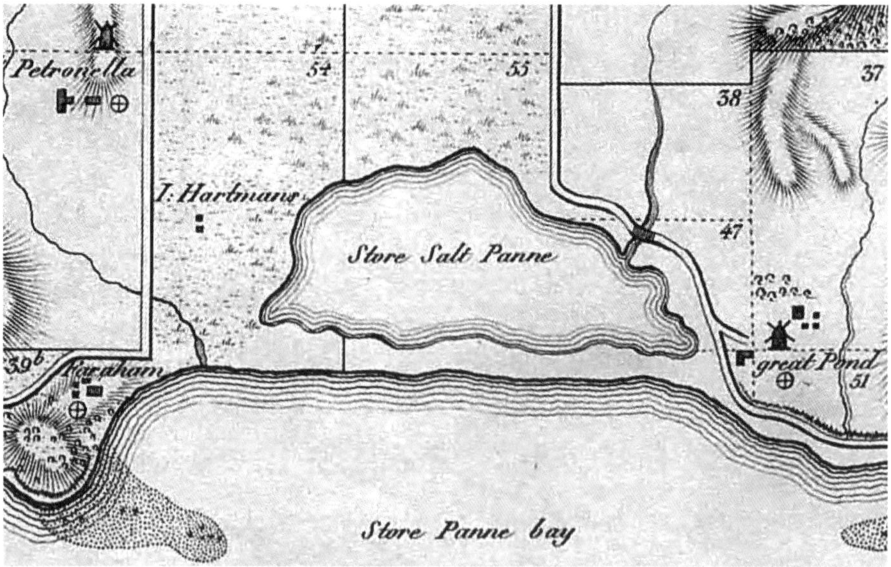

Fig. 4.4: The Great Salt Pond, in Danish Store Salt Panne, on the south coast of St Croix. Section of Oxholm (1799) from Fig. 2.3.

gigas).[576] Furthermore, the enslaved may also have eaten shellfish like lobster and shrimps from the salt ponds along the coast. These items have not left any marks on the written or archaeological sources but they are known to have been present in later periods of the island's history.[577]

Unfortunately, no detailed archaeological study has been carried out on St Croix concerning these marine food resources. Yet, on the neighbouring island of St John such a study has been conducted on Estate Cinnamon Bay. This study

576 A.E. Figueredo and George F. Tyson, *Stage I Cultural Resources Survey of two Structures in Plot 19, Estate Diamond, Prince's Quarter, St Croix, US Virgin Islands*, 1986, unpublished archaeological report, copy in St Croix Landmarks Society, Research Archive and Library, Estate Whim, St Croix, 28–30. A. E. Figueredo, *Phase I Cultural Resources Survey of a 17-acre Tract in Estate Wood Cottage, East End B Quarter, Christiansted Jurisdiction, St Croix, US Virgin Islands*, 1988, unpublished archaeological report, copy in St Croix Landmarks Society, Research Archive and Library, Estate Whim, St Croix), 36–7. Kenneth Baumgardt and George F. Tyson, *A Phase 1B Archaeological Survey of Estate Coakley Bay, St Croix, USVI*, 1987, unpublished archaeological report, copy in St Croix Landmarks Society, Research Archive and Library, Estate Whim, St Croix, II-7, II-24 and 'artefact inventory'. Donald G. Jones, *Archaeological Survey of Estate Whim Plantation Museum, St Croix, US Virgin Islands* (Boston: Boston University Office of Public Archaeology, 1990), 97.

577 Theodor Mortensen, *Om Fiskerierne paa vore vestindiske Øer* (Copenhagen, 1907) 43–44, special edition of *Atlanten*, 11.

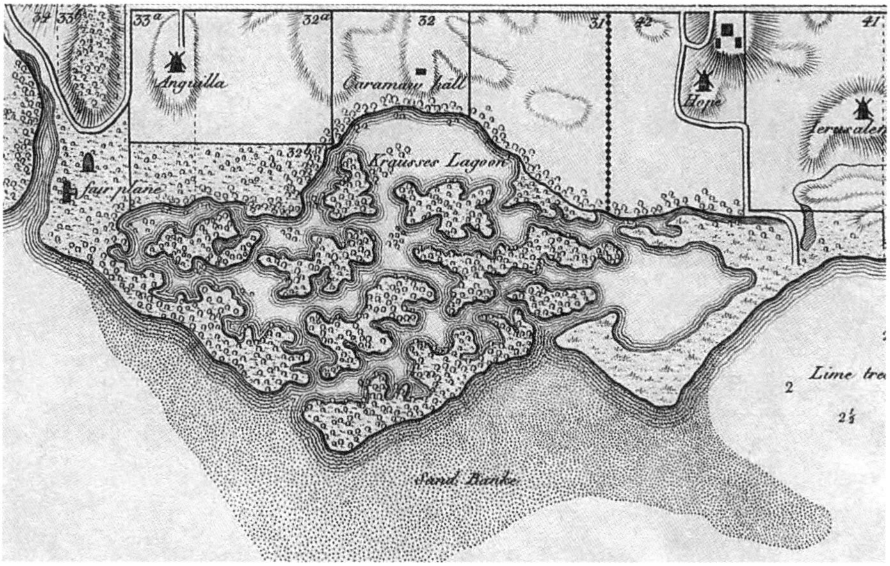

Fig. 4.5: The great Krause Lagoon on the south coast of St Croix. Section of Oxholm (1799) from Fig. 2.3.

reveals that in the period after 1819 local fish and shellfish comprised respectively 44.4 per cent and 41.7 per cent of the pieces of animal bone found.[578] However, these results cannot be directly transferred to St Croix as the geography above and below the sea is quite different between the two islands. St John and St Thomas are mountainous islands with many bays and a large common body of water with coral reefs and shallow waters, while St Croix only has fishing banks on the east end. The south and west coasts have a steep slope under the sea and on the north shore, the cliffs continue right down into the deeps. Accordingly, it is reasonable to assume that it was more difficult for the enslaved to fish on St Croix and that the enslaved workers there probably did not get quite as much food from the sea as did the enslaved on St John.

Besides fish, shellfish, birds, reptiles, and smaller mammals, nature on St Croix offered a range of wild plants, which might be used for food (and/or medicine). A good example of a wild plant with high nutritional value could be the

578 Judith A. Sichler, *Historic Period Foodways in the Danish West Indies (1718–1917): The Zooarchaeological Evidence from Cinnamon Bay and the East End, St John, US Virgin Islands* (Ph.D. dissertation, University of Tennessee, 2003), 156, 178–79.

prickly pear (*Opuntia spp.*), a species of cactus used for creating impenetrable fences around sugar fields and fortifications but also yielding a sweet fruit.[579] It is also highly likely that the enslaved filled their daily food dish, which Lieutenant Brady named 'calalue', with various green herbs and plants growing wild on the lands of the plantation.[580]

Based on the above evidence it seems that the food resources potentially available to the enslaved workers on St Croix contained large amounts of exactly those nutrients which were lacking in the rations. The low and incomplete content of protein in the ration could be complemented with protein from local fish, shellfish, reptiles, birds, and mammals. Whether the supplement was large enough is impossible to say. However, at this point it is also important to recall the pigs, goats, and chickens raised by the enslaved. They too could form an important contribution to the diet. As to vitamins and minerals, an investigation of the content of minerals in shellfish, and vitamins and minerals in local fruit and edible plants, suggests that these resources might actually have been able to meet the daily needs of an enslaved worker.[581] However, it is not possible to determine to what extent this actually happened. The only macronutrient that seems to have been chronically deficient is fat. As mentioned earlier this is a problem because some vitamins are only soluble in fat and because the body needs essential fatty acids, which it cannot produce.

It is important to stress that access to all these food resources were dependent on at least two factors. First, access was strongly dependent on geography. Not all plantations were situated close to the sea or to a lagoon, salt pond, mangrove, or forest. Accordingly, not all enslaved workers had equal access to the food resources in nature. Secondly, it took time to exploit the natural resources, and the enslaved had very little free time, especially during daylight hours. Most fishing, hunting, collection of shellfish, fruit, firewood, forage for the domestic animals etc. requires daylight. Thirdly, hunting, fishing and gathering also takes a certain level of knowhow, that is, some knowledge of technology and the environment, which was not necessarily accessible to all enslaved workers. In other words, there were limits to the extent to which the enslaved could exploit the resources offered by nature on St Croix.

579 David Kenneth Wetherbee, *An Instant Survey of St Croix, V.I., Natural History* (Boston, 1984), 33.

580 Highfield, *Observations*, 14.

581 USDA National Nutrient Database: www.nal.usda.gov/fnic/foodcomp/search/. 'Molluscs, clam, mixed species, cooked, moist heat', 'Guava', 'Orange', 'Mango' etc. (accessed 30-05-2011).

Trade and Theft

Even if an enslaved worker had obtained one or more of the food resources mentioned above, he or she did not necessarily consume it. He or she might try to sell the food on the market in one of the towns. Here the enslaved bartered corn meal, salt fish, fresh fish, meat, poultry, fruit, vegetables and other goods like firewood and forage etc.[582] What they received in return and whether this product gave them a better nutritional status or not is impossible to determine. However, we do know that all foodstuffs on Cruzian markets, indeed all foodstuffs on the island, were subject to continual quality control by the landfysikus.[583] Nonetheless, it is evident that the trade of the enslaved was also subject to geographical and temporal limitations. The distance to the nearest town could be a problem and markets were only held on Saturdays or Sundays.[584] Finally, the volume of goods one enslaved worker could carry was of course limited.

In the event that all other food resources failed or the enslaved wished to take revenge on the planter, they could try to steal the food they needed. Plantation records abound with incidences of desperate enslaved workers who out of need or anger broke into the planter's storehouse.[585] In addition, the fruit on the trees of the plantation, to which the enslaved did not usually have any right, might be the object of theft.[586] Joseph Tuckerman related from his visit in 1836/7 that locals claimed 90 per cent of all the fruit sold on the market in Christiansted to be stolen.[587]

Conclusion

The above analyses have shown that in the period 1817–48 the Danish colonial administration on St Croix played an important role in relation to the nutrition of the enslaved plantation workers. First, the administration ensured that the enslaved on both privately owned and royal plantations received a fixed weekly minimum ration. The ration was 6 quarts (around 3.75 kg) of corn meal per adult enslaved worker or the equivalent in other vegetable stables, plus most likely about six herring, though larger rations of fish were not unusual, for instance on the royal plantations. Secondly, the Danish colonial administration tried to

582 Tyson and Highfield, *The Kamina Folk*, 186–87, 204, 216–17.
583 DNA, BH, Med. rep., Danish West Indies. 1839, interim landfysikus Schlegel.
584 Hall, *Slave Society*, 114.
585 For instance: DNA, WILA, no. 2.16.8, case no. 1351, 5 September 1817.
586 DNA, WILA, no. 38.6.28, case no. 1818–40, 14 December 1818. Case concerning the theft of coconuts, which were bartered for other foodstuffs on the market.
587 Tuckerman, *Letter Respecting Santa Cruz*, 25.

ensure a stable supply of provisions just like the British occupying power had done in the years 1807–15. This intervention was of the utmost importance during the financial slump that characterised the period. After initial difficulties, the attempt seems to have succeeded since the supply of foodstuffs seems to have been stable throughout the 1830s and 1840s. The reason for the administration's control of ration sizes and supply was partly a wish for a more humane treatment of the enslaved workers, based on both moral and economic principles, yet just as important was the need to prevent unrest and rebellion among the enslaved workers with the aim of securing the continued life and economy of the colony.

The analyses have also shown that the energy content of the ration issued was too low for the estimated needs of a hardworking enslaved fieldworker. The lack of energy amounted to about one third to one fourth of the total energy requirement. To this was added a low protein content, an insufficient combination of amino acids and deficiencies in vitamins, minerals, and fat. Accordingly, there is no doubt that the enslaved had to supplement their food on their own accord to survive, which was also an idea deeply integrated in the entire rationing system.

The supplementary food came partly from plots of land assigned to each enslaved individual as provision grounds. It is not possible to determine the exact size of the provision grounds because the size was not fixed by legislation and varied due to the local quality of the soil etc. However, the analyses show that not even the largest plots found in the records, when planted with the most energy-rich crop (yams), could yield enough food to meet the estimated energy requirement of a hardworking enslaved fieldworker. Nonetheless, if planted in the usual mixture of crops, the provision grounds were capable of supplying both an important contribution of energy (mainly from carbohydrate), plus the vitamin and minerals the enslaved needed. Still, the need for protein and fat could not be covered from this source either.

Another possible source of food for the enslaved was the natural environment on St Croix. This source of protein, vitamins and minerals could probably satisfy almost all the remaining nutritional needs of the enslaved. Only one micronutrient, fat, seems to have been undersupplied in the issued ration, the cultivated crop and the natural environment. However, it is not possible to determine if the enslaved actually managed to satisfy their nutritional needs with items from the natural environment. Slave laws, geography, time, and know-how limited the enslaved workers' access to the natural resources. Accordingly, food resources in the surrounding nature can only be viewed as another supplement to the diet of the enslaved, yet an uncertain supplement that was most likely not capable of covering all the needs left by the issued ration and the crops grown on the provision grounds.

Finally, we cannot know to what extent the enslaved exchanged or sold their food resources on the markets. In this way, they may have obtained foods that could improve their nutritional status, such as fresh meat, or other goods that had no influence on nutrition, for instance a new hat.

In conclusion, there is every probability that the enslaved were malnourished, at least for part of the year. While the sugar harvest from January to August was a period of relatively abundant food, both from the sugar production and from the provision grounds of the enslaved, the autumn from October to December was characterised by very few crops from the enslaved workers' plots, by hard work in the sugar fields (holing) and rainy, windy weather (see Chapter 2). Consequently, it is likely that the enslaved were predominantly malnourished during autumn; the season with the highest incidence of disease and largest number of deaths (see Chapter 3). However, the period 1817–48 does not show any sign of widespread famine or deaths caused directly by starvation. Nonetheless, the malnutrition during the autumn may have had a great impact on mortality, especially among the enslaved children. Recent research has suggested that in present-day developing countries malnutrition is the underlying cause of about 55 per cent of all deaths among children. The direct, visible causes of death are for instance malaria, diarrhoea, respiratory diseases, and measles, but generally it is malnutrition that makes these diseases fatal.[588] On this basis, it is plausible to hypothesise that the high mortality rate (around 40 %) among enslaved children under five years of age on Cruzian plantations was also fundamentally caused by malnutrition and not by epidemic diseases or bad hygiene as such. If the nutrition had not been insufficient, these factors would not have been able to cause fatal diseases to the extent they did. Since the high child mortality rate was the main factor behind the steady annual decrease of around 1 per cent in the enslaved population, it would seem, then, that malnutrition was in fact the major factor behind the demographic decline.

The probable malnutrition of the enslaved workers points to the overarching theme in this book, the conflict and negotiation concerning power over health,

588 Richard D. Semba and Martin W. Bloem, *Nutrition and Health in Developing Countries* (New Jersey: Humana Press, 2001), 402–5.

which includes the control of food.[589] The three parties in the conflict, the Danish colonial administration, the planters, and the enslaved workers, each controlled their own part of food resources and continually negotiated this balance of power. As in other areas, the administration was successful in assuming much of the control over the rations of the enslaved, which had previously rested with the planters, because it stipulated and enforced a minimum ration and guaranteed a stable supply of provisions. So, the planter could no longer use withholding of rations as a punishment for the enslaved workers as he would use flogging or imprisonment. However, the administration could not assume full control of the size of the provision grounds of the enslaved, not even on its own plantations because of the varying quality of the soil. Accordingly, the power to decide the size of provision grounds remained in the hands of the planters and so they retained a great influence on how much of the important supplementary provisions the enslaved could produce. Finally, the enslaved workers on their side used the rules and legislation of the administration to submit complaints against the planters and so to assert themselves as a group. At the same time they continued their use of natural resources, which neither the administration nor the planters could control their access to, even though they tried.

The Nutrition of the Enslaved in a Comparative Caribbean Perspective

As mentioned, the food supply in the Caribbean slave colonies was very accurately adjusted to the immediate local conditions in terms of economy, ecology, and society. These quite diverse conditions decided each colony's individual combination of the three basic supply systems: import, cultivation for the planter, or cultivation for the enslaved worker's own consumption. For instance, the latter system was used extensively in mountainous islands like Jamaica because the mountains offered an abundance of land not suited for sugar production but adequate for the production of provisions.[590] On this basis, it is difficult to make a direct comparison of the nutritional situation among the enslaved workers in the different Caribbean colonies and the roles played by their administrations in this field. Consequently, the focus in the following

589 Archaeologist Larry McKee has investigated this aspect in 'Food Supply and Plantation Social Order: An Archaeological Perspective', in *I, Too, Am America: Archaeological Studies of African-American Life*, ed. Theresa A. Singleton (Charlottesville: University of Virginia, 1999).

590 Mary Turner, 'Slave Workers, Subsistence and Labour Bargaining: Amity Hall, Jamaica, 1805–1832', *Slavery and Abolition* 12, no. 1 (1991), 93–94.

will be on colonies that can be said to have had a certain similarity to St Croix in terms of agriculture, economy, and environment. To simplify the comparison further, the primary focus will be on the legally sanctioned sizes of rations and provision grounds employed in the British and French West Indies in the period. Obviously, the legislation was not always observed, yet nonetheless it is the most precise measure of what was the standard in the colony in question. Finally, the role of the various colonial administrations in relation to the food supply of the enslaved workers will also be compared with the role of the Danish colonial administration.

British West Indies

Among the British sugar colonies that supplied their enslaved workers with food via a combination of issued rations and allotted provision grounds were the Leeward Islands (St Kitts, Nevis, Antigua), Bahamas, Barbados, Demerara-Essequibo and Berbice.[591] In contrast, the enslaved workers on Jamaica and the four Windward Islands (Grenada, St Lucia, St Vincent and Tobago) produced all their vegetables on their provision grounds, and so they are not included in the following discussion.[592] In the former group of colonies, the components in the food supply system for the enslaved workers were generally the same as on St Croix, i.e. issued rations of a certain quantity, gardens in the slave village, separate provision grounds of a certain size, the same crops, food resources in the surrounding nature, special Christmas rations, bartering on markets etc. The legislation on the size of rations and plots, however, often differed between colonies because of their different systems of government. The older colonies, like Barbados and the Leeward Islands, had locally appointed self-governing assemblies, while many of the younger colonies, like Demerara-Essequibo, were Crown colonies subject to the control of the central authorities in London.[593] Nevertheless, in terms of the size of rations and provision grounds there seem to have been certain common features. On Barbados the emancipation laws of 1834 stipulated that each enslaved person above 10 years of age was entitled to at least 10 pints of corn, millet or equivalent vegetable foods and 2 pounds of fish per week. This corresponded fairly well with the norms that had existed

591 Turner, 'Slave Workers', 93.

592 Woodville K. Marshall, 'Provision Ground and Plantation Labor in Four Windward Islands: Competition for Resources during Slavery', in *Cultivation and Culture*, ed. Ira Berlin and Phillip D. Morgan (Charlottesville: University Press of Virginia, 1993), 203–4.

593 Higman, *Slave Populations*, 43–45.

on the island before emancipation. On the Leeward Islands, as previously mentioned, the slave law of 1798 stipulated a weekly allowance of 8 pints of corn meal (around 2.5 kg) or 9 pints of corn (3.68 kg) or equivalent foods, plus 1.25 pounds of salt fish or double that in fresh fish. On the British Virgin Islands, the closest neighbouring islands to the Danish West Indies, the standard ration around 1830 was 4–6 quarts of corn meal and six herring per week. Even in the mainland colonies of Demerara-Essequibo and Berbice, where the ecological and agricultural circumstances were quite different from St Croix, the ration in 1830 is reported to have been 9 pints of corn (around 3.68 kg) or equivalent and 2 pounds of salt fish, if the enslaved worker decided to receive rations instead of cultivating his own plot. The latter option was the most common.[594]

A quick comparison with the rules and norms on St Croix after the proclamation of 1817 clearly shows the Danish ration of corn meal to have been larger than in the British colonies. If we use the laws of the Leeward Islands as a starting point and assume that 8 pints of corn meal and 9 pints of corn amounted to the same volume of food when processed, and further assume that 8 pints of corn meal was equal to around 2.5 kg, then it is evident that not even Barbados' 10 pints of corn could contribute as much corn meal as the 6 quarts of corn meal (12 pints or around 3.75 kg) issued to the enslaved workers on St Croix. In contrast, the ration of salted fish may have been smaller on St Croix than in most British colonies. If we start with the Danish West Indian norm of 6 herring per week and maintain the above assumption that one herring weighed around 50 grams, this amounts to around 300 grams of herring per week per adult enslaved worker. This is significantly less than the 2 pounds (908 grams) on Barbados and Demerara-Essequibo and the 1.24 pounds (567.5 grams) on the Leeward Islands. The norm of six herring per week only seems to have been used in the British Virgin Islands. However, the above analyses have shown that in the 1830s both the royal and the private plantations distributed a larger quantity of fish, namely ten or eleven herring per week per adult enslaved worker. With this quantity (around 500–550 grams) the St Croix ration comes closer to that of the Leeward Islands, yet it was still significantly lower than the rations of Barbados and Demerara-Essequibo.

Even so, the size of the rations of corn meal and fish does not give any indication of the nutritional circumstances of the enslaved workers unless combined with information on the size of their provision grounds. On Barbados (1820),

594 Higman, *Slave Populations*, 205–12.

we find examples of gardens in the slave village measuring 100 square feet (9.29 square metres), but usually they were smaller. On the Leeward Islands the 1798 law stipulated that the gardens had to be at least 40 square feet (3.72 square metres). However, the size of provision grounds is not specified even if we know that such grounds were allotted to the enslaved in these colonies.[595]

As to the potential contribution from the surrounding natural environment to the diet of the enslaved workers it is evident that the possibilities were if anything even more diverse between colonies depending on the local geographical and ecological circumstances. Accordingly, it is not possible to carry out a useful comparison. However, it is likely that the minor islands with intensive sugar production like Barbados and the Leeward Islands had a surrounding natural environment similar to the one on St Croix in terms of its potential contribution to the diet of the enslaved workers.

If we attempt to compare the role of the authorities in the investigated British West Indian colonies in relation to the nutrition of the enslaved with the role of the Danish administration on St Croix, it is clear that in the British West Indies the authorities (local and central) also stipulated certain minimum standards for rations, plots etc. As shown, these standards do not seem to have been significantly different from those of the Danish West Indies. Nonetheless, there is reason to maintain that the intervention of the Danish colonial administration had a more comprehensive character than the British West Indian one. This is because the Danish administration controlled and supported the food imports and so ensured a stable supply of foodstuffs vital for both the enslaved workers and the colony. I have not found this kind of level of state control and safeguarding of the enslaved workers' food anywhere in the British West Indies.

French West Indies

Throughout the period in question, the French West Indies consisted primarily of the islands of Guadeloupe and Martinique. These islands are considerably larger than the British islands in relation to the above comparison and so their geographical and ecological circumstances are different. For instance, far more land is available for provision grounds for the enslaved workers. This makes the comparison more difficult, yet as the centralised system of government on these islands seems to have had a greater similarity to the Danish West Indian

595 Higman, *Slave Populations*, 207–9.

system than the British West Indian one did, there is reason to attempt a comparison anyway.

In contrast to the British West Indies, the colonies in the French West Indies were in principle governed by the same slave law, the *Code Noir*. The first *Code Noir* was issued in 1685 and gave all enslaved workers the right to a daily ration of a certain size plus some other benefits. Therefore, the French islands were reputed to give their enslaved workers better food than other colonies. According to the *Code Noir*, it was prohibited to exchange the food rations for plots and to give the enslaved Saturday off to cultivate their land, yet the authorities were too weak to enforce the law, and the planters preferred the old local system in which the enslaved produced their own supplies. By revisions of the *Code Noir* in the 1780s the central authorities in Paris accepted that provision grounds existed and stipulated that all enslaved workers were to receive a piece of land. Yet, the crop from this land was meant to supplement the issued rations, not to replace it.[596] From 1786 to 1846 the legally sanctioned weekly ration per adult enslaved worker was two *measures* flour of manioc (around 3.5 kg)[597] and two *livres* of fish (around 1 kg[598]).[599] After the loss of the main colony of St Domingue (1792, 1804) the problems concerning the replacement of rations with provision grounds and Saturdays off continued, and as late as 1828 the ban had to be repeated. However, it did not change the attitude of the planters, since in the 1830s almost all planters on Martinique and Guadeloupe encouraged their enslaved workers to grow their own food, and gave the enslaved all the land they could cultivate. Then in the 1840s, the authorities reached the conclusion that provision grounds were a benefit to society. Accordingly, the royal ordinance of 5 June 1846 (the Macau law) permitted the enslaved workers to choose between a provision ground and Saturdays off or issued rations. The minimum size of a provision ground was fixed at six *ares* (600 square metres)[600] on sugar plantations, but they were often as large as one or two *arpent* (1 arpent = 3,419 square

596 Dale W. Tomich, 'The Other Face of Slave Labour: Provision Grounds and Internal Marketing in Martinique', in *Caribbean Slavery in the Atlantic World: A Student Reader*, ed. Verene Shepherd and Hilary McD. Beckles (Jamaica: Ian Randle Publishers, 2000), 745.

597 *Mesure* simply means 'measure', but I assume that what is meant is in fact a French *quart* containing 3.174 litres. 2 × 3.174 litres = 6.348 litres. 6.348 litres × 550 g flour per litre = 3.4914 kg flour. Apparently, the density of corn meal, manioc flour and cassava flour were seen as equal. See Sheridan, *Doctors and Slaves*, 170.

598 Until 1795 1 livre = 489.5 g. After the establishment of the metric system in 1795 1 livre = ca. 500 g. Jørn Lund, ed., *Den Store Danske Encyklopædi* XII (Copenhagen: Nordisk Forlag, 1998), 232.

599 Leti, *Santé et société*, 155.

600 1 are = 100m². See: ' are, n.3' *The Oxford English Dictionary*. www.oed.com (accessed 30-05-2011).

metres).[601] The alternative, the weekly issued rations, were stipulated to be 6 kilograms of manioc flour or 6 kilograms of rice or 7 kilograms of corn, and 1.5 kilograms of cod or salted beef. Regardless of whether the enslaved workers chose rations or the provision ground, they had a garden by their house.[602] The enslaved workers in the French West Indies were emancipated in 1848.

Besides the above features, the elements in the French enslaved workers' supply system were generally the same as on St Croix, in the sense that they used the same crops, food resources in the surrounding nature, bartered foods on the markets etc.[603]

As stated above, a comparison of the nutrition of the enslaved workers in the French West Indies and in St Croix is difficult, because most enslaved in the French West Indies fed themselves through the cultivation of provision grounds. Accordingly, it does not make sense to compare the size of the provision grounds. However, if we compare the legally sanctioned ration sizes, it turns out that the rations stipulated from 1786 to 1846 were very similar to the ones found in the Danish and British West Indies. Admittedly, the staple was different (manioc flour), but the quantities of flour and fish were largely the same. So, there seems to have existed some kind of norm for the size of the issued provisions across national divides in the Caribbean sugar colonies. Finally, in 1846, the minimum rations in the French West Indies were increased significantly. Now at last the energy content of the issued rations reached a level that could probably cover the needs of an enslaved fieldworker. Yet, a number of vitamins and minerals, fat and possibly even protein were still lacking.

Despite the French authorities' persistent focus on the sustenance of the enslaved workers, I have not found any indication of any government intervention to ensure supply stability. This is probably due to the fact that most enslaved workers in the French West Indies produced their own food, and consequently the dependence on a stable supply of food from outside was not as strong as in the Danish West Indies and some of the British West Indies.

Conclusion

It is evident that from the last years of the eighteenth century until 1848 there existed a sort of standard, or at least a great similarity, in the quantity of rations issued to enslaved workers across the British, French and Danish West Indies.

601 See: 'Arpent', *The Oxford English Dictionary*. www.oed.com (accessed 30-05-2011).
602 Tomich, 'The Other Face', 746–51.
603 Tomich, 'The Other Face', 750–51, 755.

Despite the geographical, ecological, economic and agricultural differences between the colonies, there seems to have been a general consensus on how much food an adult enslaved worker needed to receive per week if he was not able to produce his own food. The paradoxical fact of this consensus is that this norm was too small to cover the needs of an enslaved fieldworker. This was not a problem if the majority of the enslaved workers in the colony were not fed by issued rations but produced their own food, as was the case in the French West Indies. Yet, in the Danish West Indies and some British colonies, where the majority of the enslaved workers were dependent on issued rations, the limited quantity of the rations combined with the limited size of provision grounds and limited food resources in the natural environment must have had an impact on the health of the enslaved population and its demographic development. This dependence on issued rations is also reflected in the Danish administration's increasing control of the food supply on St Croix. One might have expected something similar in those British colonies that had the same supply situation, yet at no time do the British colonial authorities seem to have tried to assume such control. Accordingly, I can conclude that the Danish colonial administration was more active in relation to the food supply of the enslaved population than comparable British West Indian colonies. The primary activity was to ensure that the legally sanctioned ration sizes were observed and to ensure a stable external supply of food under all circumstances. The incentive seems to have been a wish to preserve the health of the enslaved workers based on humane and economic considerations, but also fear of unrest and rebellion.

Smallpox, Inoculation and Vaccination[604]

Between 1803 and 1848 a unique system of vaccination against smallpox developed on St Croix. The system was based on the metropolitan Danish system but developed into a singular colonial hybrid. In the following, I will argue that the main objective of the system was to safeguard the enslaved workforce, that it achieved a degree of protection against smallpox virtually unseen anywhere else in the Caribbean, and that the fight against smallpox on St Croix reveals aspects of the struggle to control the health of the enslaved.

604 Part of this chapter has previously been published in the article 'Safeguarding Slaves: Smallpox, Vaccination, and Government Health Policies among the Enslaved Population in the Danish West Indies, 1803–1848', *Bulletin of the History of Medicine* 83, no. 1 (2009), 94–123. Copyright © 2009 The Johns Hopkins University Press.

The Smallpox

In eighteenth-century Europe, smallpox was an endemic disease. It was regularly present in the population and caused 10–15 per cent of all deaths, 80 per cent of which were children under the age of 10.[605] In the eighteenth-century Caribbean smallpox was, however, an even greater problem than in Europe. Smallpox had arrived in the Americas as early as the sixteenth century during the European conquest and caused the extermination of millions of native Americans. Yet, it was not until the seventeenth and eighteenth centuries that smallpox became a pressing problem for Europeans in the Caribbean colonies. This was because the increasing traffic of slave ships from Africa supplied a steady flow of infected enslaved workers who caused violent epidemics and high mortality among both Euro-Caribbeans and Afro-Caribbeans.[606]

In the Danish West Indies, smallpox was also a great problem. As early as 1742, only nine years after the Danish takeover of St Croix, the local administration issued a quarantine ordinance for ships in the island's harbours with the specific aim of preventing smallpox from gaining a foothold on the island. This seems to have been a very necessary safety precaution since three smallpox epidemics swept the neighbouring island of St Thomas in the 1750s alone (1749/50, 1756 and 1758) and this trend continued in the following decades.[607] However, the quarantine measures on St Croix were not totally effective; smallpox hit the island in the 1750s,[608] and at least one smallpox epidemic ravaged the island in the 1780s.[609] A quarantine system was maintained on St Croix and seems to have been functioning throughout the period 1803–48.[610]

Variolation and Vaccination

Despite its high mortality, smallpox was in fact one of the few lethal contagious diseases that could be effectively prevented in the eighteenth and early nineteenth centuries. The procedure of 'variolation', i.e. inoculation with matter

605 Kiple, *History of Human Disease*, 1010.
606 Sheridan, *Doctors and Slaves*, 249–50.
607 Oldendorp, *Historie der caribischen Inseln* II, 803, 837, 1221, 1330.
608 Jensen, *En verden til forskel?*, 68–81.
609 DNA, Private archives of Jens Michelsen Beck, archive no. 5097. Accounts for the period 1 January to 1 May 1782. Letter from Søbøtker to Beck dated 24 July 1783. Note from 19 July 1784 in accounts for the period 26 September 1782 to 29 March 1785.
610 DNA, Rentekammeret (Chamber of Revenue), Danske Kammer (Danish Chamber), 3. Departement (3. Department), 1771–1773, Vestindiske Journaler og kopibøger (West Indian Journals and Copy books), no. 2323.3: 28 October 1771 and no. 2323.2: 29 November 1771. DNA, WILA, no. 3.81.609: 1 September 1818. DNA, WILA, no. 10.2.3: 24 July 1826, 9 March 1836.

from a mild case of human smallpox, had been known in the Middle East and China for centuries but found its way to Europe in the 1720s.[611] Variolation was also known and used by Africans in some of the slave-exporting areas of Africa, and it is possible that it was in fact African enslaved workers who first introduced the technique into the Caribbean.[612] In the 1740s and 1750s, variolation began to be used in the British West Indian colonies of St Kitts, Antigua, and Barbados especially for the treatment of the enslaved populations.[613] At about the same time the technique was used to treat the enslaved in the French colony of Saint Domingue.[614] Still, variolation did not become standard practice in the British West Indies until the 1780s, which was also the time when the method was first seen on St Croix. The slow spread of variolation among both the Euro-Caribbean and Afro-Caribbean populations was most likely due to the fact that the risk of death was still 6–7 per cent. Accordingly, variolation was only used when an epidemic of natural smallpox was on the way. In addition, there was always the danger of inoculated patients unintentionally starting a smallpox epidemic by infecting non-immune individuals with natural smallpox.[615]

The revolutionary breakthrough in the fight against smallpox came in 1798 with Dr Edward Jenner's publication on the method of 'Vaccination', i.e. inoculation with matter from cowpox (*Variolae Vaccinae*). The infection produced cross-immunity against human smallpox but without the patient being dangerously ill and running the risk of disfigurement.[616] The vaccination procedure was a success from the beginning and spread with surprising speed across Europe and to the overseas colonies. Yet, the transport of vaccine matter over vast distances, for instance across the Atlantic, proved to be a persistent obstacle. Dried vaccine matter did not preserve the live vaccine well and accordingly the only way to keep the vaccine alive throughout long journeys was arm-to-arm vaccination.[617] In this way, the vaccine matter seems to have arrived first

611 Kiple, *History of Human Disease*, 1010–11.

612 Paul Erdmann Isert, *Reise nach Guinea und den Caribäischen Inseln in Columbien, in Briefen an seine Freunde beschrieben* (Copenhagen, 1788), 221.

613 Jerome S. Handler, *Africans and Creoles: Studies in Barbados Slave Life, 1627–1834* (unpublished manuscript).

614 Karol Kovalovich Weaver, *Disease in the Torrid Zone: Malady and Medicine in Eighteenth-Century Saint Domingue* (Ph.D. thesis, Pennsylvania State University, 1999), 63, 65.

615 Sheridan, *Doctors and Slaves*, 249–50.

616 Sheridan, *Doctors and Slaves*, 258.

617 Kiple, *History of Human Disease*, 1012.

in the Caribbean sometime between 1800 and 1802 by way of the British navy, which made vaccination compulsory among its personnel in 1802.[618]

Today, smallpox no longer exists naturally, but only in laboratories. According to modern medicine, the disease is caused by the virus *Variola,* which spreads through droplet infection of the respiratory tract. The virus has two strains, *Variola Major* with a mortality of 25–30 per cent and *Variola Minor* with a mortality of 1 per cent or less. The time of incubation is twelve days, after which time the disease breaks out with high fever, headache, muscle pains, and a rash. The rash spreads and develops into the characteristic blebs that burst on the eighth or ninth day and begin to dry out. Three to five weeks after the outbreak the sores heal up, the crusts fall off and the patient is cured. If the patient survives, he or she is left with the disfiguring scars after the blebs and a lifelong immunity to smallpox.[619]

The Arrival of Smallpox Vaccination in the Danish West Indies

The Danish West Indies were at the vanguard in the international race to distribute the vaccination worldwide. As early as 1802, dried vaccine matter arrived in the islands both by way of North America, where the vaccine had arrived as early as 1800,[620] and directly from Copenhagen. This timing corresponds with the recorded dispatch of sixteen vials of vaccine matter from the Royal Danish Vaccine Commission in Copenhagen on 16 February 1802.[621] The shipment was part of a government strategy for the Vaccine Commission to send vaccine matter from the newly established Vaccine Institute in Copenhagen to just about every province and colony in the Danish-Norwegian monarchy, and to some neighbouring countries as well.[622] Unfortunately, due to the problems of maintaining the live virus in dried vaccine matter, the vaccine was ineffective when it arrived in St Croix. However, in the last days of January 1803 a local doctor named John Johnston succeeded in bringing vaccine matter with living virus to the island from North America. As soon as he had vaccinated his own two children and so ascertained the efficacy of the vaccine a chain of infection from

618 Jose G. Rigau-Perez, 'The Introduction of Smallpox Vaccine in 1803 and the Adoption of Immunization as a Government Function in Puerto Rico', *The Hispanic American Historical Review* 69 (1989), 400.

619 Kiple, *History of Human Disease,* 1008–9

620 Kiple, *History of Human Disease,* 1012.

621 DNA, DC, no. G125C. Dr. W. Stedman and H. Lang, § 1.

622 Gerda Bonderup, *En kovending: Koppevaccinationen og dens udfordring til det danske samfund omkring 1800* (Aarhus: Aarhus University Press, 2001), 149.

arm to arm was set up.[623] In this way, the live vaccine was distributed to all the doctors of St Croix, St Thomas, St John, and the neighbouring Spanish island of Puerto Rico.[624]

In the course of the following two months, the Cruzian doctors vaccinated hundreds of individuals. The landfysikus J.M.F. Keutsch vaccinated the poor Euro-Caribbeans and Afro-Caribbeans without charge and published advertisements in the local newspapers to convince the populace that vaccination was both effective and harmless.[625] This was necessary because vaccination was still voluntary and not regulated by any law. Accordingly, the vaccination of the enslaved population on the plantations was carried out at the planters' discretion. It is impossible to ascertain how many enslaved workers were vaccinated in these first months or how many actually needed to be vaccinated. Landfysikus J.M.F. Keutsch suspected that many 'negro and mulatto children' did not return to the doctor for control after the vaccination to ascertain if the vaccine had taken.[626]

Despite the Cruzian doctors' efforts, it soon proved difficult to maintain the chain of infection. As early as March 1803, landfysikus J.M.F. Keutsch had to send two children to St Thomas to be vaccinated and bring back the live vaccine to St Croix.[627] According to the landfysikus, the reason for the difficulties of maintaining the vaccine was that the population on St Croix was too small to sustain a continuous chain of infection from arm to arm. Consequently, he argued that it would be necessary to have new vaccine shipped from Europe several times a year.[628] This suggestion was not followed, possibly because the shipping lines across the Atlantic were very unreliable during the Napoleonic Wars or because the virus was simply too fragile. Nonetheless, vaccination seems to have been carried out on St Croix in 1806 but the origin of the vaccine is unknown.[629] Still, it is highly likely it had been acquired from the neighbouring islands, the fastest and safest way of obtaining vaccine when an epidemic was imminent.

623 DNA, DC, no. G125C.

624 Rigau-Perez, 'The Introduction of Smallpox Vaccine', 400.

625 Notices in the local newspaper *Dansk Vestindisk Regierings Avis*,18, 22 and 25 February 1803.

626 F. Keutsch, 'Medicinalbericht des constituierten Landphysicus zu St. Croix, Dr. Med. F. Keutsch, über da Westindische gelbe Fieber und andere Gegenstände des dortigen Medicinnalwesens', *Nordisches Archiv für Naturkunde, Arzneywissenschaft und Chirurgie* IV, 2.11 (Leipzig, 1805), 97.

627 DNA, DC, no. G125C.

628 Keutsch, 'Medicinalbericht', 98.

629 *The St Croix Gazette* (alias *Dansk Vestindisk Regierings Avis*), Friday 7 April 1809. Advertisement on the front page by Dr Keutsch mentioning that a number of children were vaccinated in 1806 and 1803.

Vaccination during the Second British Occupation, 1807–15

In the years from the first vaccination in 1803 until the end of the second British occupation of the Danish West Indies in 1815 (the Napoleonic Wars), smallpox and vaccination against it were recurring problems on the islands. The British occupation authorities were very attentive to the problem of smallpox and tried to enforce regulations to support vaccination. For instance, when a smallpox epidemic threatened St Croix at the end of February and beginning of March 1809 the authorities initiated an extraordinarily ambitious plan to maintain the protective vaccine matter on St Croix for the benefit of the public. The main component of this plan was to collect information of all births on the island through weekly reports.[630] The sheer magnitude of this scheme made it practically impossible and only very few reports ever came in.[631] It appears that in 1809 the main reservoir of unvaccinated individuals on St Croix comprised the newly born children, of whom the overwhelming majority was enslaved. The adult population, both free and enslaved, was not targeted in this plan, presumably because it was already protected either by vaccination, variolation or naturally acquired immunity and so could not participate in an arm-to-arm chain of infection to maintain the vaccine. About a month later, on 7 April 1809, the landfysikus Johannes Søren Keutsch (1777–1824),[632] brother of J.M.F. Keutsch, triumphantly announced in *The Gazette* that the epidemic had been stopped by the efficacy of the vaccination. Yet, despite the success, he felt compelled to remind the public that the threat of smallpox was still present because of some parents' ignorance and prejudice. To fight these evils he announced that he and his colleague Dr Jacobs would perform a public 'counter-experiment' by inoculating some children who had been vaccinated the previous year with human smallpox. The idea was to show that the disease would not infect them because they were vaccinated and so convince any sceptical citizens of the power of vaccination. In addition, the landfysikus vaccinated all children and enslaved workers free of charge.[633]

630 *The St Croix Gazette*, Friday 10 March 1809.
631 DNA, WILA, no. 3.56.2. Lists of newborns in the Lutheran congregation in Christiansted, 1 July and 1 August 1809.
632 Carøe, *Den Danske Lægestand* III, 107 and V, 19–20, 80.
633 *The St Croix Gazette*, Friday 7 April 1809.

The Construction of the Danish West Indian Vaccination System

Despite the British authorities' efforts to promote vaccination, they had not managed to establish a comprehensive system of vaccination by the end of the occupation of St Croix in 1815. The Danish authorities immediately set out to correct this state of affairs as part of a strong focus on the Danish West Indies by the central authorities in Copenhagen and the public in Denmark.[634] The result was a process of thorough clarification and subsequent reformation of the legal and organisational structures in the Danish West Indies including the health services. This process continued up to 1848.[635]

In the health sector, the greatest importance was ascribed to vaccination. In the kingdom of Denmark itself, smallpox vaccination of the entire population had been a matter of prime concern for the government since the issuance of the law of general vaccination in 1810/11.[636] In the Danish West Indies, a similar process began as early as 1816 when the local landfysikus J.F. Bloch submitted a memorandum to the Danish West Indian government suggesting the establishment of a vaccine institute on St Croix similar to the one in Copenhagen. However, the suggestion was rejected by the Council of Citizens, who argued that an institute would be too expensive and that it was unnecessary since all plantations employed a doctor who could perform vaccinations when needed. Finally, they argued experience showed that not even vaccine institutes in great cities like Paris were successful in maintaining the live vaccine.[637] Their final decision on the matter was relayed to the central authorities in Copenhagen who, however, issued an ordinance of 30 July 1817 ordering the West Indian government to find the solution best suited to maintaining and distributing the vaccine in the Danish West Indies considering the special local circumstances.[638] The ordinance contained a plan for the establishment of a vaccine institute on St Croix. The suggested system was similar to the Danish system where a vaccine institute under the supervision of a state-employed doctor maintained the vaccine and distributed vaccine to all doctors who in turn vaccinated all the inhabitants. Yet, the Danish West Indian government again rejected the plan for

634 Vibæk, 'Dansk Vestindien, 1755–1848', 239–40.

635 Jensen, *For slavernes sundhed* (unpublished Ph.D. thesis, University of Copenhagen, 2006), 60–76, 238.

636 Petersen, *Den Danske Medicinal-Lovgivning* II, 71–78, 102–4. Law for Denmark and Norway concerning vaccination dated 3 April 1810 and Chancellery order for Denmark and Norway of 19 November 1811 containing an addition to the law of 3 April 1810.

637 DNA, WILA, no. 3.62.1. 1816, case nos. 214, 256 and 296b.

638 Petersen, *Den Danske Medicinal-Lovgivning* II, 239–40. Ordinance concerning measures to the distribution of the vaccine in the West Indies, 30 July 1817.

a vaccine institute because they felt it was based on the erroneous assumption that the vaccination had not yet reached the islands and that the entire population of enslaved workers needed to be vaccinated.[639] Contrary to this scenario, the West Indian government claimed that the majority of the population on St Croix had already been vaccinated and so the only significant group in need of vaccination were the 400–500 enslaved children born every year. Under these circumstances, the West Indian government argued: first, that a vaccine institute would be too expensive; second, that the population was in any event too small to sustain the vaccine; third, that it was too expensive to hire a doctor for the maintenance of the vaccine institute; fourth, that it was impossible to control vaccinations performed by the many foreign doctors in private practice who serviced the plantations; and finally that it would not help to vaccinate without charge because the inhabitants did not let their children or enslaved workers be vaccinated unless a smallpox epidemic was imminent.[640] Instead, the Danish West Indian government established a unique system developed especially for the local circumstances – a kind of colonial hybrid of the system in Denmark.

The local landfysikus was given the exclusive right to and responsibility for the vaccination of all enslaved workers on the island and was obliged to keep a list of all unvaccinated enslaved individuals. To perform the vaccinations the landfysikus had to travel to specific locations on the island following a fixed schedule, and to these locations the local unvaccinated enslaved workers would be summoned for vaccination and a follow-up inspection. If the enslaved individual failed to turn up for vaccination or inspection at the appointed time and place the owner would be fined. The local officials in the countryside, the Quarter Captains, supported the landfysikus in these matters. In addition, the landfysikus was responsible for obtaining the necessary vaccines and for the distribution of the vaccine to the doctors in private practice. For each enslaved person vaccinated the landfysikus received a fixed salary of two Pieces of Eight, which was actually cheaper than the then price of vaccination among the doctors in private practice. Paupers were not to be charged for vaccinations. All others (i.e. free Euro-Caribbeans and Afro-Caribbeans) were free to avail themselves of the vaccination services from any doctor they wished. However, it was stipulated that no one could be confirmed in church or go to school, and

639 DNA, WILA, no. 3.81.609, answer from Governor General Bentzon to the Danish Chancellery 1 September 1818. About the Danish vaccination system, see Bonderup, *En kovending*, 50–53.

640 DNA, WILA, no. 3.81.609, answer from Governor General Bentzon to the Danish Chancellery 1 September 1818.

no enslaved worker could be sold (i.e. in internal trade), without a certificate of vaccination or a certificate of having had natural smallpox. The landfysikus was in charge of issuing and authenticating these certificates and to this end he was to keep a register of all vaccinated individuals on the island, enslaved as well as free. Finally, the former practice of variolation with natural smallpox was banned and all citizens were instructed to report any incidence of natural smallpox to the landfysikus immediately. Those who failed to do so would be punished with imprisonment.[641]

The establishment of the Danish West Indian vaccination system took place in a way that was in many respects typical of the islands' health-related laws. First of all, it happened quickly and under external pressure. On 1 September 1818, news had arrived of smallpox cases on St Thomas. Consequently, on 5 September the new vaccination system was established by order of the Governor General. Second, the main motive behind the regulations was a concern for the preservation of the numbers of enslaved workers. The authorities in Copenhagen sanctioned the vaccination system retrospectively by a decree of 31 March 1819.[642]

The new vaccination system in the Danish West Indies was modelled on the system in the kingdom of Denmark set up in 1810/11. However, a comparison of the two systems shows differences between the metropolitan version and the colonial hybrid that reveal the implications of transplanting a health system to a very different kind of society. The first difference was the central concern in the Danish West Indian vaccination regulations for having the enslaved workers vaccinated and inspected, which was, of course, not present in the Danish legislation. The most effective control was achieved by concentrating all vaccination and registration in the hands of one person, the landfysikus. The above-mentioned obligations of the landfysikus as vaccinator included hitherto unseen interventions in the slave owner's rights of private property over his slaves. Prior to this, the Danish West Indian administration had been very reluctant to interfere in any matters related to owners' treatment of their enslaved workers. However, by utilising the unique possibility afforded by vaccination to protect the now precious enslaved workers against destructive smallpox epidemics, the

641 DNA, WILA, no. 3.81.609, Report no. 51, 5 September 1818.

642 Jacob Henrie Schou, *Chronologisk Register over de Kongelige Forordninger og Aabne Breve, samt andre trykte Anordninger, som fra Aar 1670 af ere udkomne, tilligemed et nøiagtigt Udtog af de endnu gieldende, for saavidt samme i Almindelighed angaae Undersaatterne i Danmark og Norge, forsynet med et alphabetisk Register* (Copenhagen, 1823).

Danish West Indian administration assumed a new protective role in the field of the health of the enslaved.

The free Euro-Caribbeans and Afro-Caribbeans were not subject to the same attention from the state. They enjoyed some degree of freedom in the matter of vaccination, which mirrored the metropolitan regulations. In Denmark, everyone was free to choose his own vaccinator and no one was fined for failing to be vaccinated. Yet, since no one could get married (law of 1810) or be confirmed in church (law of 1811) without having a certificate of vaccination, the legislation was effectively coercive, although in a somewhat indirect manner.[643] In the Danish West Indian regulations regarding free citizens, we find the second of these indirect sanctions but not the first. This difference was probably due to the simple fact that marriage was not a social norm in West Indian society in the way it was in Denmark. In other words, exclusion from marriage was not an effective sanction in the West Indies. Therefore, and because almost all adults had been vaccinated or immunised through natural smallpox, the administration settled for regulations concerning school and confirmation in church as indirect sanctions against the children of free citizens.

The Fight against Smallpox, 1819–28: Quarantine and Extraordinary Measures

In the years following the establishment of the vaccination system in 1818, a continuous correspondence concerning vaccination ensued between the Danish West Indies and Copenhagen, generating a growing body of legislation.[644] Here we will focus on the local regulations and measures, which afford the clearest examples of the practical problems surrounding the establishment of the state-controlled vaccination system.

On 30 March 1819, on the very day when the central authorities in Copenhagen ratified the special Danish West Indian vaccination system, a person

643 Bonderup, *En kovending*, 97.

644 DNA, WILA, no. 2.1.5., 23 January 1821: Proclamation concerning reports from all vaccinators on the progression of the vaccination. Petersen, *Den Danske Medicinal-Lovgivning* II, 2, 123, 209. 5 October 1822: Chancellery letter concerning the regulations on vaccination and the trade in enslaved individuals. 27 August 1823: Resolution concerning the West Indian governments' duty to control the compliance with the regulations of vaccination. DNA, WILA, no. 2.1.6., 19 February 1824: Regulation concerning the landfysikus' salary for the vaccination of enslaved workers. Petersen, *Den Danske Medicinal-Lovgivning* II, 2, 288, 322. 10 January 1826: Chancellery letter concerning improvements in the registration of the vaccinated. 18 May 1827: Ordinance concerning the regulations of vaccination of followers of foreign creeds (i.e. non-Lutherans).

infected with natural smallpox appeared on St Croix.[645] The situation was critical because no vaccine was at hand on the island. Yet, the vaccine was immediately requisitioned from St Thomas and the usual quarantine measures came into force in the harbours of Christiansted and Frederiksted.[646] Following Governor General Bentzon's order of 5 September 1818, landfysikus J.F. Bloch had quickly inspected and vaccinated all over St Croix, and this approach was continued by the substitute landfysikus Schlegel.[647] Due to these preventive measures no case of smallpox occurred on St Croix during the whole of 1820 even though neighbouring St Thomas suffered from a great epidemic with about 1,000 deaths (roughly 10 per cent of the population).[648] However, the weakness of this great effort was as evident as in previous instances in that landfysikus Schlegel ran out of 'vaccination subjects', i.e. non-vaccinated children. Consequently, the vaccine could not be kept alive on St Croix and new vaccine had to be brought in several times from Copenhagen, Great Britain, the USA, Puerto Rico, or other West Indian islands. Furthermore, the vaccine brought in usually turned out to be dead and ineffective unless it arrived on the arm of a recently vaccinated person. In addition to this difficulty, there were many practical and administrative problems with the registration and control of the 'vaccination subjects', who habitually failed to appear for vaccination, and the important follow-up inspection to confirm if the vaccination had taken. These problems were not limited to the West Indies but were only too familiar in the vaccination service of Denmark. Landfysikus Schlegel explained that generally most officers and planters were ready and helpful when he appeared as vaccinator, but occasionally his work was obstructed. Unfortunately, he gave no further details but the problem appears to have been more related to administrative issues than to recalcitrant planters. In other words, it does not seem that the planters opposed the greater authority assumed by the colonial administration in relation to the health of the enslaved workers.[649]

On 24 March 1824 it happened again. A person infected with natural smallpox got through the quarantine system and accordingly all owners of enslaved workers and fathers of families were urged to have their charges vaccinated immediately. However, contrary to the efforts in 1819/20, this time the govern-

645 DNA, WILA, no. 3.81.599.
646 DNA, WILA, no. 2.16.9, case no. 232, 30 March 1819.
647 DNA, WILA, no. 3.81.609, 'Draft of regulations for vaccine perquisites.'
648 Johan Peter Nissen, *Reminiscences of a 46 years' Residence in the Island of St Thomas in the West Indies* (Nazareth, Pennsylvania: Senseman and Co., 1838), 125.
649 DNA, WILA, no. 3.81.609, 'Report on the Vaccination on St Croix in the Year 1820.'

ment issued a temporary permit for all doctors in private practice to vaccinate enslaved workers under the authority of the landfysikus.[650] The reason for this deviation from the previous approach to vaccination is not evident from the announcement granting this permission. However, a royal order from the Ministry of Commerce in Copenhagen dated 25 May 1824 shows that for almost a year the Danish West Indian administration had been worrying about whether the previous vaccination effort had been thorough enough. As a result, the king ordered that if the validity of vaccination was at all doubtful with one of his subjects, he or she had to be revaccinated because the consequences could otherwise be catastrophic.[651] The reason for this heavy-handed response from the authorities in Denmark seems to have been that for the first time since the vaccination laws of 1810/11 Denmark experienced an epidemic of so-called 'mild smallpox'. Both vaccinated and unvaccinated individuals fell ill but the disease was only dangerous to the latter. The medical experts in Copenhagen were at a loss as to the cause of the epidemic and unsure whether vaccination in fact afforded the total protection they had previously thought.[652] However, the Danish West Indian government was forced to act on its suspicions before any answer arrived from Denmark and the means it chose was to include all doctors in the vaccination of the enslaved workforce. The drawback of this approach was a lower level of control over who was vaccinated because the doctors in private practice were predominantly British and known to be quite casual about their controlling obligations. While it might seem as if the administration was undermining its own objectives, apparently the situation was perceived to be so serious that there was no alternative. Luckily, the exemption had the desired effect as 2,000 enslaved workers were registered as vaccinated in 1824, the highest number registered in the entire period 1803–48 (see Fig. 4.7). The exemption was cancelled again on 25 November 1824 but had to be reactivated on 25 March 1825 because smallpox had again arrived on the island.[653] On 30 May 1825, the landfysikus resumed exclusive control of the vaccination of the enslaved workers on St Croix.[654]

In the course of the year 1826, smallpox appeared on the island of St Thomas but only caused an increased quarantine alert on St Croix.[655] In the following

650 DNA, WILA, no. 10.2.3: Announcement of 25 March 1824.
651 DNA, WILA, no. 3.81.609, letter of 25 May, 1824.
652 Bonderup, *En kovending*, 116–32.
653 DNA, WILA, no. 10.2.3: announcement of 25 November 1824 and 25 March 1825.
654 *Dansk Vestindisk Regierings Avis*, Monday 30 May, 1825, §1.
655 DNA, WILA, no. 10.2.3, letter of 24 July 1826.

year of 1827, smallpox reappeared on St Croix but this time the quarantine measures in the harbours failed and several cases of smallpox turned up on the west end of the island. Faced with this larger outbreak, which appears to have been more virulent than anything seen since the establishment of the vaccination system in 1818/19, the Danish West Indian government chose not only to repeat the temporary exemption from the monopoly of the landfysikus in matters of vaccination of the enslaved but also to wield the strongest weapon in the armoury of health: the total quarantine. As the administration apparently did not trust the entire population to be protected by vaccination, it enforced a set of rules hastily designed by landfysikus Schlegel with the aim of preventing the infection from spreading. The rules were simple quarantine laws that commanded all infected individuals, regardless of sex, colour, or class to be isolated where they were, i.e. in special accommodation either in the towns or on each plantation.[656] The enforcement of the total quarantine shows how seriously the administration took the threat of a smallpox epidemic. A couple of months after the enforcement of the new rules the Danish West Indian government added a temporary exemption to the monopoly of the landfysikus concerning the vaccination of enslaved workers.[657] On 28 March 1828, the epidemic was long gone and the exemption was revoked.[658]

The Last Smallpox Epidemic

Between 1828 and 1843 there does not seem to have been any incidence of smallpox on St Croix. The standard quarantine measures in the island's harbours warded off all threats of infection from the outside.[659] Vaccinations continued as before, yet not always with the same vigour (see Fig. 4.7). There seem to be two reasons for this variable effort. First, there was the ever-present problem of obtaining living vaccine matter from the outside to make up for the fact that the population of the Danish West Indies was too small to maintain a continuous chain of infection.[660] To this end new experiments were constantly being made,

656 DNA, WILA, no. 10.2.3, a set of quarantine regulations by Dr Schlegel dated 14 May 1827. *Dansk Vestindisk Regierings Avis*, 24 May 1827 (dated 17 May).

657 DNA, WILA, no. 2.1.6, p. 65, Announcement of 7 June 1827 concerning that all doctors authorised as such by the administration were allowed to vaccinate enslaved workers.

658 DNA, WILA, no. 2.1.6, p. 90, Announcement of 28 March 1828 revoking the temporary right of all authorised doctors to vaccinate enslaved workers.

659 DNA, WILA, no. 3.81.599, Minutes of Negotiations in the Commission of Health and Quarantine in Christiansted, 1816–1850.

660 DNA, WILA, no. 2.26.2, case no. 150 and 161. DNA, WILA, no. 2.27.12, case no. 183. DNA, WILA, no. 2.27.14, case no. 562. DNA, BH, Med. rep., Danish West Indies, 1842.

for instance using cows instead of humans as carriers of live vaccine matter from island to island.[661] Second, as previously mentioned, the population had a tendency to pay attention to vaccination only when the danger of smallpox was imminent. On the other hand, there was no resistance to the vaccination, not even on racial grounds. Given the racist nature of the society combined with the fact that the vaccine often came from Afro-Caribbean patients, this is surprising. The doctors were now convinced of the protective abilities of the vaccine, which is amply illustrated by the following quotation from one of the local doctors, Dr Hugh Morris Lang (1779–1864),[662] writing in his annual medical report of 1828:

> The safety of vaccination seems pretty well established, for with its introduction among the Negroes in the country not a case of smallpox has yet made its appearance.[663]

Despite these good results, the doctors still feared an outbreak of smallpox would claim many victims among the enslaved workers.[664] The landfysikus shared this concern and was acutely aware of the irregularities in the vaccination effort and the crucial role played by the system of quarantine in the protection against smallpox (and other communicable diseases). This unease among local medical experts became clearly visible when a royal proclamation of 1 May 1835 ordered that smallpox no longer be targeted with quarantine measures in the kingdom of Denmark.[665] On a subsequent enquiry from the Danish West Indian Governor General von Scholten to landfysikus W.S. Jacobs as to whether it was advisable to have this proclamation extended to the islands, the landfysikus answered that the consequences could be extremely dangerous. He argued that in the early period before 1821 vaccination had been conducted without proper follow-up control and so there was no certainty that the vaccinated individuals had actually acquired immunity. Consequently, quarantine was still essential for the protection of the island.[666] Apparently, the Governor General chose to listen to the landfysikus, which turned out to be a wise decision.

661 DNA, WILA, no. 2.27.12, 23 March 1836.
662 Carøe, *Den Danske Lægestand* III, 117 and V, 82.
663 DNA, BH, Med. rep., Danish West Indies, 1828.
664 DNA, BH, Med. rep., Danish West Indies, 1843. Account of the smallpox outbreak in 1843–44 by landfysikus Aagaard.
665 Petersen, *Den Danske Medicinal-Lovgivning* II, 2, 483–84.
666 DNA, WILA, no. 10.2.3, letter to Governor General Peter von Scholten of 9 March 1836.

In 1843, smallpox returned to St Croix and again the full arsenal of quarantine measures was employed to fight the disease. The epidemic started on St Croix on 18 October when a mulatto woman from St Thomas suddenly developed smallpox. On St Thomas, the epidemic had already wreaked havoc on the population. As previously mentioned, smallpox epidemics and other epidemics were far more common on St Thomas than on St Croix. Landfysikus Aagaard explained the difference between the islands:

> The interest [in smallpox] was very different on the two islands. On St Thomas, where sugar production is of minor importance, it was most important that trade was hampered as little as possible by the quarantine. On St Croix, where Negroes and the agriculture of the plantations is everything, it was most important to keep the epidemic away.[667]

In the course of the following two weeks, the infection spread and therefore Governor General von Scholten acted quickly in accordance with the above priority on St Croix. On 1 November 1843, he re-established the universal quarantine regulations of 1827 and on 11 November the doctors in private practice were granted temporary permission to vaccinate enslaved workers.[668] At about the same time a temporary smallpox hospital was established in the great house of the Mount Welcome plantation on the outskirts of the town of Christiansted. Here all enslaved and free coloured patients with smallpox were isolated, the former at their owners' expense, while Euro-Caribbean patients were quarantined in their own houses.[669] All rooms that had been occupied by smallpox patients were fumigated with chlorine vapours and the doctors tried to enforce preventive measures such as fresh air and strict hygiene. The latter measures seem to have been especially necessary in relation to the enslaved workers who were very reluctant to open windows and doors when they were ill – to the great chagrin of the landfysikus who had to endure the stench of the suppurating sores in their stuffy rooms.[670] These conflicting patterns of reaction illustrate

667 DNA, BH, Med. rep., Danish West Indies, 1843. Account of the smallpox outbreak in 1843–44 by landfysikus Aagaard. Original Danish text: 'Interessen [for kopperne] var ganske forskjellig paa de tvende Øer. Paa St Thomas, hvor Sukkeravlen er af mindre Vigtighed, gjaldt det om, at Handelen generedes saa lidt som mueligt ved Quarantainen. Paa St Croix derimod, hvor Negere og Plantagernes Dyrkning er alt, gjaldt det om at holde Epidemien borte.'

668 DNA, WILA, no. 10.2.3.

669 DNA, WILA, no. 3.81.599.

670 DNA, BH, Med. rep., Danish West Indies, 1843. Account of the smallpox outbreak in 1843–44 by landfysikus Aagaard.

the fundamentally different perceptions of disease among enslaved workers and doctors (see Chapter 2).

The epidemic lasted until April 1844. When the last patients left Mount Welcome, landfysikus Aagaard concluded that thirty-one individuals had been infected and only four had died from smallpox.[671] This was a very low number of victims compared to St Thomas where about a sixth of the population, more than 2,000 people, had been infected by the disease.[672] The number of deaths registered was 280 but the actual number was probably higher.[673]

A Comparative Caribbean Perspective: The British and French West Indies

It is difficult to give a coherent picture of how vaccination developed in the British and French West Indian colonies. The evidence is scattered and of uneven quality. Differences in governmental structures and legislative traditions shaped the various approaches and developments in the field. Yet, common trends are also visible, such as the problem of preserving the live vaccine, the reluctance of the populace and the lack of effective control.

The British West Indies

The first account of variolation being used in the British West Indian colonies dates back to 1727, only six years after it was first used in England. In the following years, the method spread at least to Barbados, Antigua, and St Kitts. On Jamaica, variolation was not recorded until 1774. It appears that the distribution followed the development of sugar production and of large populations of enslaved workers. The historian Richard Sheridan has concluded that before the end of the eighteenth century variolation had become widely used in the West Indies.[674]

It is not known when vaccination was first introduced in the British West Indies. However, vaccination was present on Barbados in 1802 and reached Jamaica in 1803.[675] On Barbados, outbreaks of smallpox seem to have been

671 DNA, BH, Med. rep., Danish West Indies, 1843. Account of the smallpox outbreak in 1843–44 by landfysikus Aagaard. DNA, WILA, no. 3.81.599.

672 Vibæk, 'Dansk Vestindien, 1755–1848', 327 (the total population on St Thomas amounted to 13,073 individuals in 1846). Donald R. Hopkins, *Princes and Peasants: Smallpox in History* (Chicago: University of Chicago Press, 1983), 227.

673 Petersen, *En historisk beretning*, 226–27.

674 Sheridan, *Doctors and Slaves*, 254–58.

675 Handler, *Africans and Creoles* (unpublished manuscript).

eliminated early in the nineteenth century, most likely due to vaccination.[676] Yet, there were many small-scale owners of enslaved workers, especially in the towns, who were reluctant to use vaccination. In the other British West Indian colonies public attention to smallpox was generally quite limited until the disease returned as a devastating epidemic in 1818/19.[677]

On Jamaica, hundreds of enslaved workers were vaccinated in the years 1803 to 1813 but vaccination spread very slowly across the island because it was difficult to obtain and sustain the live vaccine. In 1813, the islands' legislative assembly established a vaccine institute modelled on the British National Vaccine Establishment where people could be vaccinated free of charge and where vaccine matter was collected and distributed to all the doctors of the island. The demand for vaccine grew but part of the population was still against vaccination. For instance, it was a problem to get people to accept the vaccine if they did not know the person it came from. The assembly was not satisfied with the vaccine institute's results. Even though a commission proved that the vaccine institute had been successful in spreading the vaccine, it was closed down in 1822. This was possibly one of the reasons why the island was ravaged by a devastating smallpox epidemic in 1831.[678]

The great smallpox epidemic in the Caribbean in 1819 created an immense interest in vaccination in the mainland colony of Demerara-Essequibo. However, the colony's Court of Policy was of the opinion that almost all planters had vaccinated their enslaved workers and so it was not necessary to impose vaccination by law. Despite the court's decision, large parts of the population were in fact not vaccinated. The colony's administration limited its activities to encouraging the population to be vaccinated, and to public vaccinations and the establishment of a smallpox hospital in the capital. Following the next great smallpox epidemic in 1827, which wreaked havoc among the Afro-Caribbean populations in the British West Indian island colonies, Demerara-Essequibo also established a quarantine system for ships.[679]

In one single British island colony, however, the efforts to promote vaccination were much more extensive. In March 1819, the Trinidadian government ordered the compulsory vaccination of the entire population. In the capital Port of Spain, the doctors and the mayor inspected all households before issuing the

676 Handler, *Africans and Creoles* (unpublished manuscript).
677 Higman, *Slave Populations*, 278–79.
678 Sheridan, *Doctors and Slaves*, 258–62.
679 Higman, *Slave Populations*, 279–80.

required certificates of vaccination. As a result, the number of smallpox cases dropped rapidly but there was still public scepticism towards vaccination. The year 1819 also saw the establishment of a vaccine institute and a new ordinance proclaiming that all new arrivals to the colony, especially enslaved workers, were to be vaccinated within one week of arrival. All imported enslaved workers had to have a certificate of vaccination. In addition, all newborn babies had to be vaccinated within the first month after birth. The vaccine institute remained in existence after emancipation in 1834, but during the 1830s problems developed because ex-slaves did not have their children vaccinated.[680]

When smallpox returned to Barbados in 1819, the assembly decided to send away all infected ships and the population was encouraged to vaccinate, yet no vaccine institute was established. Grenada, St Vincent, Dominica, Antigua, St Kitts, and the Bahamas all suffered from a lack of vaccine institutes in the latter part of the 1820s and the beginning of the 1830s. Large parts of the population in these islands remained unvaccinated partly due to the lack of vaccine and partly because the owners of enslaved workers were reluctant to spend money on vaccination when it was not statutory. This and the uncontrolled movement of people probably contributed to the higher mortality in the smaller colonies.[681]

Richard Sheridan concludes that variolation and vaccination had a great influence on limiting the mortality rate among enslaved workers in the Caribbean.[682] Barry W. Higman agrees that the use of variolation and vaccination were the medical improvements that had the greatest impact on the health of the enslaved, but based on his extensive demographic investigations he concludes that the two procedures were not successful in significantly extending the lifespan of the enslaved.[683] This argument is also supported by Jerome Handler.[684]

The French West Indies

Until the proclamation of the Republic of Haiti in 1804, slavery and variolation developed together in the French colony of St Domingue.[685] Variolation started as early as 1725 and by 1775 it was widespread in the colony.[686] Smallpox

680 Higman, *Slave Populations*, 279–80.
681 Higman, *Slave Populations*, 279–80.
682 Sheridan, *Doctors and Slaves*, 267.
683 Higman, *Slave Populations*, 261.
684 Handler, 'Slave Medicine', 74, 82.
685 Karol Kovalovich Weaver, 'The Enslaved Healers of Eighteenth-Century Saint Domingue', *Bulletin of the History of Medicine* 76 (2002), 452–53.
686 Dominique Taffin, *Maladies et medicine á la Guadeloupe au XIXe siècle* (unpublished thesis, Ecole nationale des Chartes, Paris, 1985), 672.

claimed many victims and so variolation became a standard procedure on the plantations for the newly arrived enslaved workers and the newly born.[687]

On the island of Guadeloupe, variolation was not as widespread as it had been on St Domingue, which had a larger number of doctors. It was not until the arrival of fugitive doctors from the rebellion on St Domingue that variolation became a common phenomenon on Guadeloupe. This might also be the reason why the variolation procedure was not abandoned until 1820, many years after the arrival of vaccination. The vaccine arrived on Guadeloupe in 1802 either on French ships or via the USA. From 1804, the diffusion accelerated but until 1819 it was carried out on the basis of private initiative. After the end of the British occupation during the Napoleonic Wars (1810–16), the medical authorities on the island tried to gain control of the vaccination and make it their domain.[688] As early as 1818, the island's Council of Health claimed that vaccination was in common usage on the island and that accordingly smallpox was a rare occurrence. However, this was not supported by the facts and the following year a smallpox epidemic devastated Guadeloupe.[689] As a result, vaccine committees were established in both of the island's cities. The committees were to be in charge of vaccination and keep lists of all vaccinated individuals. They also examined all vaccinators according to the vaccination instructions issued by the vaccination committee in Paris.[690]

Despite these efforts, however, the spread of vaccination encountered great obstacles. First, it was difficult to secure a reliable source of new vaccine. The vaccine that was sent out from France was often ineffective on arrival. Therefore, the vaccinators had to limit the number vaccinated so that there would always be a group of new 'vaccine subjects' to carry on the chain of infection from arm to arm.[691] To this was added the general reluctance of the Creole population. When an epidemic was looming there was no shortage of people wanting to be vaccinated, but generally it was difficult to find enough volunteers. Often the vaccinated did not return for the follow-up check and would not allow vaccine matter to be extracted from their pustules for the next patient to be vaccinated. In their opinion, this would remove the protection given to them by the vaccination. The initial enthusiasm for the vaccination evaporated as smallpox did

687 Weaver, 'The Enslaved Healers', 452–53.
688 Taffin, *Maladies et medicine*. 677.
689 Taffin, *Maladies et medicine*, 687.
690 Taffin, *Maladies et medicine*, 671–74.
691 Taffin, *Maladies et medicine*, 676–77.

not reappear and as the problems of sustaining the vaccine grew. It was often the parents and especially the Euro-Caribbean parents who caused trouble. In their opinion, the source of the vaccine was not clean enough. Accordingly, it was Afro-Caribbean children, free and unfree, who were the first to be vaccinated. On that basis, it was possible to establish an arm-to-arm chain of vaccination but it did not solve the problem. The Euro-Caribbean parents argued that Afro-Caribbean children were not completely healthy and so they wanted their own children to be vaccinated with matter from a Euro-Caribbean child. Because of these endless difficulties vaccinations tailed off in 1838.[692]

Regardless of the many obstacles, vaccination was after all carried out with some success on Guadeloupe in the years following the 1819 epidemic. In contrast to the situation in many of the neighbouring islands at the time, Guadeloupe saw no smallpox epidemics for many years. In 1822, a vaccine institute was established with the aim of maintaining the vaccine but there were still great problems sustaining the live vaccine and new vaccine had to be requisitioned from other islands, among them St Thomas. However, because of a general feeling of security, the vaccination activities declined and by the time of the smallpox epidemic in 1849, the authorities had to recognise an almost total lack of previous vaccination.[693]

On Martinique, the development was largely similar to the one on Guadeloupe. Here vaccination was also introduced in 1803. In 1817, after the end of the British occupation, the authorities ordered the establishment of vaccination committees. Their task was the same as on Guadeloupe. However, the inhabitants continued to inoculate with natural smallpox probably due to the difficulties of obtaining live vaccine. Between 1803 and 1818, four smallpox epidemics swept the island. The difficulties of convincing the inhabitants of the efficiency of the vaccine and reluctant parents who refused to let their children be vaccinated were the same as on Guadeloupe. To sustain the vaccination programme, a vaccine institute was established and it was decreed that all children in educational facilities and orphanages had to be vaccinated. At the same time, the vaccination of the public was divided between the health officers (*Officier de Santé*) at the hospitals who vaccinated in the cities and the doctors in private practice who vaccinated in the countryside. Every third month the vaccination committee reported the number of vaccinated individuals. However, despite these

692 Taffin, *Maladies et medicine*, 681–84.
693 Taffin, *Maladies et medicine*, 685–88.

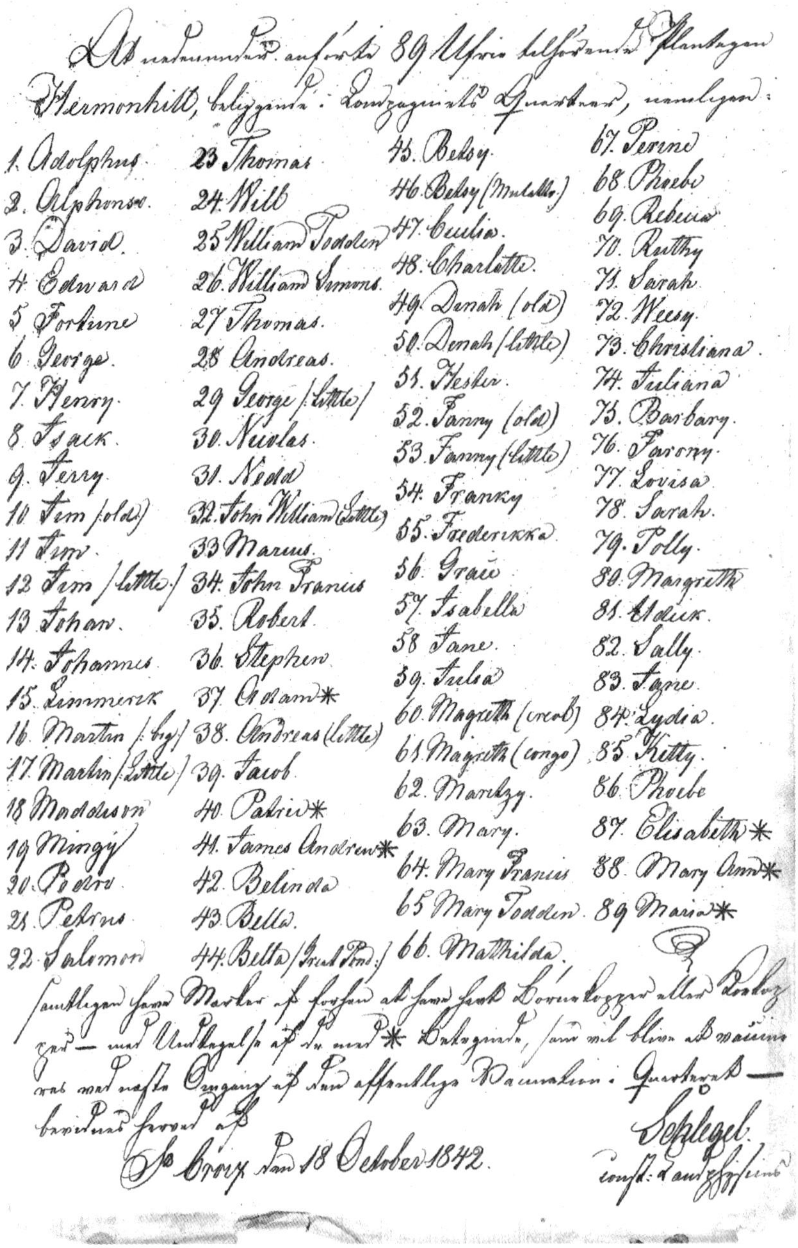

1. Adolphus
2. Alphonso
3. David
4. Edward
5. Fortune
6. George
7. Henry
8. Isack
9. Jerry
10. Jem (old)
11. Jim
12. Jem (little)
13. Johan
14. Johannes
15. Limmerick
16. Martin (big)
17. Martin (little)
18. Maddison
19. Mingy
20. Pedro
21. Petrus
22. Salomon
23. Thomas
24. Will
25. William Todden
26. William Simons
27. Thomas
28. Andreas
29. George (little)
30. Nicolas
31. Nedd
32. John William (little)
33. Marcus
34. John Francis
35. Robert
36. Stephen
37. Adam *
38. Andreas (little)
39. Jacob
40. Patric *
41. James Andrew *
42. Belinda
43. Bella
44. Bella (...)
45. Betsy
46. Betsy (Mulatto)
47. Cecilia
48. Charlotte
49. Dinah (old)
50. Dinah (little)
51. Hester
52. Fanny (old)
53. Fanny (little)
54. Franky
55. Frederikka
56. Grace
57. Isabella
58. Jane
59. Julia
60. Magreth (creol)
61. Magreth (congo)
62. Maritzy
63. Mary
64. Mary Francis
65. Mary Todden
66. Matthilda
67. Perine
68. Phoebe
69. Rebecca
70. Ruthy
71. Sarah
72. Weesy
73. Christiana
74. Juliana
75. Barbary
76. Farony
77. Lovisa
78. Sarah
79. Polly
80. Margrethe
81. Aldick
82. Sally
83. Jane
84. Lydia
85. Ketty
86. Phoebe
87. Elisabeth *
88. Mary Ann *
89. Maria *

St Croix den 18 October 1842.

Schlegel

Fig. 4.6: Vaccination list from the royal plantation Hermon Hill, 18 October 1842. The names marked with a asterisk (*) indicate that the enslaved worker in question still needs to be vaccinated. Issuing officer was interim landfysikus P.E.W. Schlegel. DNA, WILA, no. 46.17.33.

efforts, the government did not succeed in convincing the population of the effectiveness of vaccination and so vaccination was not common on the island. Consequently, in 1831 it was an epidemic of smallpox and not the usual suspect of dysentery that caused the greatest number of deaths.[694] In 1836/7 and again in 1848 new epidemics of smallpox swept the island.[695]

Conclusion

With respect to the impact of the efforts of the administration on St Croix on the fight against smallpox a clear development is evident. Until the use of vaccination, the administration's efforts towards smallpox were no different from those taken towards other contagious diseases. The administration attempted to establish protection through quarantine measures but did not involve itself with variolation with natural smallpox. This was a private matter for the owners of enslaved workers. The discovery of vaccination did not at first change this state of affairs. Even if the health authorities in Denmark dispatched vaccine to the islands it was a doctor in private practice who managed to bring the live vaccine from North America in 1803. In the following years, local doctors seem to have continued vaccination as part of their private practice. This might be due to the somewhat unstable circumstances surrounding the British occupation of the islands, but in any case the landfysikus and the public health service did not get involved until 1809, and then with the strong support of the occupation authorities. How many individuals were actually vaccinated during these years is unknown and neither do we know if variolation with natural smallpox continued.

From 1809 to 1818, and so up to the restoration of the Danish administration, there is a lacuna in the existing materials on the development of the vaccination effort. However, it is evident that the public vaccination system, which was developed in 1818 and expanded through to 1848, was not modelled on a British system but shows clear affinities with the metropolitan Danish system. Yet, at the same time, the Danish West Indian system was also unique because of its effective control of the vaccination of the enslaved workers. The landfysikus, the local colonial administration, the local Commission of Health and the quarantine measures all worked together to form an effective system of barriers within barriers. As stated above, no devastating smallpox epidemics appeared

694 Leti, *Santé et société*, 412–20.
695 Leti, *Santé et société*, 122.

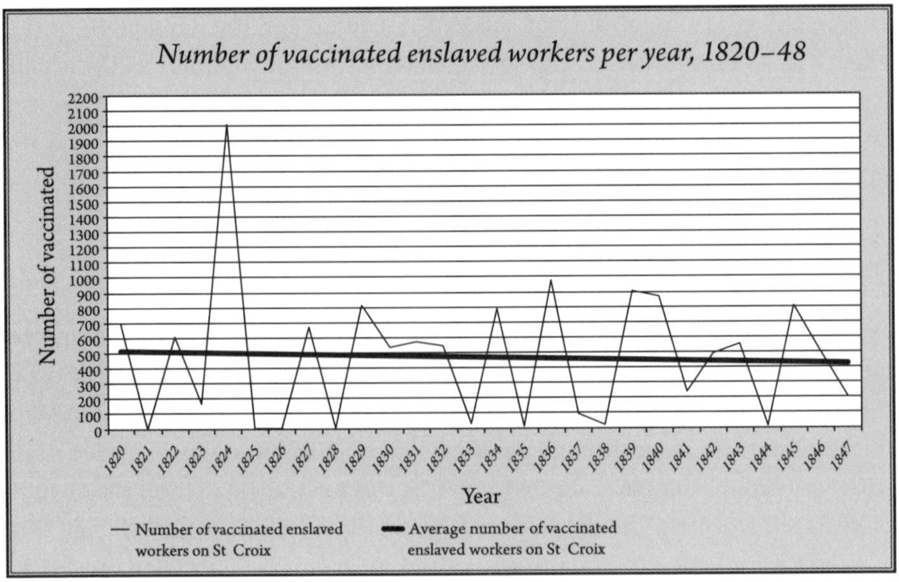

Fig. 4.7. Source: Table 4.4.

on St Croix from the introduction of vaccination in 1803 up to 1848. The island was often threatened by epidemics from the outside and several times smallpox turned up on the island itself but the number of infected and dead was always extremely limited.

So, the measures against smallpox seem to have worked together exceptionally well, but what was the significance of vaccination in this positive result? Fortunately, the registration of all vaccinated individuals makes it possible to establish a better picture of just how great the vaccination effort was.

As can be seen from Fig. 4.7 the number of vaccinated enslaved workers fluctuated significantly from year to year. Generally, it seems that a year with a high number of vaccinations (usually 500–1,000) was often followed by a year with a very low number (fewer than 100). This pattern was most likely due to two factors. First, the population on St Croix was not large enough to support a continuous chain of infection from arm to arm. As early as 1818 just about all adult inhabitants seem to have been protected against smallpox because of naturally acquired immunity, variolation or vaccination. Accordingly, it was in fact only each year's newly born enslaved children who required vaccination and their numbers were generally estimated at 400–500 per year. Because of the limited number of vaccinations, the landfysikus often ran out of vaccine, which then had to be brought in from the outside with the associated problems of keeping it alive during transport. The second factor was that the free population only allowed their children and enslaved workers to be vaccinated when an epidemic was imminent. This must have caused some minor fluctuations in the numbers of people vaccinated. Only the year of 1824 deviated from the pattern with the unusually high number of 2,011 vaccinated. This variation must be explained partly by the royal order of 25 May 1824 to revaccinate all suspicious cases and partly by the exemption allowing all doctors in private practice to vaccinate enslaved workers.

Despite the great yearly variation in the number of vaccinated enslaved workers, it is striking that the linear tendency line in the chart indicates the average yearly number to be about 500 individuals falling towards 400 at the end of the period. This corresponds to the estimated number of enslaved children born per year. Hence, it seems that vaccination did cover just about all enslaved children born in a particular year, yet occasionally with a delay of one year. The conclusion must be that between 1820 and 1848 vaccination achieved a very high coverage on St Croix and that this was the main reason for the very few incidents of smallpox. The conclusion is supported by the above description of events on St Croix where incidents of smallpox penetrating the system of quarantine and the ensuing outbreaks of smallpox on the island itself only caused very few infections and deaths.

The state-controlled vaccination system on St Croix, which was based on the Danish model and with the specific aim of protecting the enslaved workers against smallpox, worked as intended despite many practical difficulties. However, the success of the system was dependent on a high level of government control and exercise of power over the enslaved workers who were also private property. Prior to 1803, the administration had avoided interfering with the planters' rights to private property. With the establishment of the vaccination system, the Danish West Indian administration appropriated a part of the control of the health of the enslaved workers through the health regulations. Whereas free citizens were only coerced indirectly, the owners of enslaved workers were not asked if they wanted to have their slaves vaccinated. The administration perceived vaccination to be a benefit to the public, but as this boon was only possible if everyone participated there was no room for discussion. It is a fact, however, that the administration established a vaccination system with the tightest controls possible while it made inroads into the planters' freedom. This approach ensured the efficiency and success of the vaccination programme.

In this negotiation of power between the administration and the planters, the enslaved workers were not heard. They were vaccinated, inspected and registered but their understandings of and attitudes towards vaccination are, regrettably, not visible anywhere at all in the archival documents from the Danish West Indies. Still, running the risk of arguing ex silencio, one could hypothesise that the reason for this absolute silence was that the vaccination procedure was very similar to variolation, which was familiar to the enslaved, perhaps even from their ancestral West Africa.

If we compare the development of vaccination in the Danish West Indies with its development in the British and French West Indies many similarities are identifiable. It seems that vaccination originally came to all colonies as a private initiative riding on a wave of enthusiasm among private 'enlightened' individuals. All colonies experienced the same problem of keeping the vaccine matter alive and there were attempts to establish systems to maintain the vaccine, preferably chains of infection from arm to arm. However, this rarely met with success and often new vaccine had to be brought in from other colonies, from the USA or from Europe with the ensuing problems of sustaining the vaccine during transport. In the first years, administrators in all colonies were reluctant to force vaccination on their inhabitants. In the British and French West Indies, the population harboured a common scepticism towards vaccination. The problems did not stop when people were vaccinated as they often failed to return for the important follow-up check. In most colonies (except Barbados and Jamaica), the great epidemic of 1818/19 seems to have been a turning point because drastic improvements and reorganisations were subsequently initiated in relation to the vaccination systems. A contributing factor behind this development was undoubtedly the end of the Napoleonic Wars and their sequels in the Caribbean area.

Efforts to evaluate the success of the various colonies in using vaccination (and quarantine) to ward off smallpox suggest that it was only in some parts of the Danish and British West Indies that citizens and their enslaved workers were properly protected. In the French West Indies and most of the British West Indian colonies, the majority of the population remained unvaccinated and so the attempt to ward off devastating smallpox epidemics was not successful. Based on the materials presented here, the success of vaccination in the colonies mentioned seems to be based on two factors. Most important was statutory vaccination supported by an efficient apparatus of state control (certificates and registers) and an efficient quarantine system for ships. On St

Croix, and apparently on Trinidad too, this system was the prerequisite for an effective vaccination programme. However, for the system to work efficiently another factor was also crucial, namely the colony's geography. It is obviously far easier to distribute and control vaccination on a relatively small and flat island with a well-developed network of roads such as St Croix than on larger, mountainous islands like Jamaica or Guadeloupe or in a densely forested landscape of rivers and swamps like Demerara-Essequibo. On Trinidad, all inhabited areas were accessible by ship and as colonisation did not accelerate until after the British takeover in 1797 the administrators had the advantage of being able to vaccinate all enslaved workers, and so the majority of the population, when they arrived. In other words, the combination of a strong central administration and geographical circumstances afforded St Croix an unusual level of protection against smallpox. The same protection was not extended to the other Danish West Indian islands of St Thomas and St John because of their different commercial focus. The Danish West Indian vaccination system was rooted in the Danish laws of general vaccination and in the physiocratic and cameralistic administrational traditions of the absolutist Danish-Norwegian monarchy, which meant that the regulations of vaccination on St Croix were stricter than in almost any other Caribbean colony. The geographical circumstances and the apparent support from the planters allowed the vaccination system on St Croix to be more efficient than elsewhere in the Caribbean. The fundamental aim of this effort was to protect the valuable enslaved workers against the lethal smallpox and so to preserve the livelihood of the colony.

Midwives, Obstetrics and Births[696]

Like the system of smallpox vaccination, the policies concerning midwifery developed on St Croix between 1803 and 1848 also formed a hybrid colonial system. No other Caribbean colony seems to have had a similar system of government-sanctioned training and authorisation of enslaved women as plantation midwives. In the following, I will examine the efforts to construct this system and the multiple clashes of power and culture involved in it. The central argument is that in early nineteenth-century Cruzian society, midwifery among

696 Part of this chapter has previously been published in the article '"For the Benefit of the Planters and the Benefit of Mankind": The Struggle to Control Midwives and Obstetrics on St Croix, Danish West Indies, 1818–1848', in *Health and Medicine in the Circum-Caribbean, 1600–1900,* ed. Juanita De Barros, Steve Palmer and David Wright (London: Routledge, 2009), 19–39. Copyright © 2009 Routledge.

the enslaved population constituted a contested field of medicine. Neither the colonial administration nor the planters or the enslaved workers had complete control of practices and perceptions. Consequently, the field of midwifery was the scene of a continual negotiation of power.

The System of Midwifery in the Danish West Indies

In the period 1803–48, the Danish administration on the island of St Croix set out to expand and develop the system of midwives. The aim was to improve the care of the labouring enslaved women and their newborn babies. In theory, the system was designed like a hierarchical pyramid. The top was made up of two royally appointed and state-employed midwives stationed in each of the towns of Christiansted and Frederiksted. This arrangement had existed since 1768 when the first two midwives received licences as royal midwives.[697] In the hierarchy of the Danish West Indian colonial health system, the royal midwives were under the supervision and control of the landfysikus. They were always trained at Den Kongelige Fødsels- og Plejestiftelse (the Royal Birth and Nursing Foundation) in Copenhagen and of Danish extraction. Their licences were exact copies of midwives' licences in Denmark and so the obligations listed in them were the same. First of all the midwives were required to serve all women on St Croix – the poor for free and the wealthy at a fixed moderate rate. The enslaved were not mentioned in the licence, which is only natural as it was based on conditions in Denmark. However, the two royal midwives were obviously not able to serve the thousands of enslaved women on St Croix, and accordingly the following obligation in the licence becomes of interest:

> to assign to themselves [i.e. the royal midwives] such local subjects whom they might find suitable and willing and whom, when in time they become sufficiently capable to pass examination by the landfysikus, may also be allowed to practise as midwives…[698]

In other words, the royal midwives were allowed to employ local women and train them in midwifery and if the apprentices passed examination by the landfysikus they were allowed to work as midwives. However, apparently the royal

697 DNA, WILA, no. 3.40, Register of instructions, 1723–1784. Kirstine Nyestæd and Kirstine Stær.

698 DNA, WILA, no. 3.40. Original Danish text: '… at adjungere sig saadanne Subjecta sammestæds, som de dertil maatte finde beqvemme og villige, hvilke, naar de med Tiden bliver dygtige nock til at udstaae af Landphysico den sædvanlige Examen, ogsaa maae tillades at practicere som Jordemødre…'.

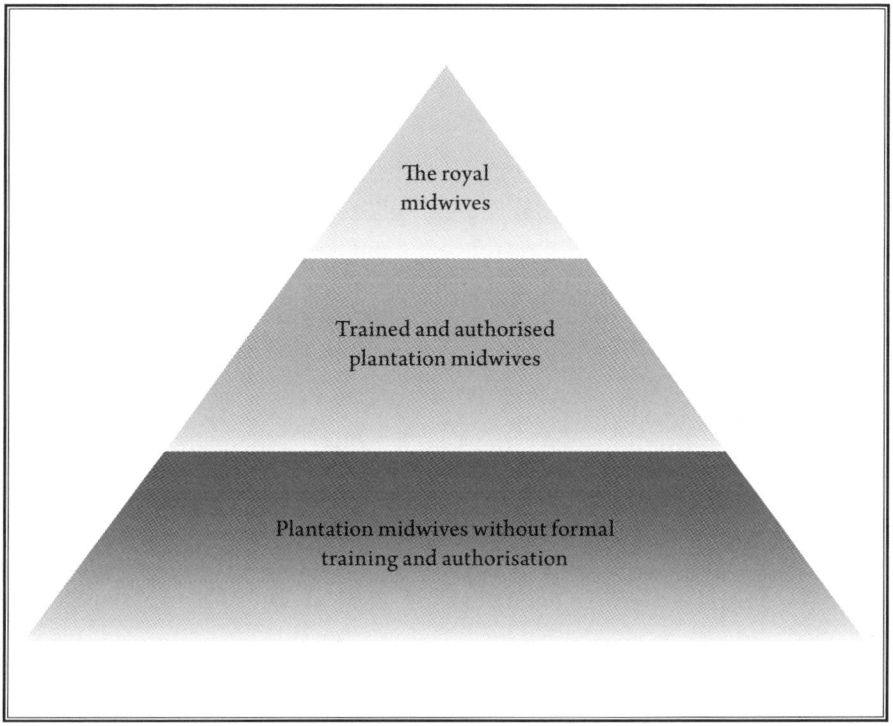

Fig. 4.8: The hierarchy of midwives in the Danish West Indies.

midwives did not observe this obligation in the years prior to 1803. In that year, landfysikus J.M.F. Keutsch wrote in the first medical report from the Danish West Indies that in the countryside of St Croix (i.e. on the plantations) births were only attended by old, untrained enslaved women. To alleviate this condition, Keutsch suggested that the royal midwives, and possibly the landfysikus too, undertook the task of training six to eight enslaved women as plantation midwives.[699] Two years later the prominent St Croix planter Peter Lotharius Oxholm (1753–1827)[700] expanded on this view by claiming that it was these old, untrained, enslaved midwives who were responsible for the high mortality among the newborn enslaved children. According to Oxholm, the untrained plantation midwives did no harm in 'natural births', i.e. births without com-

699 DNA, DC, no. G125C. Medical report, 1804. J.M.F. Keutsch.
700 Bricka, *Dansk biografisk Lexikon* XII, 507–8.

plications, but in difficult cases they did not call on the plantation doctor or a trained midwife fast enough. Furthermore, Oxholm added, the plantation midwives often tried to get the baby out by force, which caused the death of the child.[701]

The call to train enslaved plantation midwives does not seem to have been followed by any action until after the second British occupation ended in 1815 and the issuance of *Instruks for Stifts- og Landphysici* (Instructions for Physicians of Dioceses and Lands) of 4 March 1818. These instructions required that 'in places where no examined midwife is to be found', i.e. on the plantations, the landfysikus had to see to it that untrained midwives obtained the necessary guidance.[702] During the 1820s, the royal midwives began to apprentice young enslaved women from the plantations of St Croix.[703] The planters funded the training individually and afterwards the apprentices returned to their home plantations and took over as plantation midwives. The duration of the apprenticeship seems to have been two to three years during which time the apprentice assisted the royal midwife in her daily work.[704] At the end of the apprenticeship, the royal midwife received a fee for the apprenticeship[705] and the landfysikus and another local authorised doctor examined the apprentice.[706] If she passed the exam, the apprentice was authorised as a plantation midwife. These trained and authorised plantation midwives came to form an intermediate stratum in the hierarchy of midwives.

However, not all plantations obtained a formally trained and authorised plantation midwife – quite the contrary in fact. In the medical reports from the 1820s and onwards the doctors in private practice commented in unison that nearly all plantations had an enslaved woman who assisted as midwife but that only a few of them had received formal training with royal midwives or doctors.[707] So these plantation midwives without training and authorisation remained the third (lowest) and numerically largest stratum in the hierarchy of midwives.

From the years prior to 1848 there exists no precise information as to how

701 Oxholm, *Nogle Anmærkninger*, 27.

702 Schou, *Chronologisk Register*, section XVIII, 38. Original Danish text: 'Paa de Steder, hvor ingen examinerede Giordemødre haves eller kan faaes…'.

703 DNA, BH, Med. rep., Danish West Indies, 1826.

704 DNA, BH, Med. rep., Danish West Indies, 1837.

705 DNA, WILA, no. 10.2.1. 31 May, 1837. DNA, DSD, no. 1129. Estate Longford, 1828.

706 DNA, BH, Med. rep., Danish West Indies, 1826, 1844.

707 DNA, BH, Med. rep., Danish West Indies, 1825, 1826, 1828, 1829, 1830, 1834, 1835, 1836, 1837, 1838, 1844, 1846.

many plantation midwives there were on St Croix or what kind of training they had received. However, a register from 1852 shows that in the western jurisdiction of Frederiksted (town and plantations) there were twenty-five midwives of whom four were trained by a royal midwife or doctor.[708] A comparable register from 1864 shows that in the central district of the island (Kingshill) there were eight plantations with midwives trained and examined by royal midwives and authorised doctors, twenty-nine plantations with midwives without formal training and thirty-eight plantations with no midwife at all. Finally, a third register from the same year shows that in the eastern town of Christiansted there were four midwives examined by doctors and in the country district of Christiansted there were a total of eleven plantation midwives none of whom were formally trained.[709] Based on this evidence it is clear that in the years following emancipation only about a fifth of all plantation midwives in the three districts of St Croix had received formal training or been examined. As previously mentioned the medical reports from the doctors in private practice give no reason to believe that the situation was any better before the emancipation.

In 1826, the interim landfysikus Schlegel noted in his medical report that the planters were less inclined than previously to apprentice their bondswomen to the royal midwives. In Schlegel's opinion legislation would not have any effect on this, but he called for the royal plantations to set a good example by sending their enslaved midwives for training.[710] To what extent the private leaseholders of the royal plantations followed this call is not clear, yet it is certain that some of the royal plantations had an enslaved woman registered as a 'midwife'.[711] So, she was not just an ordinary 'sick-nurse' who could be found at any plantation hospital. However, only a few of the midwives on the royal plantations were formally trained.[712]

Many reasons can be suggested for the decreasing number of apprentices with the royal midwives. However, in view of the fact that in the period between around 1820 and 1848 the plantations on St Croix suffered from increasing economic strain due to bad harvests, falling sugar prices and lack of manpower, the

708 NARA, RG55, Entry 82, Box 220.

709 NARA, RG55, Entry 82, Box 319.

710 DNA, BH, Med. rep., Danish West Indies, 1826.

711 DNA, WILA, no. 46.21, Estate Retreat, 1839. DNA, WILA, no. 46.21, Estate Work and Rest, 1833. DNA, WILA, no. 46.17.45, Estate Longford, 1843, 1846. DNA, WILA, no. 46.17.32, Estate Hermon Hill, 1835. NARA, RG55, Entry 1109, Box 2435, Estate Jolly Hill, 1840. DNA, BH, Med. rep., Danish West Indies, 1826. Appendix to the medical report by landfysikus Schlegel.

712 DNA, DSD, no. 1129. Estate Longford, 1828. DNA, WILA, no. 46.17.32, Estate Hermon Hill, 1835.

planters had strong economic motives for keeping all hands on the plantation and save the fee for an apprenticeship with the royal midwife. Yet, the planters' expenses from having one enslaved woman trained and examined were negligible compared to what they spent each year on doctors' bills, the plantation hospital, and other health-related expenses.[713] Naturally, it was cheaper in the short run to neglect the training of a midwife and carry on the tradition of relying on the experience of old enslaved women – especially since no law prohibited it. Another contributing cause might have been the problem of making the enslaved women accept the European birth practices introduced by the trained midwives. Later we shall see that these practices of European obstetric science went against the enslaved women's traditional notions of taboos and rites of passage during labour.

On plantations that did not have a midwife at all, there were several ways of acquiring one. If the plantation was situated near one of the towns, the royal midwife could be called in. A cheaper alternative was to fetch one of the free coloured townswomen who seem to have practised midwifery as a business on the side.[714] A third possibility was to hire or borrow a midwife from a neighbouring plantation in the same way that planters hired or borrowed enslaved men trained in various trades.[715] In the very few instances when this hired plantation midwife was trained she often carried out midwifery on several plantations in the neighbourhood.[716] The use of external midwives is revealed in account books from several plantations. It is not possible to discern if the midwives in question were royal midwives or plantation midwives from the neighbouring plantations but the latter case is the more likely. Only very rarely do the accounts show a doctor functioning as an accoucheur (man-midwife) among the enslaved.[717]

Concerning the royal plantations it is curious that the government body in charge of them, the *Likvidationskommissionen* (The Liquidation Commission), did not heed landfysikus Schlegel's call to make a good example of them by stipulating a demand for the training and examination of plantation midwives in the lease contracts. In fact, the reproductive field is absolutely absent in the lease contracts and regulations despite the administration's interest in the field

713 DNA, DSD, no. 1129. Accounts for 1828.
714 DNA, BH, Med. rep., Danish West Indies, 1839, 1842, 1846.
715 DNA, BH, Med. rep., Danish West Indies, 1825, 1826.
716 DNA, BH, Med. rep., Danish West Indies, 1844.
717 NARA, RG55, Entry 1109, box 2438, Estate Mount Victory, 1828.

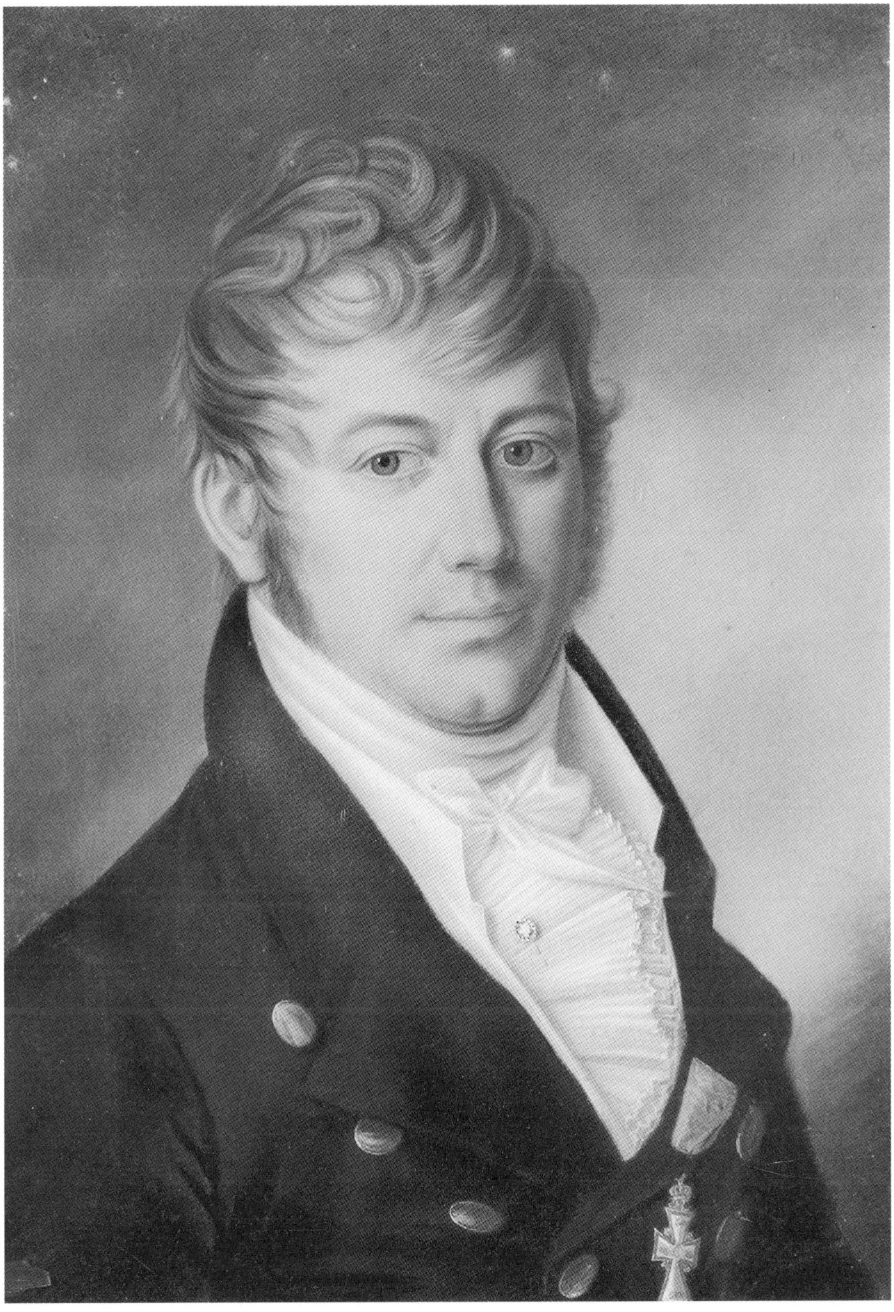

Fig. 4.9: Painting of interim landfysikus and garrison surgeon in Christiansted, Poul Elias Wintmöhl Schlegel. Artist unknown, undated, Danish National Museum, Copenhagen, Denmark.

in these years. Among other approaches in the reproductive field that the *Likvidationskommissionen* might have tried to use to improve fertility and the survival of newborn babies was rewarding mothers by reducing their workload or by offering them gifts. In the last years of the 1820s, Lieutenant Brady described the use of this reward system on private plantations on St Croix:

> At births and deaths, the families in which they occur generally receive about ten pounds of sugar and two gallons of rum. At [Estate Mannings Bay] and upon some other estates, lying-in women receive two bottles of Madeira wine, and other comforts.[718]

It is not clear how common it was to reward enslaved mothers but it does not seem to have been practised on the royal plantations.

The Danish Model

Based on the above it is evident that the local colonial administration's attempts to structure the system of midwifery in the Danish West Indies were modelled on the system in Denmark. In the period 1803–48, the Danish system of midwifery developed into a fine-meshed and efficient system, which covered all of Denmark and had a significant impact on the lowering of neonatal mortality. The system was based on the Midwife Ordinance of 21 November 1810, which applied to the kingdom of Denmark (and to the kingdom of Norway until its independence from Denmark in 1814) but not to the Danish West Indies. Following this ordinance, Denmark was subdivided into midwife districts with one royal midwife in each district. In 1850, there were 686 such districts in Denmark outside Copenhagen.[719] All state-employed royal midwives were trained at the Royal Birth and Nursing Foundation in Copenhagen, but if no trained midwife was to be found in a district a local woman could be trained and authorised by the local landfysikus. This midwife was then put in charge of midwifery in the district while another local woman was chosen to be sent for training in Copenhagen. If a woman in labour chose to use an unauthorised midwife, she still had to pay a fixed fee to the royal midwife in the district. Finally, in cases of difficult labour, the royal midwife was obliged to call for her superior, the landfysikus.[720]

718 Highfield, *Observations*, 13.

719 Anne Løkke, 'Did Midwives Matter? 1787–1845', in *Pathways of the Past: Essays in Honour of Sølvi Sogner*, ed. Hilde Sandvik, Kari Telste and Gunnar Thorvaldsen (Oslo: Novus Forlag, 2002), 71–72.

720 Petersen, *Den Danske Medicinal-Lovgivning* I, 81–89. 21 November 1810.

Accordingly, the formal and traditional role of Danish doctors was to supervise the midwives not to act as accoucheurs.[721]

On St Croix one can recognise the hierarchy of the Danish system in the division between the Danish trained state-employed royal midwives, the locally trained and authorised plantation midwives (enslaved women) and the untrained plantation midwives (enslaved women). But in contrast to the situation in Denmark where the trained state-employed midwives seem to have gradually replaced the untrained midwives by the first half of the nineteenth century,[722] the situation on St Croix does not seem to have changed after 1826. Neither the number of Danish trained and state employed midwives on the island nor the number of locally trained and authorised plantation midwives seems to have increased.

Midwives, Doctors and Administration: Conflicts of Knowledge, Training, and Economy

Despite their privileged position, the royal midwives did not have a legally sanctioned monopoly on midwifery. This created problems from the very beginning as is apparent from the fact that the royal midwives accused the unauthorised enslaved plantation midwives and free coloured midwives of stealing their customers.[723] As an example, the royal midwives Madam Biørn (Christiansted) and Madam Clark (Frederiksted) complained in 1815 to the local government that Afro-Caribbean women practised midwifery without authorisation.[724] The government rejected the complaint and declared in an ordinance of 9 December 1815 that since it was impossible for the two royal midwives to assist at all births on the island, other authorised midwives were permitted to set up business on the island if they subjected themselves to licensing for practice.[725] The authorised midwives referred to by the government were probably midwives who might arrive from Denmark, but to Danish midwives only the positions of royal midwives were economically attractive. In 1820, the government reminded the doctors of their duty to supervise all midwives[726] and to report any whose behaviour gave cause for complaint.[727] Finally, in 1821 the govern-

721 Nyland, *De praktiserende læger*, 247.
722 Løkke, 'Did Midwives Matter?', 61–66.
723 DNA, WILA, no. 3.30. Pro Memoria by midwife A.C. Lindefield in Christiansted, 1786.
724 DNA, WILA, no. 2.2.1. DNA, WILA, no. 2.16.5.
725 DNA, WILA, no. 2.1.6. p. 634.
726 DNA, WILA, no. 3.18, 1820, no. 59.
727 DNA, WILA, no. 10.2.1, 26 October 1821.

ment stressed that midwives were only allowed to practise if they had passed examination by the landfysikus or another local authorised doctor.[728] These regulations seem to have been aimed primarily at the unexamined free coloured midwives who, however, did not change their behaviour. They practised in the towns and so were the closest competitors in the royal midwives' primary market. Despite the government's attempts to address the matter the problems continued. In 1835, the royal midwife in Christiansted filed a new complaint concerning unauthorised persons practising midwifery.[729] In 1837, landfysikus Schlegel proposed a new procedure to control the practice of the plantation midwives. His idea was to put the plantation doctors in charge of issuing written certificates documenting the practical skills of plantation midwives and by whom they had been taught. If the certificate supported it, the landfysikus could issue an authorisation to practice on plantations other than the one where the midwife lived.[730] However, the government did not approve the proposal.

As is evident from the above, the problem was not to find a midwife but ascertaining what knowledge she had, or, rather, did not have. Most of the doctors entertained not the slightest confidence in the skills of the plantation midwives and described them as generally ignorant of obstetrics because only a few of them had received formal training.[731] In 1829, for instance, the interim landfysikus W.S. Jacobs powerfully expressed this attitude in his medical report:

> The state of midwifery on estates is miserable, very few having been instructed. I frequently attend with the Danish midwifes in difficult and tedious cases, and I have the same fault to find with them all, which is, that they are always in a hurry, and anxious to have the business terminated, and are too desirous of having instruments used, when only a little patience is necessary.[732]

In addition to this alleged ignorance, the plantation midwives kept stubbornly to their own traditional knowledge and practices, and they were unwilling to listen to the exhortations of the plantation doctors.[733] However, the doctors' critique was not founded solely on strictly professional concerns. Many of them were themselves accoucheurs with the wealthy Euro-Caribbean citi-

728 DNA, WILA, no. 3.18, 1821: no. 15.
729 DNA, WILA, no. 10.2.1, 23 January 1835.
730 DNA, WILA, no. 10.2.1, 31 May 1837.
731 DNA, BH, Med. rep., Danish West Indies, 1825, 1828.
732 DNA, BH, Med. rep., Danish West Indies, 1829.
733 DNA, BH, Med. rep., Danish West Indies, 1834.

zens in accordance with British traditions.[734] In other words, there was some degree of professional and economic competition between the doctors and the entire group of midwives. By contrast, the relationship between doctors and midwives in Denmark was much better. This was because legislation and tradition separated the domains of doctors and midwives and the state controlled the professional skills of both groups. Because there were many more midwives than doctors in the Danish countryside, and as the midwives enjoyed the trust of the locals, the doctors were forced to maintain a good relationship with the midwives.[735]

To counter the dangerous situations that might occur due to their lack of training, the plantation midwives were obliged to call for the plantation doctor, another accoucheur (doctor in private practice) or the royal midwife in the event of problems during labour.[736] This was in accordance with the above-mentioned instructions for landfysici in Denmark, which demanded that all midwives seek the help of a doctor if a difficult labour arose.[737] Nevertheless, calling the doctor was generally the last resort to prevent mother and child from dying. The special means which only the doctor had at his disposal was, firstly, his knowledge of how to turn the baby manually. Secondly, he had a range of instruments, which the midwives were not allowed to use. There were instruments for delivery by forceps, for surgical removal of the child through the birth passage and, as a last resort, caesarean section.[738] The first known incidence of caesarean section on St Croix was performed by the above-mentioned landfysikus Schlegel on an enslaved woman named Sophia in 1821.[739] Thirdly, the doctor disposed of pharmaceuticals like Secale cornutum, which causes uterine contractions. The enslaved women in labour were aware of the effect of the drug and asked for it if they felt the labour took too long.[740]

As previously mentioned, the idea of lowering the neonatal mortality rate through improvements in the standard of the plantation midwives had been around since it was aired by Keutsch and Oxholm at the beginning of the century. Since then, the administration had tried to 'raise the standard' by having

734 DNA, WILA, no. 10.2.1. Draft from landfysikus Schlegel, 31 May 1837.
735 Nyland, *De praktiserende læger*, 247–49.
736 DNA, BH, Med. rep., Danish West Indies, 1834, 1836, 1838.
737 Schou, *Chronologisk Register*, section XVIII, 38.
738 DNA, BH, Med. rep., Danish West Indies, 1832, 1834, 1842, 1843.
739 Poul Schlegel, 'Beskrivelse af en Sectio Cæsarea foretaget paa negerinden Sophia paa St Croix i Christiansstæds Bye d. 6te Febr. 1821', *Bibliothek for Læger* 3 (1823), 140–49.
740 DNA, BH, Med. rep., Danish West Indies, 1842.

apprentices trained in the art of midwifery. However, success had been limited. It was not until 1832 that the administration turned the idea into a real plan for action. On February 4 of that year, Governor General von Scholten sent a memorandum to landfysikus Schlegel containing a draft for a new ordinance employing ten new examined midwives on St Croix. Von Scholten explained the reason for the draft in this way:

> I will only point to one reason for this decrease [in the enslaved population], which we have been taught from experience, namely the death of the Negro children in the first 9 days after birth. The reason for this seems to be the bad midwives who, with only a few exceptions, are employed at the plantations…[741]

Accordingly, the purpose of the draft was to stop the decrease in the enslaved population by lowering the neonatal and infant mortality rates. The task of the new examined midwives was to strengthen the supervision of the women in labour on the plantations and to increase the knowledge of obstetrics through education of the plantation midwives and enslaved women. Because the government was not able to pay a salary substantial enough to attract midwives from Denmark, von Scholten wanted to select ten Afro-Caribbean women, presumably free coloured women, and send them for a one-year internship at the Royal Birth and Nursing Foundation in Copenhagen. After their examination, the midwives were to return to their new positions in the Cruzian countryside where specially built official residences would await them.[742] Von Scholten's draft shows that at this time, if not earlier, the administration was aware of the potential importance of educated midwives. The draft also shows that the administration did not focus on the longstanding and popular Euro-Caribbean presumption that it was the promiscuity and self-inflicted venereal diseases of the enslaved that caused the decrease in the population.

However, nothing came of von Scholten's draft. An analysis of the apprentices at the Royal Birth and Nursing Foundation in Copenhagen shows that in the period 1806–48 only one woman from the Danish West Indies was admit-

741 DNA, WILA, no. 10.2.1. Original text in Danish: 'Jeg vil blot udpege en Aarsag til denne Aftagen [i slavepopulationen], som Erfaringen har lært, nemlig Negerbørnenes Død i de 9 første Dage efter Fødselen. Grunden hertil maa vist søges i de daarlige Giordemødre, som paa nogle faae Undtagelser nær, haves paa Plantagerne…'.

742 DNA, WILA, no. 10.2.1.

ted and she was of Danish extraction.[743] The main reason why the draft was not made into an ordinance seems to have been that it was economically inconvenient at the time. According to a memorandum from landfysikus Schlegel dated 1837, the plantation owners were unable to pay the additional tax on each enslaved worker, which was the economic basis of von Scholten's draft. Furthermore, Schlegel pointed out, because of the emancipation of the enslaved in the British West Indies in 1834 the enslaved population in the Danish West Indies would also have to be emancipated within the foreseeable future. As it was unlikely that the former slaves would be able to afford to pay for the services of trained midwives, and so to maintain a new elaborate system of midwives, Schlegel advised against the idea. In addition to these economic arguments, Schlegel also stated a number of other reasons in support of the existing, time-honoured system of plantation midwives. First, he claimed that cases of difficult labour were rare on St Croix due to the warm climate, and that when they occurred all plantations had a doctor on contract whose services could be called upon. Second, Schlegel claimed that tetanus among the enslaved newborn babies was not as common as previously, and that this was because the system of midwifery was working quite well. Finally, he noted that the plantation midwives had the confidence of the enslaved women, which the royal midwives did not.[744] So, he hinted that the enslaved women might not accept midwives trained in European obstetrics. In conclusion, Schlegel was of the opinion that even if the system of midwifery was not perfect, it was adequate.

About ten years later, in 1846, the idea of improving the training of midwives re-emerged. This time it was the doctor of the garrison in Frederiksted, Rasmus Pedersen Worm (1786–1863),[745] who used his annual medical report to complain about the ignorance of the plantation midwives. He claimed that he was often called out to cases of enslaved women in labour, which any trained midwife would have been able to handle on her own. Therefore and 'for the benefit of the planters and the benefit of mankind', he called for more trained midwives on the island.[746]

743 DNA, The Royal Birth and Nursing Foundation. Copybook of matron's instructions and a protocol on apprentices, 1806–1838, no. 186.

744 DNA, WILA, no. 10.2.1. Draft from landfysikus Schlegel, 31 May 1837.

745 Carøe, *Den Danske lægestand*, III, 233 and V, 100.

746 DNA, BH, Med. rep., Danish West Indies, 1846. Original Danish text: '... til fordel for Plantageejerne, og til fordel for Menneskeligheden...'.

Based on the statements by von Scholten, Keutsch, Worm, Schlegel, and Jacobs a picture emerges of three conflicting views among doctors and administration as to how the system of midwifery was to be structured. Von Scholten, as a representative of the administration, and Keutsch and Worm as representatives of both administration and state doctors, were all in favour of the 'Danish' model, i.e. the training of midwives to take care of births on the plantations. Schlegel, who as landfysikus was both a doctor and member of the administration, positioned himself in a pragmatic middle position in as much as he found the existing system to be time-honoured and difficult to change due to the weak economy. Finally, the interim landfysikus Jacobs expressed the opinion of the majority of the doctors on the island, namely that the plantation midwives were incompetent. Training or improvement was not an issue at all. Seen against the background of the national affiliation which Jacobs himself and the majority of the doctors on St Croix had to the Anglophone world (Britain, its colonies and the USA) and the disdain with which doctors in this world regarded midwives at the time, it is no wonder that many of the doctors shared this view. Jacobs' temporary appointment as landfysikus did not change his opinion of midwives. No greater wonder is it that von Scholten and the doctors trained in Denmark and employed by the administration showed the same attitude as the medical establishment in Denmark, namely that midwives ought to be trained. More interesting is landfysikus Schlegel's middle position. As the premier officer for many years in the medical hierarchy of the colonial administration and as a doctor trained in Denmark, one would have expected him to support the 'Danish' model. However, he chose a pragmatic line. As mentioned, his reasons were primarily economic ones, yet it may also have been a matter of responsibility. As landfysikus for many years, Schlegel was himself responsible for the proper functioning of the midwifery system and so not likely to admit that it did not work.

In the end, the administration shelved the question of improving the system of midwifery. The reason for this reticence after the draft of 1832 may be found, if we are to believe Schlegel's account, in the events of the year 1834. This was the year of the emancipation in the British West Indies and the administration in the Danish West Indies could no longer harbour any doubt that something similar would take place in the Danish islands sooner or later. The only question was how long the emancipation could be postponed before the enslaved revolted. The administration needed time to study the British example and to see what happened afterwards so as to prepare better for emancipation and minimise the economic damages.[747] In this situation, it was not opportune, as Schlegel remarked in 1837, to experiment with costly improvements to the system of midwives, which in all probability could not be maintained after emancipation. This was especially the case since the economy of the plantations was ailing. However, Schlegel's suggestions for almost cost-free improvements of the existing system do not seem to have been heeded either.[748]

The Struggle over Births: Enslaved 'Superstition' versus Doctoral 'Science'

Descriptions of practices surrounding births and midwifery among the enslaved population on St Croix are rare. However, in the first medical report from the Danish West Indies of 1803 some of the doctors on the island described the 'superstition' in the reproductive field, which they claimed existed among the enslaved, and its harmful consequences.[749] As mentioned, child mortality among the enslaved, including neonatal and infant mortality, was high, and throughout the period doctors consistently pointed to lockjaw as the most important cause.[750] In the medical report of 1803, Drs W. Stedman and H.M. Lang listed three possible causes of 'nine day lockjaw', i.e. deaths among newborn babies caused by tetanus in the first nine days after birth: retention of meconium (child's first stools), wrong treatment of the umbilical cord, and polluted air. According to Stedman and Lang, the first cause was immaterial because all plantation midwives gave the newborn an enema of castor oil. The second factor, however, was far more serious, because of the 'superstition' connected to the umbilical cord. Stedman and Lang claimed that normally the plantation midwives did not examine the cord until the seventh or eighth day after birth, which was the reason why it generally became infected and caused nine-day lockjaw. To this can be added landfysikus J.M.F. Keutsch's description from the same medical report:

> the Negroes' nasty habit of binding the umbilicus with a thick and long string, wrapping it in a large piece of coarse linen and afterwards binding one, maybe two, coarse umbilicus-cloths around the child's abdomen as tightly as

747 Vibæk, 'Dansk Vestindien, 1755–1848', 271–73.
748 DNA, WILA, no. 10.2.1. Draft from landfysikus Schlegel, 31 May 1837.
749 DNA, DC, no. G125C. Medical report, 1804.
750 DNA, BH, Med. rep., Danish West Indies, 1830, 1831, 1838, 1846.

possible, must absolutely cause the umbilicus to become squeezed, the tissue irritated and inflamed...[751]

Landfysikus Keutsch considered this treatment of the umbilical cord to be wrong and the sole reason for the tetanus deaths. Since it was not possible to treat tetanus effectively, he asserted that one should try to prevent tetanus by bathing the child every day and gently dress the umbilicus. However, it was even more important to try to educate the enslaved midwives. Only through them could the treatment of the children be improved.

To Stedman and Lang the third factor was also connected to the 'superstition' of the enslaved. They explained that

> it is a common practice among Negroes not to allow the smallest particle of free air to be admitted into the chamber of a lying-in woman for 4 or 5 days after delivery ... That impure air is one of the most frequent causes of this complaint we are led to believe from many circumstances.[752]

To remove the impure air (miasma) Stedman and Lang recommended that all planters build a special airy maternity ward where the children could be bathed in cold water every day. They claimed that these procedures had been tested with great success on one of the plantations they attended as contracted plantation doctors.[753]

The occurrence of such maternity wards on the plantations seems to have become more common during the 1820s and 1830s. When new plantation hospitals were constructed, a maternity ward was often added. However, it cannot be said to have become a general trend.[754] This description of the situation is supported by Lieutenant Brady. Writing in the late 1820s, he described how births on some plantations took place in maternity wards and on others in the house of the woman in labour.[755] Whether women also gave birth on plantation hospitals

751 DNA, DC, no. G125C. Medical report, 1804. Landfysikus J.M.F. Keutsch. Original Danish text: '... den slemme Vane af Negerne, at binde Navlen med en tyk og lang Stræng, svøbe samme ind i et stort stykke ofte grovt Lærred, og derefter at binde et, maaske to, ligeledes grove Navle Klæder rundt om Barnets Underliv, saa tæt som det er dem mueligt, maae absolut foraarsage at Navlen bliver trykket, Vævet irriteret og inflammeret...'.

752 DNA, DC, no. G125C. Medical report, 1804. Drs Stedman and Lang.

753 DNA, DC, no. G125C. Medical report, 1804. Drs Stedman and Lang.

754 DNA, WILA, no. 3.81.690, 46.17.5, 46.17.6, 46.17.15, 46.17.30, 46.17.32, 46.17.33, 46.17.44, 46.17.45, 46.17.53, 46.17.54, 46.17.72, 46.20, 46.21. DNA, DSD, no. 1113.

755 Highfield, *Observations*, 24.

without maternity wards is not certain, but in any case they do not seem to have spent their days of maternity leave either before or after the birth in the hospital. It appears that after the birth they were excused from work for three to six weeks, during which time they stayed in their own houses.[756] Despite the new maternity wards and the good intentions of the doctors, it seems to have been difficult to make the enslaved women change their ways and use the new facilities. In the previously mentioned article by Oxholm from 1805, he explains that when the planters forced the enslaved women to abandon the tightly sealed slave houses or huts, they became 'dissatisfied',[757] and only slowly did they change their habits.[758] This resistance on the part of the enslaved women is especially interesting because the reactions of the enslaved to the government or private health initiatives concerning them are rarely visible in the existing source materials. The enslaved women's dissatisfaction with their removal from the closed houses or huts is understandable in the light of how the enslaved understood the newborn child. In his book *Various Remarks Collected on and about the Island of St Croix in America* (1788) Dr Johan Christian Schmidt (1728–1807) explained that the enslaved were afraid their newborn babies would be stolen or eaten by witches. If a witch had the opportunity to look into the eyes of the child during the first eight days after birth, she could steal its breath and so kill it.[759] This was possibly the reason why the house or hut had to be locked tight in the first nine days after birth. Another explanation with similar features comes from early twentieth-century West Africa (the Akan tribe of Ghana amongst others) which was the ancestral home of many slaves in the Danish West Indies. Here the newborn baby was perceived as belonging to the spirit world for eight to nine days after birth and so ritually non-existent. Not until nine days had passed were the newly born counted among humans and if the child died before then it had never existed.[760] In other words, there seem to have been perceptions of childbirth both in their ancestral West Africa and among the slaves on St Croix in the period just prior to the one dealt with here that included a tabooed rite of passage with a duration of about nine days. The above quotation from Stedman and Lang shows that a similar perception still existed in the period 1803–48. The clash between this magico-religious perception of birth and the

756 For instance DNA, WILA, no. 45.17.55, 45.17.5.
757 The Danish word is *misfornøjede* which translates as 'displeased' or 'dissatisfied'.
758 Oxholm, *Nogle Anmærkninger*, 27.
759 Schmidt, *Various Remarks*, 29.
760 Barbara Bush, *Slave Women in Caribbean Society, 1650–1838* (London: James Curry Ltd., 1990), 146.

newborn child on one side and on the other the physiological European perception of the diseases of the newborn child and the treatment of nine-day lockjaw was inevitable.

Judging from this, it seems to have been necessary for the planters, at least initially, to force the enslaved women to use the maternity wards. By depositing the women in the wards, they achieved two goals: removing the women from the village of the enslaved, where 'superstition' allegedly ruled with destructive force, and securing the conditions and facilities for treatment demanded by the doctors. In addition, it became easier for doctors and managers to monitor and control both the pregnant women and those in labour, as well as the suspicious activities of the plantation midwives. On this basis, it is possible to view enslaved births as a field in which a conflict between an Afro-Caribbean and a European perception and practice of health was played out. As mentioned earlier, this conflict was not located exclusively in the maternity wards but also took place between the European doctors and royal midwives on the one side and the suspicious unexamined midwives in alliance with women in confinement on the other. Judging from the slowly increasing number of maternity wards on the plantations it would appear plausible that the victors in this struggle were the doctors and by extension European medical science. However, as the unexamined plantation midwife was still in charge of the large majority of births among the enslaved it is not evident that the practices surrounding births became European because some enslaved women were removed to maternity wards.

In this perspective, I see the resistance of the enslaved women towards the European conception and practice of birth as a part of a negotiation of power in which none of the parties were in charge but all engaged in a continuous process of compromise and change. The planter and the plantation doctor could decide the framework of the birth, i.e. the maternity ward, but the content, the practice, was far more difficult to control. Ideally, it required the plantation doctor to be in charge of the birth itself and for this to happen he had to overcome the taboos of the enslaved surrounding confinement. If the relocation of women in labour to the well-ventilated maternity ward could create 'dissatisfaction', it is beyond doubt that the doctor's takeover of the birth itself could create a high degree of 'dissatisfaction', not just among the labouring women but also among the entire enslaved population at the plantation. Notwithstanding the planters' economic calculations in relation to the doctor's salary, the risk of unrest may have been a significant reason why the plantation doctors did not take over the domain of the plantation midwives. The number of doctors on St Croix was in fact large enough to make this scenario possible but nonetheless it did not happen.[761] To avoid making the enslaved population even more uncooperative and sabotaging it was in the interest of the planter only to send for the doctor when there was no other alternative lest both mother and child were to die. In other words, a compromise had to be established between the regard for the economy of the plantation, the survival of the newly born and the views of the enslaved.

Such a compromise could have been personified by the trained and examined plantation midwife. As she was both woman, enslaved, known by the locals and trained in European obstetrics she could potentially mediate the contrasts surrounding births between the norms of the doctors and the planter on one side and the enslaved on the other.[762] However, as mentioned there were only very few of these trained plantation midwives. This can be due to the economical strategy of the planters or due to the fact that not even the trained plantation midwives had an easy job being accepted by their enslaved sisters.

Conclusion

The system of midwives on St Croix is central in answering the question of what the Danish colonial administration did to maintain and improve the health of the enslaved population. In the period 1803–48, the administration tried to expand and improve the hierarchical system of midwifery in the Danish West Indies in an effort to lower the child mortality rate. The model for both the design and the improvements was the successful system of midwives in Denmark. However, the efforts of the colonial administration were not successful, presumably because they were not supported by legislation. The training and examination of plantation midwives seem to have been opted out of in the economic strategies of the planters, possibly due to problems with integrating the European birth practices of the trained midwives into the cultural norms of the enslaved. Governor General von Scholten's proposal to train district midwives foundered on the bad financial situation in the 1830s and on the expected emancipation of the enslaved. Accordingly, it was not because the administration failed to see the possibilities of an efficient system

761 A total of approximately 600 births per year divided among 15 doctors equals about 40 births per doctor per year. In addition, the royal midwives took care of births.

762 A similar mediating function between local practice and authorised obstetrics can be seen among midwives in Denmark. See: Løkke, *Døden i Barndommen*, 309–10.

of midwifery. Von Scholten's draft shows that the colonial administration was aware of the connection between child mortality and a decreasing enslaved population. So the importance of this field was not neglected because of the prevailing perception that the declining population was due to the promiscuity of the enslaved.

Because the administration's initiatives fell through, the untrained plantation midwives remained in charge of large parts of the system of midwifery. Between the untrained midwives, the doctors, and the royal midwives there existed several related conflicts of interest: economic competition, professional antagonism, and cultural opposition. The doctors' criticism of the plantation midwives' lack of abilities was not just a sign of professional egoism and jealousy but also of the cultural antagonisms between on the one hand the doctors and the Danish royal midwives and on the other the Afro-Caribbean plantation midwives. Between the royal midwives and the plantation midwives the cultural antagonisms expressed themselves in the enslaved women's lack of confidence in the former and confidence in the latter. The plantation midwife was part of the same Afro-Caribbean culture as the women in labour and she knew the traditional practices and the English-Creole language. Conversely, the royal midwives were both culturally and linguistically foreign to the world of the enslaved. Accordingly, the enslaved women's trust in their conduct of something as intimate as births almost inevitably had to be low.

The doctors met the enslaved women's distrust of the royal midwives with a similar professional and cultural distrust. They criticised the birth practices of the enslaved as being rife with harmful superstition, which raised the child mortality rate and so had a negative effect on the important growth of the enslaved population. The doctors wanted the births of the enslaved to be subject to European medical perceptions and practices, and so under the supervision of the doctors themselves. To achieve this end, the enslaved women in confinement were moved to special maternity wards. The existence of such wards in some plantation hospitals may indicate that the doctors were successful in this conflict between the two perceptions of health over the control of the place of birth. However, the birth itself was generally carried out by uneducated plantation midwives. The reason for this was not just economic considerations but also the 'dissatisfaction' in the enslaved population of the plantation which would result from the doctor taking over the domain of birth.

Midwives, Obstetrics and Births in a Comparative Caribbean Perspective

British West Indies

In the British West Indies, attempts to improve the fertility of the enslaved workers, including improvements of the system of midwives, did not gain momentum until after 1790. This happened because of the threat of a ban on the slave trade and the resulting problem of maintaining the enslaved population. The plantation doctors argued for better treatment of the mothers, including the construction of maternity wards and houses, and better education of the midwives who were generally perceived to be incompetent and negligent.[763] So in 1811, the planter Gilbert Mathison of Jamaica wrote that the plantation midwife was in most cases an old, invalid enslaved woman who could not carry out any other work. Among these midwives, it was standard practice to cut the umbilical cord with rusty scissors and neglect to change the child's clothes for the first nine days after birth. Mathison argued that if every plantation had a maternity ward and a well-educated midwife, the number of tetanus cases would no longer curb the growth of the enslaved population.[764]

However, in reality not much appears to have been done to improve the proficiency of the midwives. Around 1817, Dr John Williamson suggested in his manual of slave medicine *Medical and Miscellaneous Observations Relative to the West India Islands* that Jamaica should establish a system of public hospitals designed to educate the midwives. The suggestion was never implemented.[765] A couple of years later the previously mentioned Dr Collins suggested a course of action in his manual, which was probably more in line with the planters' way of thinking. According to Collins, the individual planter should employ a doctor or a well-educated midwife to give the plantation midwife some lessons in how to carry out births properly. The reason for the minimal instruction was that the midwife was only supposed to be in charge of the 'natural', i.e. normal, births. At the slightest anomaly, the plantation doctor should be called in and accordingly the planter had to contract the doctor for that specific purpose.[766] In some places, for instance Barbados, the doctors seem to have assumed the function of the plantation midwife completely.[767] This view of the role of the midwife in

763 Bush, *Slave Women*, 135.
764 Sheridan, *Doctors and Slaves*, 230.
765 Sheridan, *Doctors and Slaves*, 95.
766 Collins, *Practical Rules*, 137–38.
767 Higman, *Slave Populations*, 262.

relation to the doctor was in line with the view in Britain, the USA and other British colonies where doctors acting as accoucheurs increasingly displaced midwives from their domain during the eighteenth and nineteenth centuries.[768]

As part of the effort to decrease neonatal mortality, maternity wards began to be constructed on plantations. In Jamaica, maternity wards were even sanctioned by law in 1790. Nonetheless, many plantations never received a maternity ward and the enslaved women gave birth in their own houses as they had always done, which was also what they preferred.[769] In general, the enslaved women were reluctant to change their birth practices, especially if the maternity ward was located in or close to the plantation hospital.[770] Consequently, the women were often at odds with the plantation doctors who had a vested interest in locating births within their domain, the plantation hospital. However, the planters' reluctance to interfere in this conflict could indicate that they were not wholly convinced of the positive effect of the maternity wards.[771]

Instead, the planters concentrated on improving fertility by paying the mothers with money and amenities, just as in the Danish West Indies. For instance, they reduced the working hours for the pregnant enslaved women and women with small children, they provided special medical treatment for mothers and children, and gave material benefits to the enslaved who married and established a family within the plantation. The planters also tried to reduce the period of breastfeeding with the aim of enhancing the possibility of a new pregnancy, and they tried to prevent partnerships between enslaved couples from different plantations.[772]

French West Indies

During the eighteenth century, the plantation surgeons in the French West Indies also had to take over control of births at the expense of the midwives. From 1773, St Domingue had a system for training and authorisation that required the midwives to follow a special course and pass an exam to obtain a licence to practise.[773] However, this system only seems to have affected the mid-

768 Harriet Deacon, 'Midwives and Medical Men in the Cape Colony before 1860', *Journal of African History* 39 (1998) 272–74.
769 Higman, *Slave Populations*, 352.
770 John Williamson, *Medical and Miscellaneous Observations Relative to the West India Islands* II (Edinburgh, 1817), 202, 205.
771 Higman, *Slave Populations*, 349, 352.
772 Higman, *Slave Populations*, 349.
773 Weaver, *Disease in the Torrid Zone*, 161–64.

wives in the towns, because on the plantations it was still the enslaved midwife who assisted during births. Actually, it was illegal for enslaved and free coloured people to partake in any medical work (i.e. as doctors, nurses, midwives, apothecaries etc.), but on the plantations economics and geography made it impossible to fetch the plantation surgeon for all enslaved workers who were sick or in labour. Accordingly, the government suggested that the free coloured midwives should submit themselves to formalised training in obstetrics under the control of the doctors. Yet, the suggestion came to nothing.[774]

After 1804, the situation in the French West Indies is known from Guadeloupe and Martinique. On the former island, the Council of Health appointed a Dr Loreillard as a professor of obstetrics as early as 1817. He was to reside and work in the town of Basse-Terre, and all other quarters on the island were to send their midwives for a three-month course with him. However, this project came to nothing because only the surgeons from the town's hospital attended the course and soon Dr Loreillard died. In 1821, the government made a new attempt in as much as two state-employed surgeons held a three-month course, which all women who occupied themselves with obstetrics were bound to attend. It is doubtful if this system was a success, since the central government in Paris does not seem to have heard of it. In any case, the system was changed in 1829 when Paris installed a Madame Riby as a teacher of obstetrics on Guadeloupe. However, it proved difficult to maintain her teaching because of disagreements between her and the Council of Health regarding remuneration. Madame Riby taught until 1835 when the post was taken over by a Madame Lacroix, who had previously taught on Martinique. However, Madame Riby continued to work on a private basis for a while to the great annoyance of the high-handed Council of Health. Madame Lacroix was also unfortunate enough to annoy the Council of Health, which led to the closure of the training in obstetrics in 1841.[775]

On Martinique, just as in Guadeloupe, uneducated midwives and birth attendants ('*sage-femmes, ventrières et matrons*') attended most births. The doctor was only called in if it was a difficult birth or if it was necessary to do a forceps delivery. The doctors accused the midwives of being ignorant of the female anatomy, of being the cause of the high infant mortality, and of battering the labouring woman if the birth was not progressing fast enough. These midwives

774 Weaver, *Disease in the Torrid Zone*, 198–203.

775 Marie-Antoinette Menier, 'Hommes sages contre sages-femmes à la Guadeloupe (1829–1842)', *Bulletin de la Societe d'Historie de la Guadeloupe* 87–90 (1991), 4, 5, 12, 23, 26, 27.

(*ventriéres*) had been trained by the local midwife or by their mothers. In 1828, a Dr Garnot started the first state-supported training in obstetrics, which took the form of a free course for local women who could read and write. However, the course only lasted until Dr Garnot left three years later. The cause of Dr Garnot's departure was probably that his teaching met with resistance from the colonial assembly, where some members did not believe midwives were capable of understanding obstetrics.[776] In 1834, the French state sent a trained and authorised midwife, a widow Lacroix, to Martinique to teach obstetrics. However, the colonial assembly would not pay her salary, partly because the colony lacked funds and partly because the members felt there was no need for training in obstetrics, since the untrained midwives could call for a surgeon if they needed help. In the following year, the French minister in charge of the colonies suggested the establishment of free training in obstetrics on Martinique, in the same way as on Guadeloupe (Madame Riby). The argument was that the ignorance and prejudice of the Afro-Caribbean birth attendants (*matrons*) had catastrophic consequences. Nonetheless, the local authorities did not heed the advice.[777] Only in 1847 did the governor of Martinique issue an order, which authorised Madame Lacroix to start free training in obstetrics. The students were required to be able to read and write, they had to be between 18 and 35 years of age and able to give proof of a moral life. The training took two years and was supervised by the health commission of the island, which also examined the students.

In conclusion, in the period 1802–48, the vast majority of midwives in the towns and country districts of Martinique were trained in the way they had always been and not formally educated in obstetrics.[778]

Conclusion

It is evident that in the period in question the system of midwives in the Danish West Indies was subject to a much higher degree of control, organisation, and training than the systems in either the British or French West Indies. Admittedly, the majority of plantation midwives in the Danish West Indies were uneducated, just as in the British and French West Indies, but the Danish colonial administration enforced its control through the landfysikus, the doctors, and the royal midwives and repeatedly tried to ensure a better training of the plan-

776 Leti, *Santé et société*, 84–85.
777 Leti, *Santé et société*, 85–86.
778 Leti, *Santé et société*, 86–87.

tation midwives. In the British West Indies, the lack of effective training and control of midwives seems to have been almost total. In the French islands of Guadeloupe and Martinique the situation does not seem to have been much better, though the authorities made several attempts at introducing formalised training of midwives, and finally succeeded in the last years of the period.

The reason for the difference between the colonies is probably to be found in fundamental differences in the development and organisation of the midwife systems in the mother countries. From the middle of the eighteenth century, Britain saw a development where doctors/surgeons gradually took over control of the obstetric field from the midwives. There was no formalised training of midwives, legislation, or control of the field until 1902, and the doctors regarded midwives as generally ignorant.[779] In contrast, France had had a hierarchical system of state-controlled midwives since the first part of the eighteenth century. As mentioned previously, similar systems existed in Denmark and other continental and northern European countries, for instance Sweden and the Netherlands. These countries had formalised training in obstetrics for midwives supported by state control and authorisation.[780] In Denmark, craft traditions and few doctors/surgeons meant that the doctors did not begin to compete with the midwives until the latter part of the nineteenth century.[781]

However, in the Danish West Indies the medical coverage, i.e. the number of doctors, was far better than in Denmark, so it would not have been a surprise if the doctors there, of whom the majority belonged to the British professional tradition, had taken over the obstetric field following the British example. Yet, they did not. The reason was probably the planters' economic strategies in as much as a plantation midwife, trained or untrained, was always cheaper than the doctor. Still, the perpetual attempts of the Danish colonial administration to regulate the field may also have had an impact. The same kind of problems can be seen in colonies on other continents where the continental and the British medical traditions faced each other.[782] The common problem for the midwifery systems in the Caribbean sugar colonies seems primarily to have been the regard for the economy of the planters. In those cases where the respective administrative

779 Porter, *Ve og Vel*, 381–82.

780 Irvine Loudon, *Death in Childbirth: An International Study of Maternal Care and Maternal Mortality, 1800–1950* (Oxford: Clarendon Press, 1992), 398–427.

781 Anne Løkke, 'The "Antiseptic" Transformation of Danish Midwifes, 1860–1920', in *Midwives, Society and Childbirth: Debates and Controversies in the Modern Period*, ed. Hilary Marland and Anne Marie Raffery (London: Routledge, 1997), 106–8.

782 Deacon, 'Midwives and Medical Men', 284 et passim.

systems had a tradition for controlling the midwifery system, as in the case of France and Denmark, the control, organisation, and training often foundered on lack of funds (and commitment) with the local economic and political elite: the planters.

Finally, obstetrics was a field in which not only European administrative traditions faced each other, but which also saw a continual struggle or negotiation between European and Afro-Caribbean perceptions and practices. Because of this conflict, it is possible that the Danish colonial administration would have had problems creating a successful midwifery system on St Croix anyhow, regardless of the economic strategies of the planters, because the enslaved workers would not summarily accept Euro-Caribbean interventions in the reproductive field.

Chapter 5

Conclusion

The Medical World, Morbidity, and Mortality among the Enslaved Workers on St Croix

The Structure of the Medical World on St Croix

The first of the initial questions for this book was how the medical world surrounding the enslaved on St Croix was structured in the period 1803–48. As outlined in the introduction using Arthur Kleinman's model, the medical world was structured in three sectors: the professional, the folk, and the popular sector. The professional sector was the Euro-Caribbean plantation health system with plantation doctors in private practice and plantation hospitals. This system had a lot in common with similar systems in the British and French West Indies. The safeguarding of the health of the enslaved was rarely based on or sanctioned by legislation, yet in the French and particularly in the Danish West Indies, the plantation doctors were authorised and their conduct controlled by local and central health authorities. Such systems were rarely found in the British West Indies. Furthermore, the plantation doctors in the French and particularly the Danish West Indies were supported by a public health system controlled by the government (landfysikus, royal midwives etc.), which did not exist in the British West Indies. The reason for the higher level of control of the health system in the Danish and French West Indies seems to be the hierarchical structures inherited from the health systems in the mother countries.

The folk medical sector was the domain of Afro-Caribbean healers, enslaved and free, and can be further divided into performers of Obeah and herbalists. Both groups worked according to the general African/Afro-Caribbean perception of health and disease, which was of a magico-religious and holistic character and so clearly distinguishable from the European/Euro-Caribbean perception of health and disease. Whereas the practice of Obeah was regarded as superstition and problematic by the Euro-Caribbeans on St Croix, they did not regard the practice and skills of the herbalists as a problem – except in the case of the use of vegetable poison. Parallel to the folk sector, and probably closely integrated with it, was the popular sector. However, the source materials of this

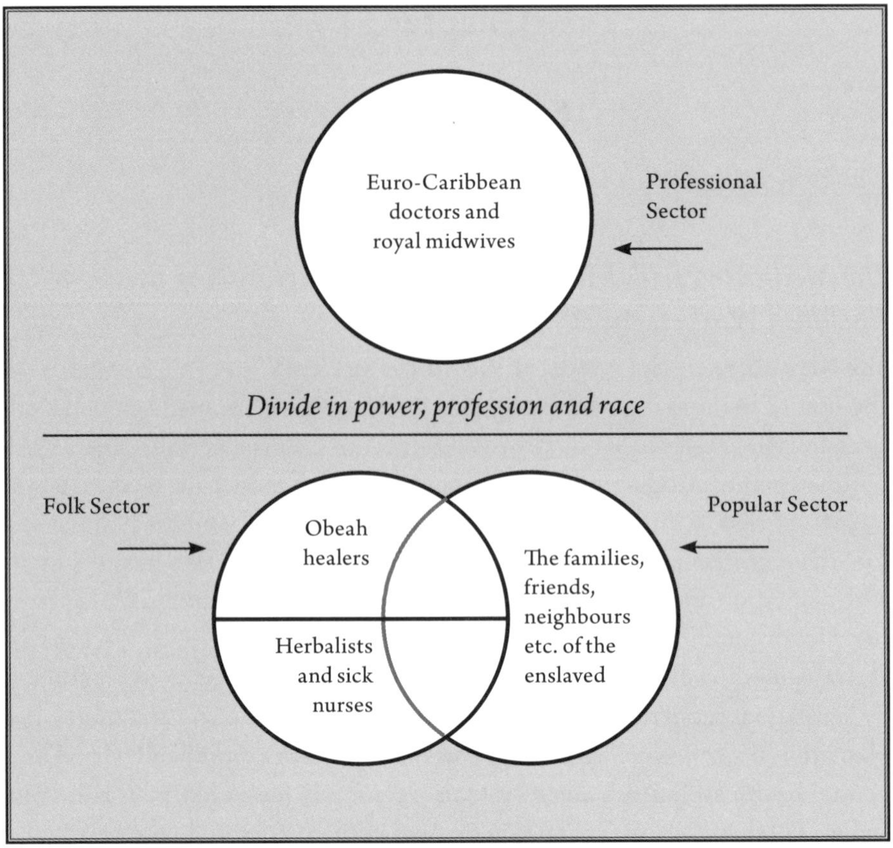

Fig. 5.1: Health workers on St Croix, 1803–48, based on Arthur Kleinman's model for sectors in health care systems in developed societies.

investigation have not yielded any indication of the divisions and treatments in this sector. However, we must assume that the majority of the enslaved workers' treatments of themselves were carried out in the sector composed of family, friends and neighbours.

If we compare this image of the health care system surrounding the enslaved on St Croix with Kleinman's original model of the three sectors a clear structural difference emerges. In Kleinman's model, the sectors are overlapping because the healers can belong to more than one sector at the same time, but on St Croix there was a clear division between the professional sector on one side and the folk and popular sectors on the other (see Fig. 5.1). The professional sector was, formally speaking, reserved for Euro-Caribbean doctors (and the royal midwives), whose position and power was sanctioned and controlled by the colonial administration. On the other side of this divide in power, profession, and race, the folk and popular sectors contained only Afro-Caribbeans. Accordingly, the structure of the Cruzian health care system was largely an expression of the social structure and the power relations in the society as such. Nonetheless, there was a small group of health workers who transcended the divide between the three sectors. This will be further discussed in the following.

Morbidity, Mortality and the Factors behind Them

The second initial question in this book concerned which diseases the enslaved workers on St Croix suffered and died from in the period in question, and which factors were behind the diseases and mortality causing the negative demographic trend.

The investigations in Chapter 3 have shown that the enslaved workers on Cruzian plantations suffered from a number of diseases. The four most common disease categories were 'Fever', 'Pains and Injuries', 'Gastrointestinal diseases' and 'Boils and Sores'. On four selected royal plantations, these four disease categories accounted for 60 to 95 per cent of all admissions to the plantation hospitals. Furthermore, there were a number of diseases that caused far fewer admissions, but in some instances with a much longer duration. It is significant to note the extent to which the diseases of the enslaved workers were caused by their living conditions. The pains and injuries generally originated from the hard and draining fieldwork, boils and sores were related both to the work and bad hygiene, whereas gastrointestinal complaints were connected to poor water supply, nutrition, and hygiene. If we compare the diseases among the enslaved workers of Cruzian plantations with information from the British and French West Indies, it appears that the spectrum of diseases was almost identical. However, the ranking of the diseases according to their incidence and severity among the enslaved was occasionally somewhat different, which has not been adequately explained.

Previous investigations from the British West Indies (Higman) of the seasonal mortality of the enslaved workers have indicated that the morbidity followed a certain annual rhythm caused by the changing workload in the sugar production and climatic and nutritional factors. The investigation in Chapter 3 confirms this pattern of seasonal morbidity and the influence of the climatic and nutritional factors, yet they cannot confirm the decisive role attributed to the workload.

Also in Chapter 3, the investigation of the most important causes of death among the enslaved workers on St Croix (measured per 1,000 enslaved at risk) has shown that in the 1840s it was respectively 'Fever', 'Bowels and Dysentery', 'Consumption and Lungs', and 'Old Age, Debility and Infirmity'. The two former categories correspond with the diseases causing the highest morbidity among the enslaved. The total mortality and frequency of the different causes of death varied strongly according to the age of the enslaved. In contrast, there were no significant gender differences to be found in the causes of death. The change in mortality throughout the year turned out to be seasonal in the same way as the morbidity, because the lowest number of deaths occurred in August and the highest in December. This seasonal pattern of mortality was different from the British West Indies (Higman), yet the factors causing the deaths seem largely to have been the same, namely workloads, bad hygiene, and bad weather in the months from September to January. However, the materials from St Croix cannot confirm Higman's hypothesis about an indirect and delayed effect of the workload during harvest time. Finally, there were great similarities between the frequency of different causes of death on St Croix and in the British West Indies respectively (similar data is not available from the French West Indies).

On this basis, I can now answer the last part of the second initial question concerning which factors were behind the diseases of the enslaved workers, their mortality and by extension the negative demographic development. Previous investigations in other sugar producing colonies have shown that the main cause was the workload. The amount of work was the single most important factor that could be manipulated in sugar production and so also in the economy of the planters and the health of the enslaved workers. Nevertheless, the above investigation indicates that the workload did not carry sole responsibility. It was a larger complex of synergic factors behind the living conditions of the enslaved on the sugar plantations that caused the morbidity and mortality. In addition, the investigation of the Danish West Indian administration's efforts in relation to the workload of the enslaved shows that generally these efforts were not as pronounced as in the British and French West Indies. This reluctance probably illustrates the fundamental importance of the work of the enslaved workers for the economy and the very existence of the Danish West Indies. Apparently, the Danish colonial administration did not find it opportune, or else lacked the necessary strength, to intervene in this central field. However, in terms of efforts towards a number of other factors, i.e. housing, clothing/shoes, the Danish West Indian administration was in line with the British and French West

Indies. Still, in one area the administration's efforts were significantly stronger, namely concerning the nutrition of the enslaved workers. In my opinion, this order of priorities on the Danish administration's behalf illustrates the power relation between the administration and the planters, and it shows what kind of health policy it was possible for the administration to implement considering this power relation.

The Health Policy of the Danish Colonial Administration and the Power over the Health of the Enslaved

The aim of this book was to answer two central questions: first, what health policy initiatives did the Danish administration instigate to deal with the excess mortality in the enslaved population, and second, what do these initiatives reveal about the power relations between the administration, the planters and the enslaved workers concerning the health of the enslaved? To answer these questions, I undertook three case studies of the administration's most central health policy initiatives in the period: nutrition, vaccination, and midwifery. These cases illustrate the efforts of the administration in three very different fields related to the health of the enslaved workers. Nutrition was the broadest and most fundamental field, deeply integrated with both the local environment and numerous other factors in the daily lives of the enslaved workers. In contrast, vaccination was a prophylactic procedure aimed at one disease, yet unique because it was the only effective prophylactic treatment known at the time. Finally, the system of midwives and birth practices was related to the reproductive health of the enslaved, which was of prime importance because of the high child mortality.

CASE ONE: *The Nutrition of the Enslaved Workers*

The Danish colonial administration on St Croix came to play an important role in relation to the nutrition of the enslaved plantation workers. First, from 1817 the administration ensured that the enslaved workers received a fixed weekly minimum ration. Subsequently, and despite several crises, the administration was successful in securing a stable supply of food for the colony, and particularly for the enslaved workers. The reason for this assumption of control of the main part of the nutrition of the enslaved rested on two factors. On the one hand the administration wanted a more humane treatment of the enslaved, both on moral and economic grounds. On the other hand, and just as importantly, the administration wanted to prevent unrest and rebellion among the enslaved workers, and thereby ensure the continuation of the economy and life of the colony. In a comparative perspective, there was no noticeable difference between the legally sanctioned minimum weekly rations per adult enslaved worker in respectively the British, French, and Danish West Indies. Instead, the difference was the degree to which the administration controlled the food supply. Neither the British nor the French West Indies administration seems to have been as active in securing the food supply of the enslaved workers as the administration in the Danish West Indies.

However, regardless of the administration's enforcement of minimum rations, the present investigations have shown that the energy content in the issued rations was too low to satisfy the needs of hardworking enslaved fieldworkers. I have estimated that the issued rations only contributed three quarters to two thirds of the required energy. In addition, the rations' content of proteins, fat, vitamins, and minerals was insufficient. Accordingly, the enslaved workers had to supplement their diet on their own accord to survive, which was also the intention behind the size of the rations. This supplementary food came partly from the provision grounds of the enslaved, yet the present investigations indicate that these plots could not supply enough food to cover the energy needs of an enslaved fieldworker either. Another possible source for supplementing the food of the enslaved was the surrounding natural environment. However, it is not possible to determine if this supplementing actually took place. Consequently, the food resources from the natural environment can only be viewed as an uncertain supplement to the enslaved workers' diet, which at times could and at other times could not cover the remaining nutritional needs of the enslaved. A similar uncertainty concerns the contribution of food from trade and theft. So, overall, there is every probability that the enslaved workers were malnourished for at least part of the year. Since the autumn (October–December) was characterised by few crops in the provision grounds and hard work, it is most likely that the enslaved workers were malnourished during this time of year. This corresponds with the above investigations showing the highest number of sicknesses and deaths among the enslaved workers during the autumn. It was not a matter of outright famine or that the enslaved died of hunger per se, but undernourishment and/or malnutrition may nonetheless have had a great impact on the mortality of the enslaved workers, especially among the children. Recent research has shown that in present-day developing countries malnutrition is the fundamental cause of around 55 per cent of all deaths among children. It must be regarded as very likely that something similar was the case among the enslaved on Cruzian plantations. Accordingly, I shall propose the cautious hypothesis that the primary cause of the excess mortality in the enslaved population on Cruzian plantations may very likely have been insufficient nutrition, and only secondarily poor hygiene and epidemic diseases.

The centrality of nutrition to the safeguarding of the health of the enslaved made it a field in a larger struggle for power. The three parties in the conflict, the administration, the planters and the enslaved workers, each controlled part of the food resources and continuously negotiated their positions of power. Insofar as the colonial administration succeeded in establishing and enforcing a minimum ration and guaranteed stable food supplies, it assumed part of the control the planters had previously had over the rations of the enslaved, so the planters could no longer use withholding of provisions as punishment. It was not a given that such an encroachment on the planters' rights of private property was even possible, since the administration's power vis-à-vis the planters was in many ways limited (cf. the absence of an actual slave law, see Chapter 3). However, the size of the provision grounds remained the domain of the planters and in this way they retained great influence on how much of the important supplementary food the enslaved were capable of growing. Hence, the struggle or negotiation resulted in the planters retaining control of a strategically important part of the food supply while they surrendered another part. The enslaved on their part fought the planters' power over the rations by allying themselves with the administration, in as much as they used the new legislation as a basis for complaints to the administration. At the same time the enslaved workers continued to exploit the natural resources, which neither the administration nor the planters could control the access to – although they tried. From this it becomes apparent that the administration and the planters did not necessarily form one unified power block in opposition to the enslaved. Admittedly, the administration and the planters had a common objective in maintaining the health of the enslaved workers and by extension maintaining the economy and existence of the colony, yet apparently they had different views on how to accomplish this objective. The administration tried to assume and exercise a centralised control of the health of the enslaved workers, an endeavour supported by the enslaved, while the planters tried to retain their rights of private property over the enslaved.

Finally, it is difficult to conclude if the nutrition of the enslaved improved in the course of the period in question. As the excess mortality among the enslaved workers continued at the same level throughout the period, it is not known whether the administration's efforts to improve the health of the enslaved in the field of nutrition had any effect, or if the effect was only cancelled out by other factors, for instance an increasing workload.

CASE TWO: *The Vaccination and the Enslaved*

Another field where the colonial administration on St Croix instigated initiatives in health policy to improve the health of the enslaved workers was vaccination against smallpox. Here, the Danish administration succeeded, despite numerous and continuous practical problems, in establishing a public vaccination system on St Croix. The model for this system was Danish, but it received a unique Danish West Indian design. This system succeeded in keeping smallpox epidemics away from St Croix (though not from St Thomas) and so warded off one of the most serious omnipresent threats against the health and lives of the enslaved workers.

The reasons for the success of vaccination on St Croix become apparent in a comparative Caribbean perspective. It seems that it was only in some parts of the Danish and British West Indies (St Croix and Trinidad) that the citizens and their enslaved workers received efficient protection against smallpox. In the French West Indies and the major part of the British West Indies, a large part of the population remained unvaccinated and consequently smallpox epidemics were not prevented. There were two reasons for the success. First, there was the statutory vaccination of all inhabitants, supported by an efficient and centralised government control apparatus (licences and registers) plus a well-run quarantine system. However, for these systems to function effectively, the administration was dependent on another set of circumstances, namely the geography of the colony and the infrastructure. It is evident that it was far easier to disseminate and control vaccination on a relatively small and relatively flat island with a well-developed network of roads like St Croix than on larger mountainous islands like Jamaica and Guadeloupe. In other words, a combination of an effective centralised government and geographical circumstances made it possible for St Croix to achieve an apparently unusually high level of protection against smallpox. The Danish West Indian vaccination system's origin in the Danish legislation on vaccination and in the administrative traditions of the absolutist Danish monarchy meant that the legislation on vaccination on St Croix was stricter than in virtually any other Caribbean colony. The geographical circumstances and the planters' apparent support for vaccination permitted the vaccination system on St Croix to become more efficient than it was in almost any other Caribbean colony. A comparison with the vaccination system on St Thomas clearly shows that the objective of this effort was to protect the precious enslaved workers against the lethal smallpox: to protect the health of the enslaved.

The success of the vaccination system was also dependent on a high level of government control. Given that the majority of the inhabitants on St Croix were enslaved workers, the main thrust of this successful exercise of power by the administration was directed towards individuals who were private property. Accordingly, with the establishment of the vaccination system, the administration assumed yet another part of the control of the health of the enslaved, which had previously belonged to the planters. So, in this field of health policy there also appears to have been a conflict and negotiation of the power over the health of the enslaved. Nonetheless, in this case there does not seem to have been any noticeable disagreement between the administration and the planters. The attitude of the enslaved workers towards vaccination is absent from the source materials. Possibly, they viewed vaccination in the light of the familiar practice of variolation and so did not object to vaccination, control, and registration.

CASE THREE: *The Enslaved, the System of Midwives and the Practices of Births*

The third field where the colonial administration on St Croix instigated health policy initiatives to promote the health of the enslaved population was in relation to the system of midwives and obstetrics. In the period 1803–48, the administration tried to expand and improve the hierarchical system of midwives in the Danish West Indies with the aim of bringing down the high level of child mortality among the enslaved workers. The model for the structure and the improvements was the efficient system of midwives in Denmark. However, the administration's efforts to obtain trained and examined enslaved midwives for the plantations met with very limited success. There were probably several reasons for this outcome, but the regard for the planters' economy and in the longer term for the enslaved workers' ability to pay for such a service after the expected emancipation seems to have prevented the introduction of legislation in the field. Consequently, large parts of the system of midwives on St Croix remained in the hands of untrained enslaved plantation midwives.

However, in a comparative Caribbean perspective, the system of midwives in the Danish West Indies appears to have been subject to a higher degree of control, organisation, and formalised training than in the British and French West Indies. The Danish colonial administration enforced its control via the landfysikus, the doctors in private practice and the royal midwives and attempted repeatedly to ensure a better training of the enslaved plantation midwives. The reason for the difference between the colonies is probably to be found in fundamental differences in the organisation of the systems of midwives in the mother countries. In Britain, there was no formalised training for midwives, no legislation, and no control, while France and Denmark had hierarchical systems of midwives controlled and authorised by the government dating back to the eighteenth century. When the control, the organisation, and the training of the latter countries nevertheless foundered in their West Indian colonies, the cause was usually lack of support from the local economic and political elite: the planters.

In keeping with the two former case studies, the system of midwives and the associated obstetric practices also became a field in the struggle for and negotiation of the power over the health of the enslaved. However, here the contest took place on another level, that is to say between on the one side the plantation doctors and the royal midwives as representatives of the Euro-Caribbean power (the administration and the planters) and on the other side the enslaved women and the enslaved midwives. The focus was on the obstetric practices of the enslaved women and midwives. The doctors criticised these practices as being based on harmful superstition and accordingly they increased infant mortality, which again had a negative effect on the crucial growth in the enslaved population. To eradicate the alleged superstition and lower the infant mortality the doctors wanted the births of the enslaved to be submitted to European medical perceptions and practices and so to the doctors' control. Some planters tried to accomplish this objective by removing the enslaved women in confinement to specially constructed maternity wards, even if this triggered strong objections from the enslaved. The maternity wards were not sanctioned by law but their existence could be interpreted as if the doctors, and so the Euro-Caribbean side, had been capable of assuming control of the area. However, the birth itself was still to a large extent overseen by untrained plantation midwives and accordingly it is not certain whether the maternity wards had any impact on birth practices. The persistently high level of infant mortality might suggest that it did not.

The struggle for power over births indicates that under any circumstances the Danish colonial administration would have had difficulties establishing a successful system of midwives on St Croix. Regardless of how the planters' attitude to such a system would have been, the third party in the affair, the enslaved workers, just did not accept Euro-Caribbean intervention in their

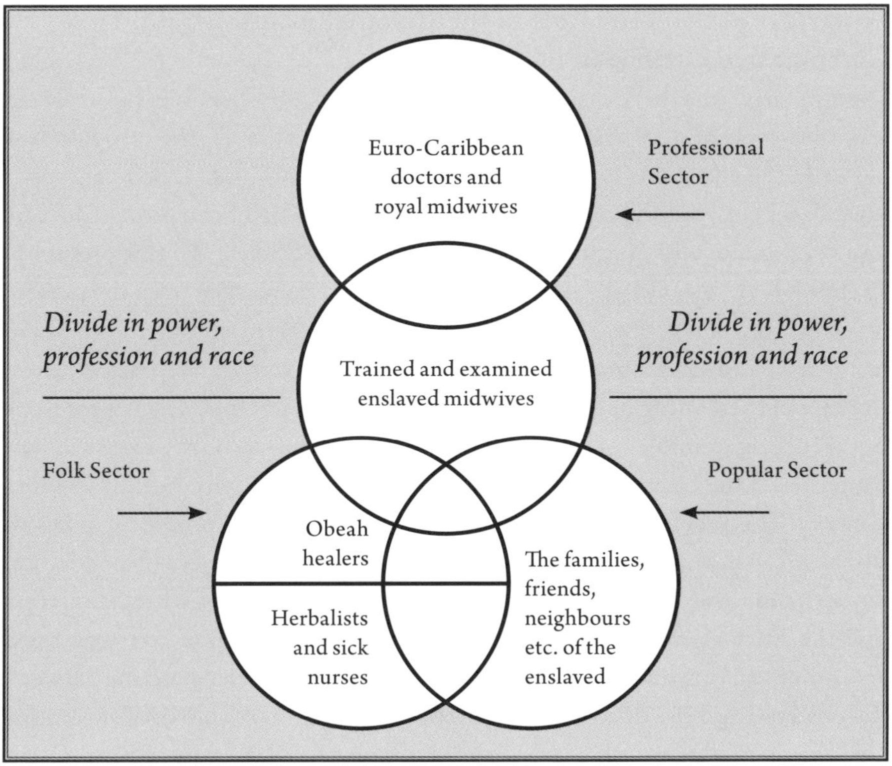

Fig. 5.2: The health workers on St Croix with the trained and examined enslaved midwives in the divide between Euro-Caribbean and Afro-Caribbean health workers.

perceptions and practices in the reproductive field. The only group that had the potential of mediating the conflict was that of the trained and examined enslaved midwives, whom the administration had tried to provide, but without much luck. The examined enslaved midwives were positioned between both the traditional enslaved midwife with knowledge of Afro-Caribbean perceptions and birth practices and the perceptions and practices of European medicine regarding births. If we try to place this group in the previously presented model of the structure of the medical world on St Croix, it will stand at the intersection between the Euro-Caribbean doctors' professional sector, the folk sector of the Obeah men and the herbalists, and the enslaved workers' popular sector (see Fig. 5.2). This mediating position might possibly have afforded them great importance in the reduction in infant mortality, yet, as mentioned, the number of trained and examined enslaved midwives remained extremely low.

Power, Health and the Role of the Colonial Administration in a Comparative Caribbean Perspective

To summarise, the three case studies have shown that the health of the enslaved was the scene of a struggle for power. On a general level, the struggle was between the administration, the planters, and the enslaved workers and on a lower level between the representatives of the Euro-Caribbean power (doctors and royal midwives) and the enslaved workers respectively. To this picture of the lower level, we may add other examples that have emerged from the present investigations. First, the investigation of disease patterns among the enslaved workers on Cruzian plantations showed that the enslaved did not passively leave the care of their ailing bodies to the Euro-Caribbean doctors. There were weak but recurring examples of enslaved workers perceiving certain illnesses or conditions, and the treatment of them, to be domains that were not the doctors' concern. This was for instance the case with scabies, dental problems, venereal diseases, birth, and death (autopsy). The enslaved workers' rejection of doctoral authority in these domains led to confrontations and friction with the doctors and the Euro-Caribbean authorities they represented. These confrontations also point to a continuous negotiation for power over health occurring between the enslaved and the doctors. Second, the investigation of the disease patterns also exemplified the clash of worldviews, which could be a part of Euro-Caribbean doctors' treatment of their enslaved patients, because the enslaved interpreted the use of anaesthesia during surgical operations very differently from Euro-Caribbean patients.

The three case studies also showed that the colonial administration and the planters did not necessarily act as a unified power block towards the enslaved regarding health care. What divided the administration and the planters seems to have been the balance between the planters' rights of private property over the enslaved against the importance of the health of the enslaved for the economy and the very existence of the colony. The administration tried and succeeded in assuming a minor part of the planters' power over the health of the enslaved. In return for the limitation of their rights, the planters gained an increase in the protection of the health of the enslaved, which could only be supplied by the superior central control and coordination of a health policy.

Viewed in a comparative and general Caribbean perspective, the health of the enslaved workers on St Croix in the period 1803–48 was neither substantially better nor worse than in the British and French West Indian colonies. The diseases the enslaved suffered from were broadly the same and this was also true for the causes of death. The factors behind disease and death respectively were also the same despite great geographical and environmental differences. This situation is reflected in the fact that the negative demographic trend was a condition of life for the majority of enslaved workers in the Caribbean in this period.

Instead, what made St Croix different was the degree of government control of the health of the enslaved. This is not to say that control was always stronger than in the British or French West Indies. For instance, the control of workloads seems to have been weaker. Yet, concerning food supply, vaccination against smallpox and the system of midwives, the Danish West Indian administration initiated health policies with relatively greater effectiveness than in the British and French colonies. In my opinion, the reason for this stronger central control of the health services in the Danish West Indies was that the health services in the mother country were under strong, centralised control. The Danish administration on St Croix tried to implement a similar central control of health in a society with a very different structure, which, as I have shown, was not always altogether a success. The problem of this manoeuvre was that the majority of the population in the Danish West Indies was enslaved workers, and as such not just ordinary citizens subject to the control of the colonial administration (the state) but private property. Consequently, the health policies of the Danish colonial administration regarding the enslaved had to cause conflict with the planters concerning power over the health of the enslaved. Of course, the enslaved themselves also participated in various ways in the struggle for power over their own health. In the daily interaction with the representatives of the health policy of the administration and the planters, the enslaved did not accept interference without opposition. In various areas and ways they were capable of maintaining their own perceptions and practices in the struggle for power over health.

Appendix

Table 2.1: The enslaved population in each quarter, 1804–46

Quarter	1804	1815	1825	1835	1841	1846	Index 1804 1846
Company's	2,049	1,864	1,471	1,474	1,496	1,232	60
Queens's	4,153	4,027	3,696	3,458	3,229	3,043	73
King's	2,476	2,223	1,956	1,828	1,779	1,672	68
Northside B	1,217	1,119	927	774	786	746	61
Prince's	3,988	3,944	3,752	3,489	3,377	3,366	84
West End	3,456	3,122	2,854	2,527	2,399	2,195	64
Northside A	2,373	2,282	2,190	2,098	1,935	1,913	81
East End A	1,692	1,461	1,263	1,152	854	797	47
East End B	672	646	393	368	333	346	51
Total	22,076	20,688	18,502	17,168	16,188	15,310	69

Source: Asmussen, *Slavedemografi*, 36, table 3.1, appendix I, II and III.

Table 2.2: The population of free Afro-Caribbeans, 1792–1834[1]

Year	1792	1815	1834
Total of free Afro-Caribbeans	1,164	2,480	3,411

Source: Bergsøe, *Den danske Stats Statistik* IV, 611.

1 In 1835, the registration of descent for free citizens was discontinued. This is the reason why we do not have any data on the number of free Afro-Caribbeans after 1834. Bergsøe, *Den danske Stats Statistik* IV, 611.

Table 2.3: Number of inhabitants per doctor in the Danish West Indies and Denmark, ca. 1800–50

Inhabitants per doctor in the Danish West Indies			
Year	1800	1830	1846
Total population	40,000[2]	41,275[3]	39,588[4]
Total doctors	21[5]	23[6]	18[7]
Inhabitants per doctor	1,905	1,795	2,199

Inhabitants per doctor in the kingdom of Denmark[8]			
Year	1808		1850
Total population	944,751		1,443,710
Total doctors	279		529
Inhabitants per doctor	3,386		2,729

2 Hornby, 'Kolonierne i Vestindien', 189.

3 Stanley L. Engerman, 'A Population History of the Caribbean', in *A Population History of North America*, ed. Michael R. Haines and Richard H. Steckel (Cambridge: Cambridge University Press, 2000), 497.

4 Bergsøe, *Den danske Stats Statistik* IV, 600.

5 Jensen, *En verden til forskel?*, appendix 3.

6 Jensen, *En verden til forskel?*, appendix 3.

7 DNA, BH, Med. rep., 1848.

8 V. Falbe-Hansen and Dr. W. Scharling, *Danmarks Statistik* V (Copenhagen, 1881), 81.

Table 2.4: Sick nurses and midwives on the royal plantations, 1830–43

Name of estate	Year	Sick nurses and/or midwife
North Star	1833[9]	Sick nurse: healthy, able, 39 years old
	1838[10]	Sick nurse: healthy, able, 39 years old
	1843[11]	Sick nurse: healthy, able, 45 years old
Longford	1836[12]	Midwife: not effective, sickly, 42 years old
	1843[13]	Sick nurse: good, able, 54 years old Midwife: good, able, 34 years old
Boetzberg	1838[14]	Sick nurse: sickly, useful, 65 years old
Hermon Hill	1835[15]	Sick nurse: infirm, 55 years old Midwife: effective, 40 years old
	1836[16]	Sick nurse: healthy, effective, 40 years old
Cotton Grove	1839	Sick nurse: 65 years old
Grange	1835	Sick nurse: healthy, effective, 52 years old
Upper Love	1835	Sick nurse: healthy, very useful, 50 years old
Retreat	1839	Sick nurse: healthy, superannuated, 65 years old Midwife: healthy, able, 32 years old
Humbug	1839	Sick nurse: indifferent, not efficient, 37 years old
Work and Rest	1833	Sick nurse: Sickly, still useful, 61 years old Midwife: strong and healthy, 41 years old
Rust up Twist	1838	Sick nurse: healthy, not efficient (blind), 42 years old
Work and Rest	1830	Sick nurse: healthy and strong, 45 years old

9 DNA, WILA, no. 46.21.
10 DNA, WILA, no. 46.17.54. Original Danish text: 'Sygevogterske, sund, dygtig, 39 år'.
11 DNA, WILA, no. 46.17.54.
12 DNA, WILA, no. 46.17.45.
13 DNA, WILA, no. 46.17.45.
14 DNA, WILA, no. 46.17.6. Original Danish text: 'Sygevogterske: sygelig, nyttig, 65 år'.
15 DNA, WILA, no. 46.17.32.
16 This entry and all the following: DNA, WILA, no. 46.21.

Table 3.1: Estate North Star, 1830–33:
Number of hospitalisation days, patients and incidence rate

Disease category	Hospitalisation days	Patients	Average no. of hospitalisation days per patient	Per cent of all hospitalisation days	Incidence rate per 1,000 person-years at risk [(2)]
Pains and injuries	1,298	156	8	19.14	674.84
Gastrointestinal complaints	1,140	160	20	16.81	692.14
Fever and ague	775	152	5	11.43	657.53
Boils and sores	885	36	42	13.05	155.73
Rose	594	80	7	8.76	346.07
Swellings	190	7	27	2.80	30.28
Pregnancy, birth and lying in	657	8	82	9.69	34.61
Venereal disease	137	4	34	2.02	17.30
Genital complaints	23	6	4	0.34	25.96
Cold and cough	278	48	6	4.10	207.64
Sore throat	30	5	6	0.44	21.63
Old age, weakness and incapable of working	390	10	39	5.75	43.26
Whooping cough	278	4	70	4.10	17.30
Dental and oral complaints	27	7	4	0.40	30.28
Other complaints	79	7	11	1.17	30.28
Total	6,781	690		100.00	2,984.85
Total no. of person-years at risk [(1)]					231

Source: DNA, WILA, no. 46.17.55.
(1) = 91,157 person-days at risk minus 6,781 admission days / 365 days per year
(2) = (patients/total person-years at risk)*1,000

Table 3.2: Estate Longford, 1829–35:
Number of hospitalisation days, patients and incidence rate

Disease category	Hospi-talisation days	Patients	Average no. of hospi-talisation days per patient	Per cent of all hospi-talisation days	Inci-dence rate per 1,000 person-years at risk [(2)]
Fever	541	42	13	28.47	63.61
Pains and injuries	488	37	19	25.68	56.04
Sores and boils	227	4	57	11.95	6.06
Dropsy (edema) and swelling	133	4	28	7.00	6.06
Rose	52	3	17	2.74	4.54
Yaws	90	1	90	4.74	1.51
Vomiting and purging	46	7	7	2.42	10.60
Consumption	183	1	183	9.63	1.51
Venereal	42	1	42	2.21	1.51
Pregnancy	43	1	43	2.26	1.51
Chicken pox	27	1	27	1.42	1.51
Shingles	12	1	12	0.63	1.51
Cold	11	1	11	0.58	1.51
Old age and weakness	4	1	4	0.21	1.51
Dental complaints	1	1	1	0.05	1.51
Total	1,900	106		100.00	160.54
Total person years at risk [(1)]					660

Source: DNA, WILA, no. 46.17.46.
(1) = 242,906 person-days at risk minus 1,900 hospitalisation days / 365 days per year
(2) = (patients/total person-years at risk)*1,000

Table 3.3: Estate Boetzberg, 1832–33: Number of hospitalisation days, patients and incidence rate

Disease category	Hospitalisation days	Patients	Average no. of hospitalisation days per patient	Per cent of all hospitalisation days	Incidence rate per 1,000 person-years at risk (2)
Fever	379	114	3	31.30	1,229.25
Pain in head, back, sides, arms, legs, feet and hands	208	50	4	17.18	539.14
Gastrointestinal complaints	156	48	3	12.88	517.58
Sores and boils	398	16	25	32.87	172.53
Rose	8	2	4	0.66	21.57
Sore eyes	26	4	7	2.15	43.13
Venereal	32	1	32	2.64	10.78
Teeth	1	1	1	0.08	10.78
Other	3	1	3	0.25	10.78
Total	1,211	237		100.00	2,555.54
Total person years at risk (1)					93

Source: DNA, WILA, no. 46.17.5.
(1) = 35,061 person-days at risk minus 1,211 hospitalisation days / 365 days per year
(2) = (patients/total person-years at risk)*1,000

Table 3.4: Estate Hermon Hill, 1830:
Number of hospitalisation days, patients and incidence rate

Disease category	Hospitalisation days	Patients	Average no. of hospitalisation days per patient	Per cent of all hospitalisation days	Incidence rate per 1,000 person-years at risk (2)
Fever	237	12	77	32.87	287.97
Pain	178	8	16	24.69	191.98
Gastrointestinal complaints	146	4	37	20.25	95.99
Sores	125	1	125	17.34	24.00
Swellings	3	2	2	0.42	47.99
Yaws	7	1	7	0.97	24.00
Cough	25	1	25	3.47	24.00
Total	721	29		100.00	695.92
Total person-years at risk (1)					42

Source: DNA, WILA, no. 46.17.31.
(1) =15,931 person-days at risk minus 721 hospitalisation days / 365 days per year
(2) = (patients/total person-years at risk)*1,000

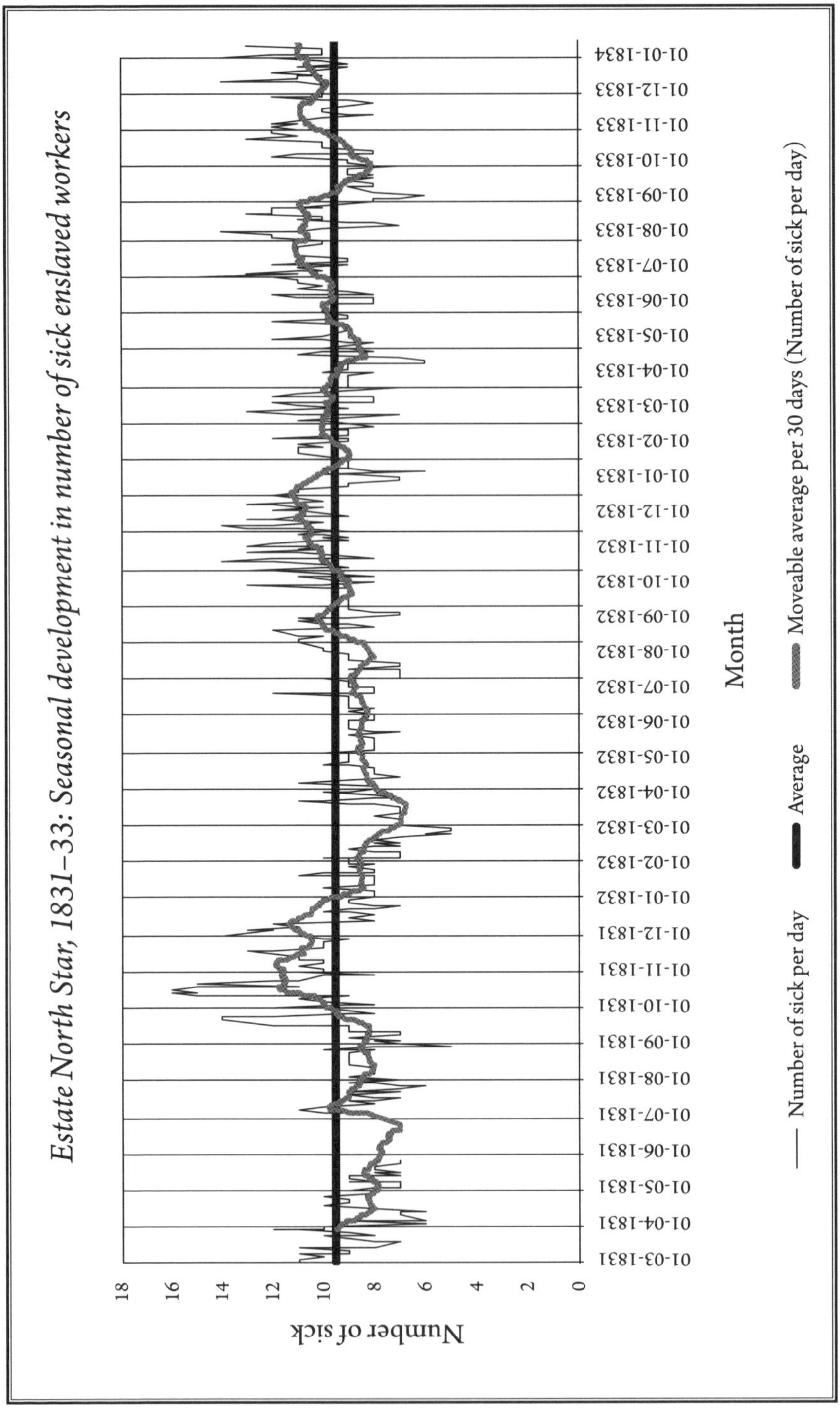

Fig. 3.2. Source, DNA, WILA, no. 46.17.55.

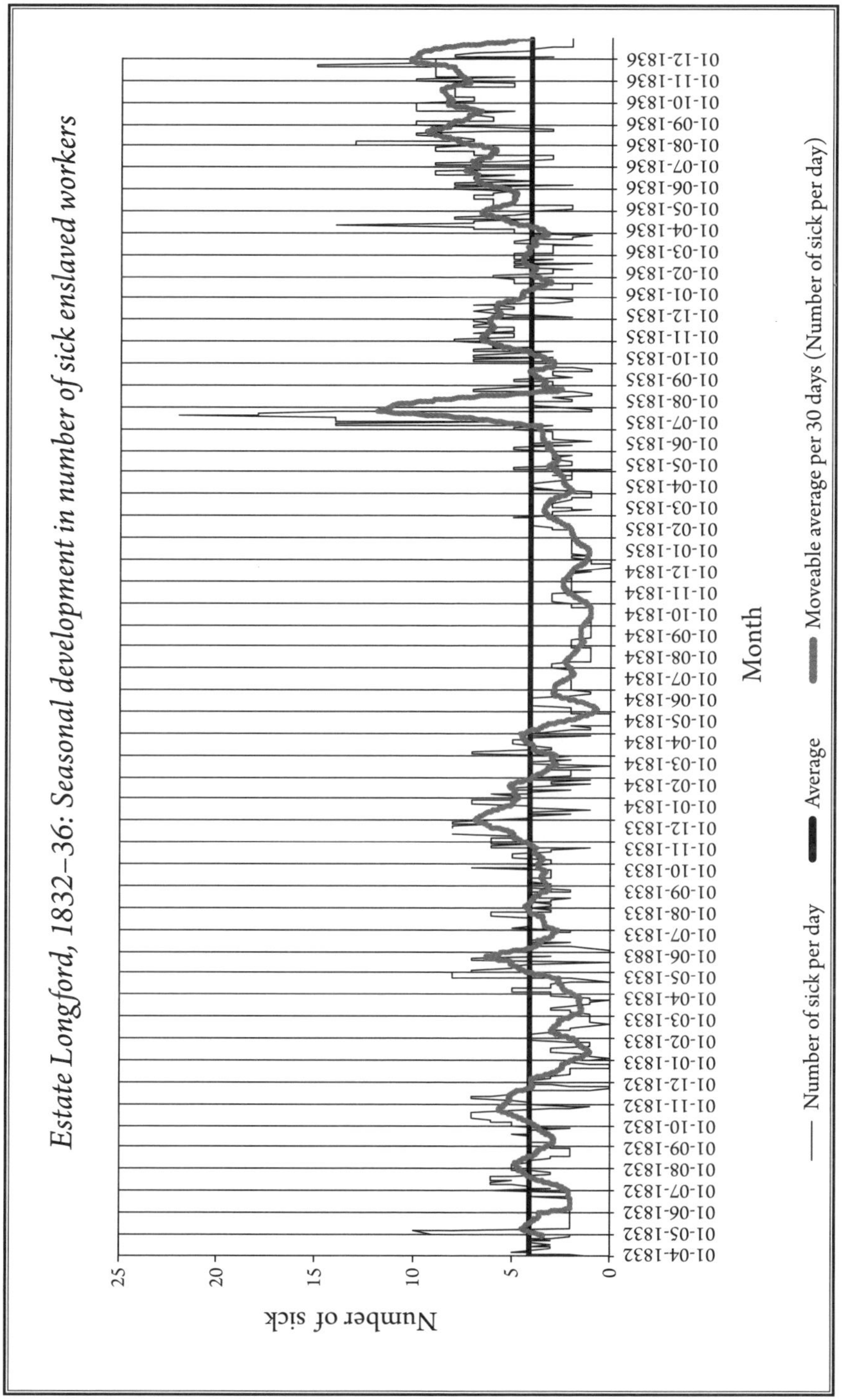

Fig. 3.3. Source, DNA, WILA, no. 46.17.46.

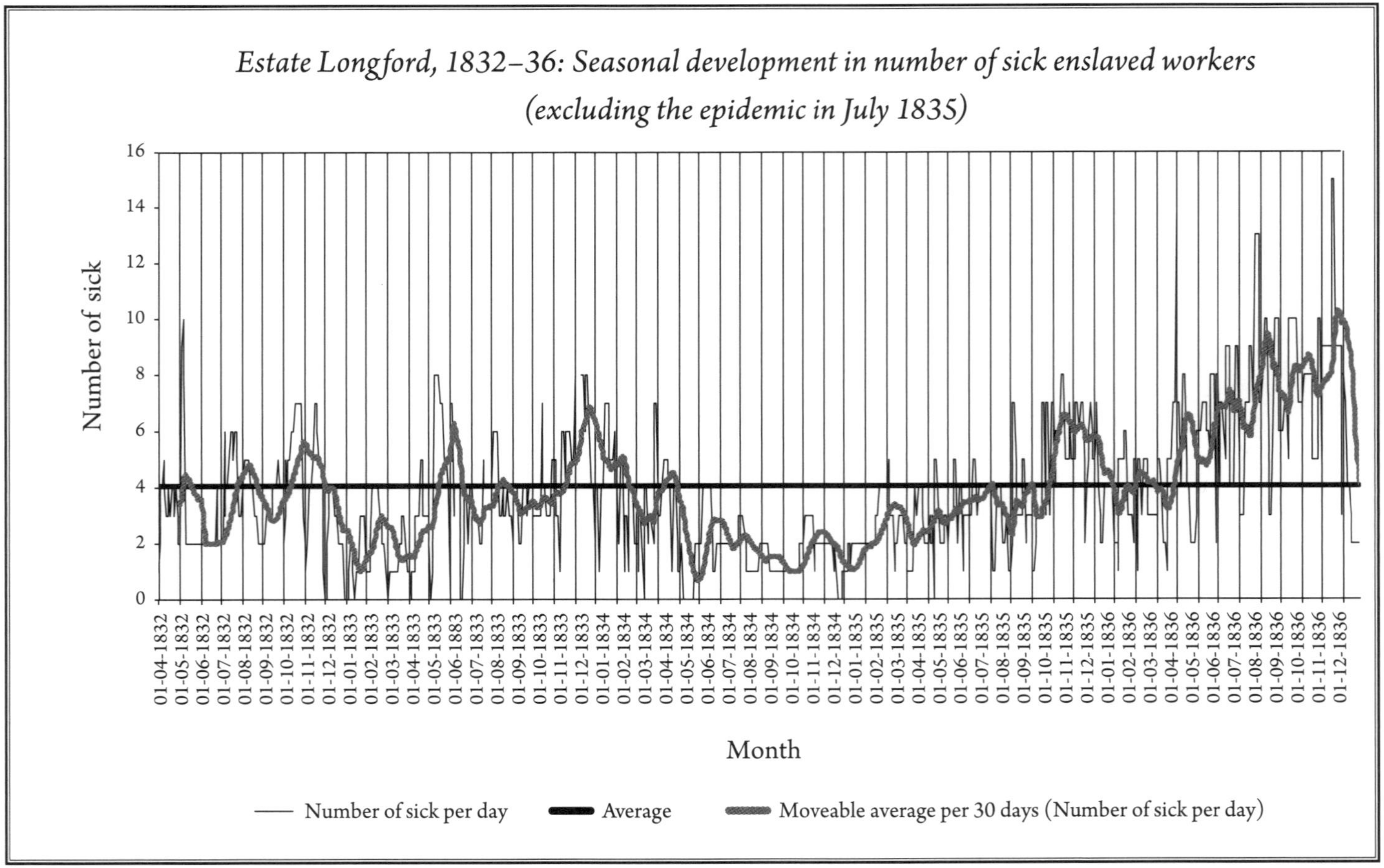

Fig. 3.4. Source, DNA, WILA, no. 46.17.46.

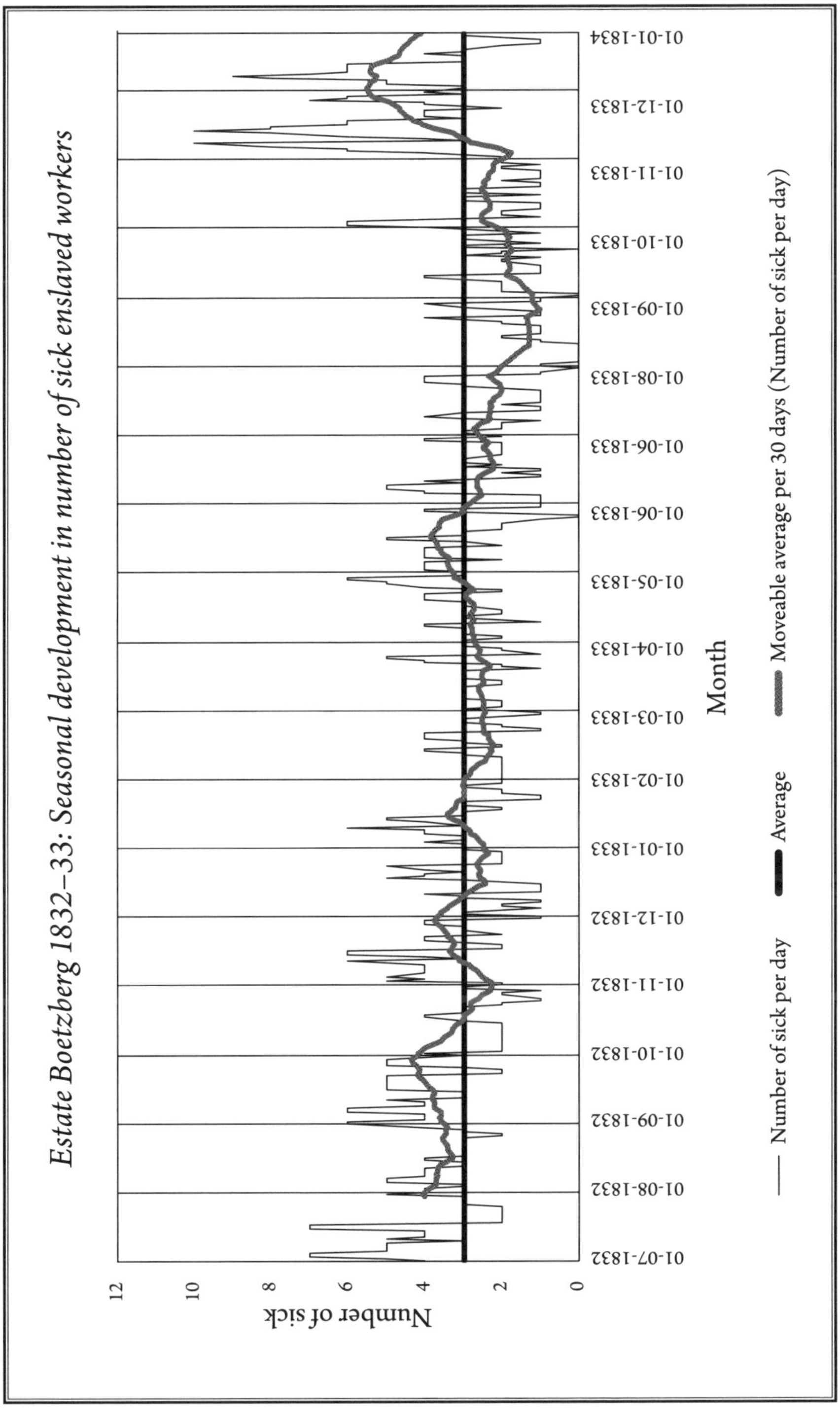

Fig. 3.5. Source, DNA, WILA, no. 46.17.5.

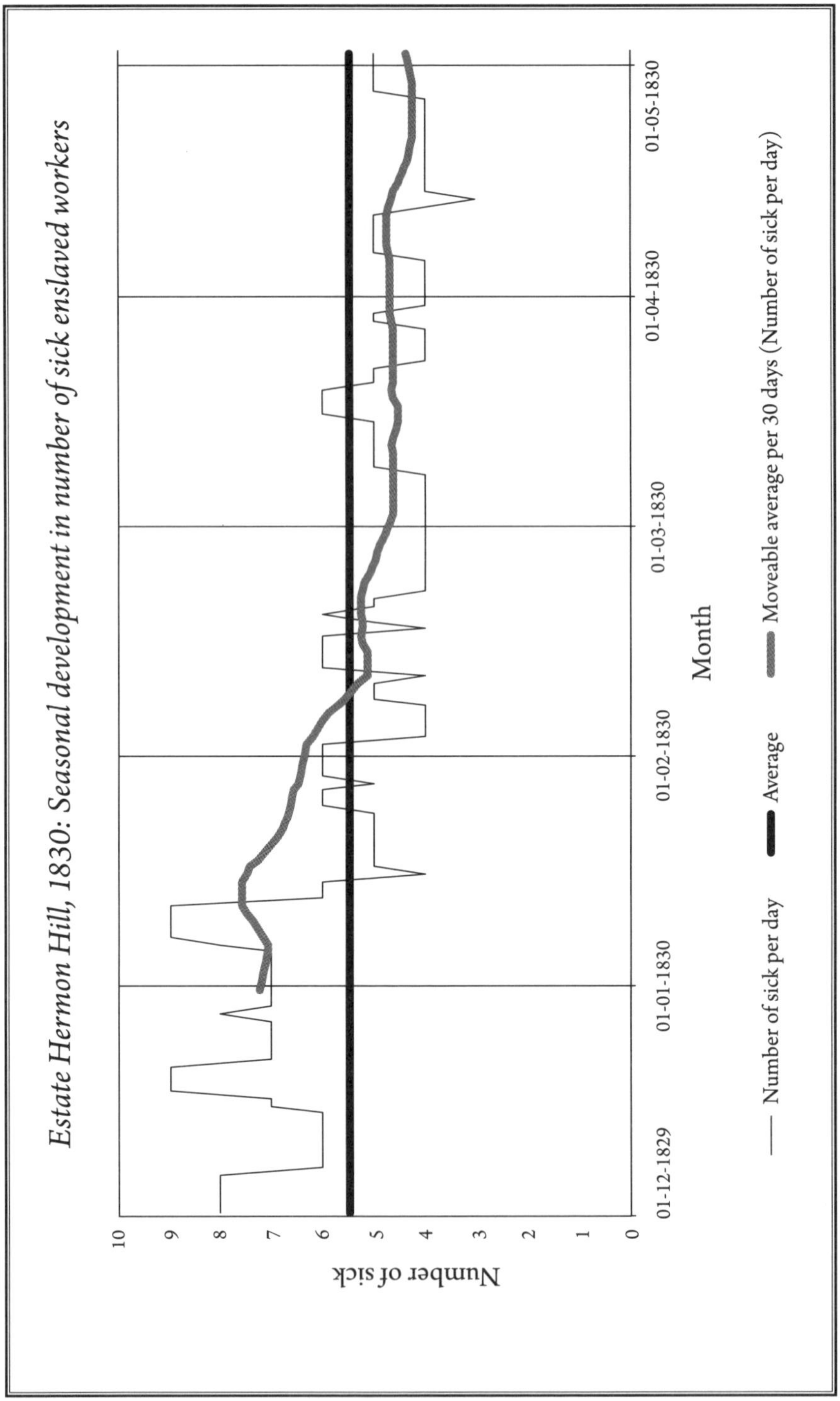

Fig. 3.6. Source, DNA, WILA, no. 46.17.31.

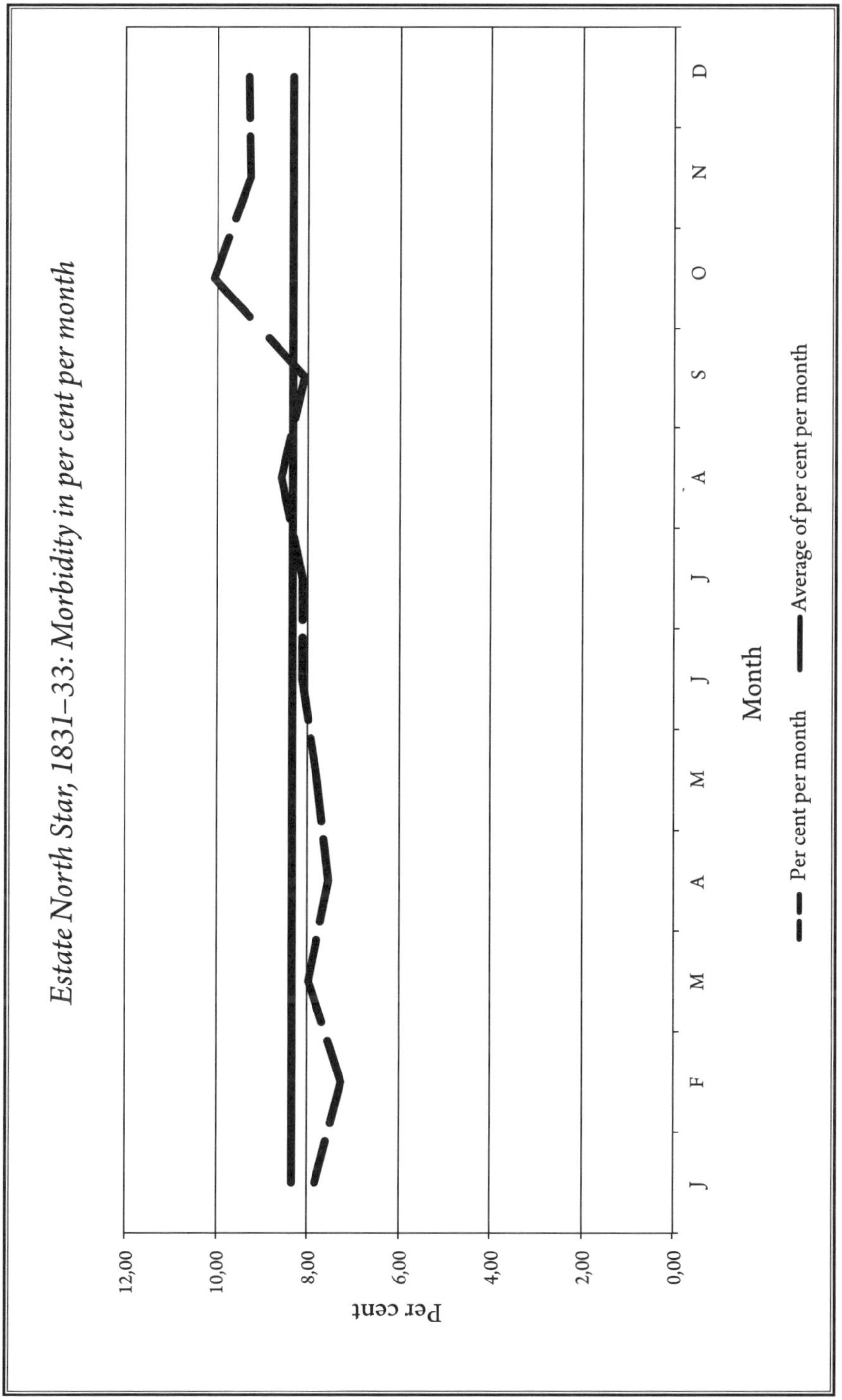

Fig. 3.7. Source: Table 3.6.

Table 3.6: Estate North Star, 1831–33:
Average number and percentage of sick enslaved per month

Months	Total number of sick per month 1831	1832	1833	Total per month 1831–33	Per cent sick per month of the whole year
January	218	266	310	794	7.84
February	238	225	273	736	7.26
March	296	225	287	808	7.97
April	242	253	268	763	7.53
May	227	264	299	790	7.80
June	234[17]	264	325	823	8.12
July	241	253	329	823	8.12
August	267	316	289	872	8.61
September	283	271	266	820	8.09
October	359	325	336	1,020	10.07
November	314	321	306	941	9.29
December	315	310	318	943	9.31
Total	5,065	5,125	5,439	10,133	100.00
Average	270	274	301	844	8.33

Source, DNA, WILA, no. 46.17.55.

17 Data is not available for June 1831, but 234 is the average of the previous and the following month (227 and 241).

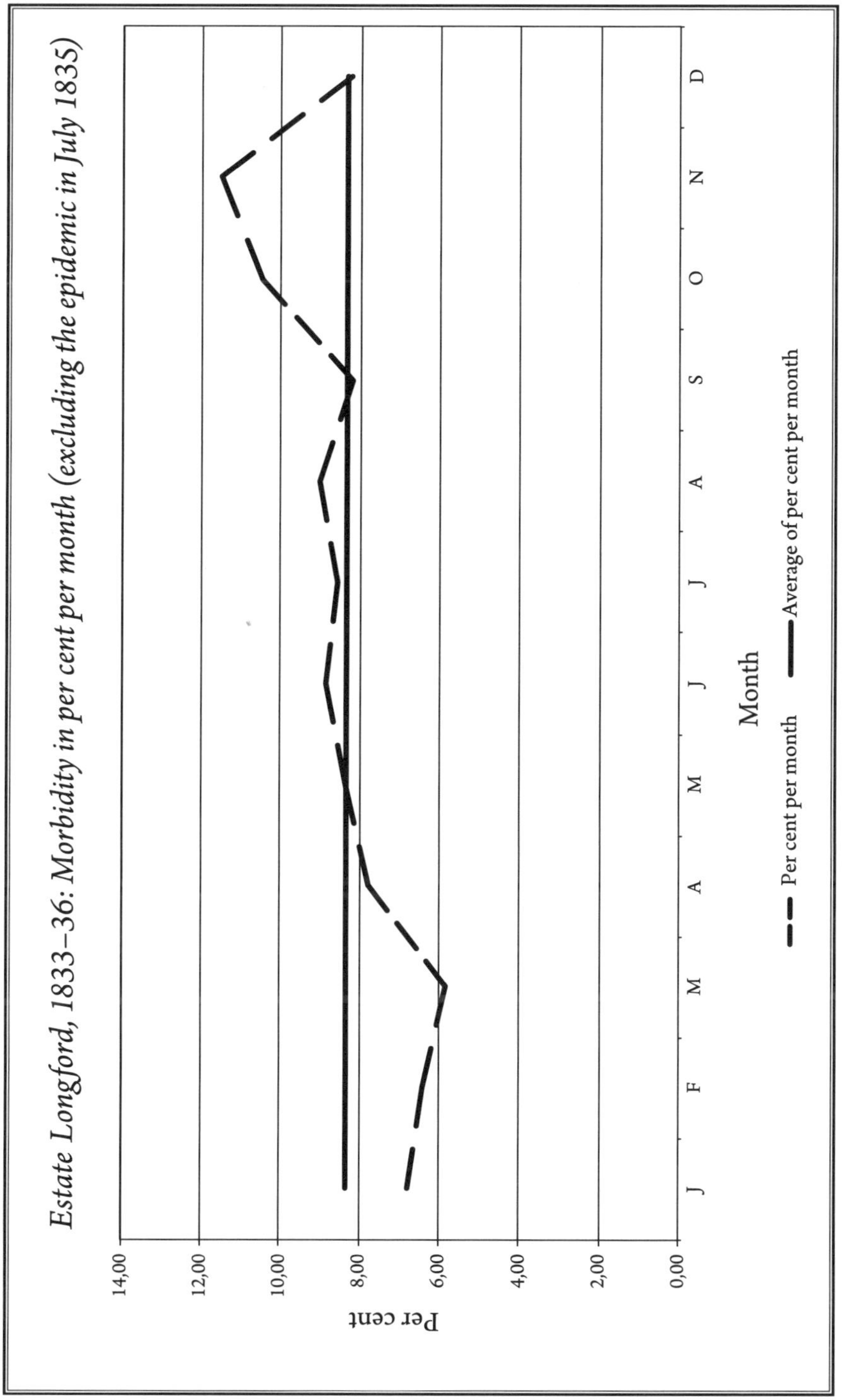

Fig. 3.8. Source: Table 3.7.

Table 3.7: Estate Longford, 1833–36:
Average number and percentage of sick enslaved per month

Months	Total number of sick per month					
	1833	1834	1835	1836	Total per month, 1833–36	Per cent sick per month of the whole year
January	50	157	62	125	394	6.78
February	75	79	97	122	373	6.42
March	48	122	64	104	338	5.82
April	77	89	92	194	452	7.78
May	183	46	99	157	485	8.35
June	93	73	128	220	514	8.85
July	112	67	116[18]	202	497	8.56
August	112	46	104	261	523	9.00
September	99	30	98	249	476	8.20
October	117	61	205	226	609	10.49
November	127	61	174	307	669	11.52
December	167	34	139	138	478	8.23
Total	3,093	2,699	3,213	4,141	5,808	100.00
Average	105	72	115	192	484	8.33

Source, DNA, WILA, no. 46.17.46.

18 Originally, July 1835 had a total of 319 sick, presumably because of an epidemic of some unknown disease (see Fig. 3.3). Accordingly, the data has been corrected to an average of the previous and the following month (see Fig. 3.4).

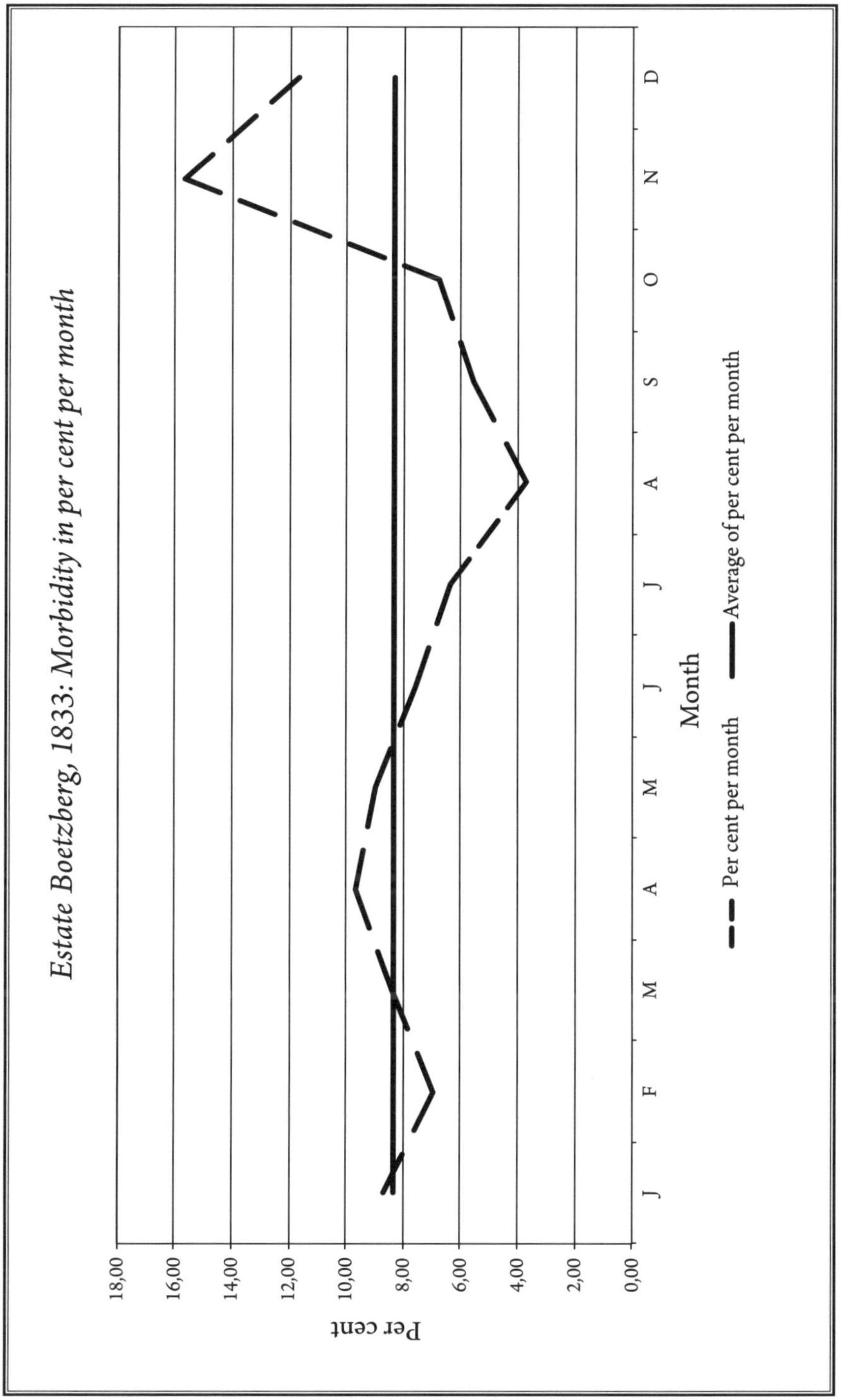

Fig. 3.9. Source: Table 3.8.

Table 3.8: Estate Boetzberg, 1833: Average number and percentage of sick enslaved per month

Months	Total number of sick per month, 1833	Per cent sick per month of the whole year
January	87	8.67
February	70	6.98
March	84	8.37
April	97	9.67
May	90	8.97
June	76	7.58
July	64	6.38
August	37	3.69
September	56	5.58
October	68	6.78
November	157	15.65
December	117	11.67
Total	1,003	100.00
Average	84	8.33

Source, DNA, WILA, no. 46.17.5.

Table 3.9: Estates North Star (1831–33), Longford (1833–36), Bọetzberg (1833): Morbidity per month in per cent of whole year

	North Star, 1831–33	Longford, 1833–36	Boetzberg, 1833	
Months	Per cent sick per month of whole year	Per cent sick per month of whole year	Per cent sick per month of whole year	Average of all plantations per month
January	7.84	6.78	8.67	7.76
February	7.26	6.42	6.98	6.89
March	7.97	5.82	8.37	7.39
April	7.53	7.78	9.67	8.33
May	7.80	8.35	8.97	8.37
June	8.12	8.85	7.58	8.18
July	8.12	8.56	6.38	7.69
August	8.61	9.00	3.69	7.10
September	8.09	8.20	5.58	7.29
October	10.07	10.49	6.78	9.11
November	9.29	11.52	15.65	12.15
December	9.31	8.23	11.67	9.73
Total	100.00	100.00	100.00	100.00

Sources: Table 3.6, 3.7 and 3.8.

Table 3.10: Causes of death per 1,000 enslaved workers, 1842–47

Year	1842	Deaths per 1,000	1843	Per 1,000	1844	Per 1,000
Population at risk (36 % of all enslaved)	5,701		5,536		5,444	
Total number of dead	217	38.1	289	52.2	170	31.2
Fever	14	2.5	30	5.4	30	5.5
Bowels and Dysentery	40	7.0	49	8.9	14	2.6
Consumption and Lungs	18	3.2	33	6.0	37	6.8
Old Age, Debility and Infirmity	13	2.3	33	6.0	23	4.2
Not stated, Unknown and Sudden death	47	8.2	16	2.9	4	0.7
Dropsy and Water in chest/brain	10	1.8	18	3.3	12	2.2
Leprosy	11	1.9	8	1.4	2	0.4
Convulsions	7	1.2	6	1.1	4	0.7
Measles	2	0.4	30	5.4	0	0.0
Worms	2	0.4	0	0.0	4	0.7
Rose	9	1.6	8	1.4	2	0.4
Inflammation	5	0.9	6	1.1	4	0.7
Ulcers	6	1.1	1	0.2	3	0.6
Accident and Drowned	1	0.2	6	1.1	6	1.1
Lock jaw	3	0.5	2	0.4	1	0.2
Teething	4	0.7	2	0.4	2	0.4
Cold	1	0.2	4	0.7	1	0.2
Apoplexy	3	0.5	2	0.4	3	0.6
Child bed	1	0.2	1	0.2	1	0.2
Eating dirt	2	0.4	4	0.7	2	0.4
Whooping cough	0	0.0	8	1.4	0	0.0
Cough	0	0.0	6	1.1	1	0.2
Liver complaint	2	0.4	4	0.7	1	0.2
Asthma	4	0.7	1	0.2	1	0.2
Epilepsy	2	0.4	0	0.0	1	0.2
Rupture	1	0.2	1	0.2	0	0.0
Abscess	0	0.0	0	0.0	2	0.4
Paralysis	1	0.2	2	0.4	0	0.0
Cancer	0	0.0	1	0.2	1	0.2
Heart disease	1	0.2	1	0.2	0	0.0
Insane	1	0.2	0	0.0	1	0.2
Drunkenness	0	0.0	0	0.0	3	0.6
Thrush	0	0.0	1	0.2	0	0.0
Brain fever	0	0.0	0	0.0	1	0.2
Delirium	0	0.0	0	0.0	1	0.2
Influenza	2	0.4	0	0.0	0	0.0
Tumours	2	0.4	0	0.0	0	0.0
Scurvy	1	0.2	1	0.2	0	0.0
Jaundice	0	0.0	1	0.2	0	0.0
Suicide	0	0.0	1	0.2	0	0.0
Rheumatism	0	0.0	1	0.2	0	0.0
Urinal	0	0.0	0	0.0	1	0.2
Loss of blood	0	0.0	0	0.0	1	0.2
Internal haemorrhage	0	0.0	0	0.0	0	0.0
Poison	0	0.0	1	0.2	0	0.0
Headache	1	0.2	0	0.0	0	0.0

Source: Church records, St Patrick, St Paul and St John, St Croix, 1842–47. Tax records, 1842–47, no. 86.69-74.

1845	Per 1,000	1846	Per 1,000	1847	Per 1,000	Total	Death per 1,000, average 1842–47	Per cent of deaths per 1,000
5,432		5,379		5,314		32,806		
171	31.5	192	35.7	173	32.6	1,212	36.9	100.0
43	7.9	59	11.0	40	7.5	216	6.6	17.8
11	2.0	27	5.0	22	4.1	163	5.0	13.4
17	3.1	20	3.7	26	4.9	151	4.6	12.5
34	6.3	28	5.2	19	3.6	150	4.6	12.4
7	1.3	0	0.0	2	0.4	76	2.3	6.3
11	2.0	13	2.4	7	1.3	71	2.2	5.9
12	2.2	7	1.3	4	0.8	44	1.3	3.6
5	0.9	2	0.4	10	1.9	34	1.0	2.8
0	0.0	0	0.0	0	0.0	32	1.0	2.6
5	0.9	8	1.5	10	1.9	29	0.9	2.4
2	0.4	1	0.2	4	0.8	26	0.8	2.1
4	0.7	1	0.2	3	0.6	23	0.7	1.9
2	0.4	5	0.9	4	0.8	21	0.6	1.7
5	0.9	3	0.6	0	0.0	21	0.6	1.7
3	0.6	4	0.7	4	0.8	17	0.5	1.4
2	0.4	1	0.2	2	0.4	13	0.4	1.1
2	0.4	1	0.2	2	0.4	11	0.3	0.9
1	0.2	0	0.0	1	0.2	10	0.3	0.8
1	0.2	4	0.7	2	0.4	10	0.3	0.8
0	0.0	1	0.2	1	0.2	10	0.3	0.8
0	0.0	0	0.0	0	0.0	8	0.2	0.7
0	0.0	0	0.0	1	0.2	8	0.2	0.7
0	0.0	0	0.0	0	0.0	7	0.2	0.6
0	0.0	0	0.0	1	0.2	7	0.2	0.6
2	0.4	1	0.2	0	0.0	6	0.2	0.5
0	0.0	0	0.0	3	0.6	5	0.2	0.4
1	0.2	1	0.2	1	0.2	5	0.2	0.4
0	0.0	0	0.0	1	0.2	4	0.1	0.3
0	0.0	2	0.4	0	0.0	4	0.1	0.3
0	0.0	0	0.0	2	0.4	4	0.1	0.3
0	0.0	0	0.0	1	0.2	3	0.1	0.2
0	0.0	0	0.0	0	0.0	3	0.1	0.2
0	0.0	1	0.2	0	0.0	2	0.1	0.2
0	0.0	1	0.2	0	0.0	2	0.1	0.2
0	0.0	1	0.2	0	0.0	2	0.1	0.2
0	0.0	0	0.0	0	0.0	2	0.1	0.2
0	0.0	0	0.0	0	0.0	2	0.1	0.2
0	0.0	0	0.0	0	0.0	2	0.1	0.2
0	0.0	0	0.0	0	0.0	1	0.0	0.1
0	0.0	0	0.0	0	0.0	1	0.0	0.1
0	0.0	0	0.0	0	0.0	1	0.0	0.1
0	0.0	0	0.0	0	0.0	1	0.0	0.1
0	0.0	0	0.0	0	0.0	1	0.0	0.1
1	0.2	0	0.0	0	0.0	1	0.0	0.1
0	0.0	0	0.0	0	0.0	1	0.0	0.1
0	0.0	0	0.0	0	0.0	1	0.0	0.1

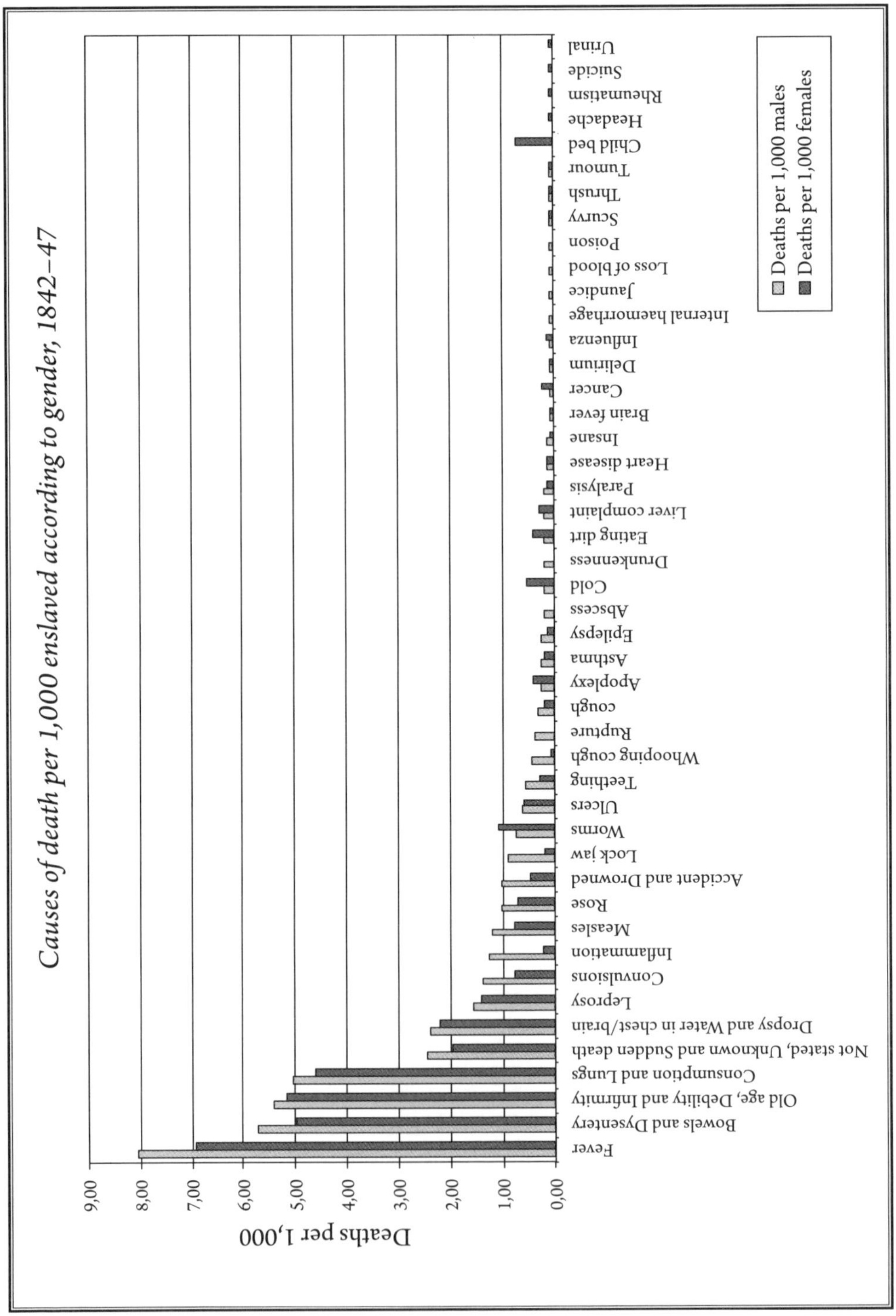

Fig. 3.12. Source: Table 3.11.

Table 3.11: Causes of death per 1,000 enslaved according to gender, 1842–47

Gender	Male	Deaths per 1,000 males	Female	Deaths per 1,000 females	Sex unknown
Population at risk (36 % of all enslaved)	15,903.72		16,900.2		
Total number of dead	688	43.26	615	36.39	16
Fever	128	8.05	117	6.92	0
Bowels and Dysentery	91	5.72	84	4.97	0
Old Age, Debility and Infirmity	86	5.41	87	5.15	0
Consumption and Lungs	80	5.03	78	4.62	3
Not stated, Unknown and Sudden death	39	2.45	33	1.95	8
Dropsy and Water in chest/brain	38	2.39	37	2.19	0
Leprosy	25	1.57	24	1.42	0
Convulsions	22	1.38	13	0.77	1
Inflammation	20	1.26	4	0.24	1
Measles	19	1.19	13	0.77	0
Rose	16	1.01	12	0.71	0
Accident and Drowned	16	1.01	8	0.47	0
Lock jaw	14	0.88	3	0.18	2
Worms	12	0.75	18	1.07	0
Ulcers	10	0.63	10	0.59	1
Teething	9	0.57	5	0.30	0
Whooping cough	7	0.44	1	0.06	0
Rupture	6	0.38	0	0.00	0
Cough	5	0.31	3	0.18	0
Apoplexy	4	0.25	7	0.41	0
Asthma	4	0.25	3	0.18	0
Epilepsy	4	0.25	2	0.12	0
Abscess	3	0.19	0	0.00	0
Cold	3	0.19	9	0.53	0
Drunkenness	3	0.19	0	0.00	0
Eating dirt	3	0.19	7	0.41	0
Liver complaint	3	0.19	5	0.30	0
Paralysis	3	0.19	2	0.12	0
Heart disease	2	0.13	2	0.12	0
Insane	2	0.13	1	0.06	0
Brain fever	1	0.06	1	0.06	0
Cancer	1	0.06	4	0.24	0
Delirium	1	0.06	1	0.06	0
Influenza	1	0.06	2	0.12	0
Internal haemorrhage	1	0.06	0	0.00	0
Jaundice	1	0.06	0	0.00	0
Loss of blood	1	0.06	0	0.00	0
Poison	1	0.06	0	0.00	0
Scurvy	1	0.06	1	0.06	0
Thrush	1	0.06	1	0.06	0
Tumour	1	0.06	1	0.06	0
Child bed	0	0.00	12	0.71	0
Headache	0	0.00	1	0.06	0
Rheumatism	0	0.00	1	0.06	0
Suicide	0	0.00	1	0.06	0
Urinal	0	0.00	1	0.06	0

Source: Church records, St Patrick, St Paul and St John on St Croix, 1842–47. Tax records, 1842–47, no. 86.69.

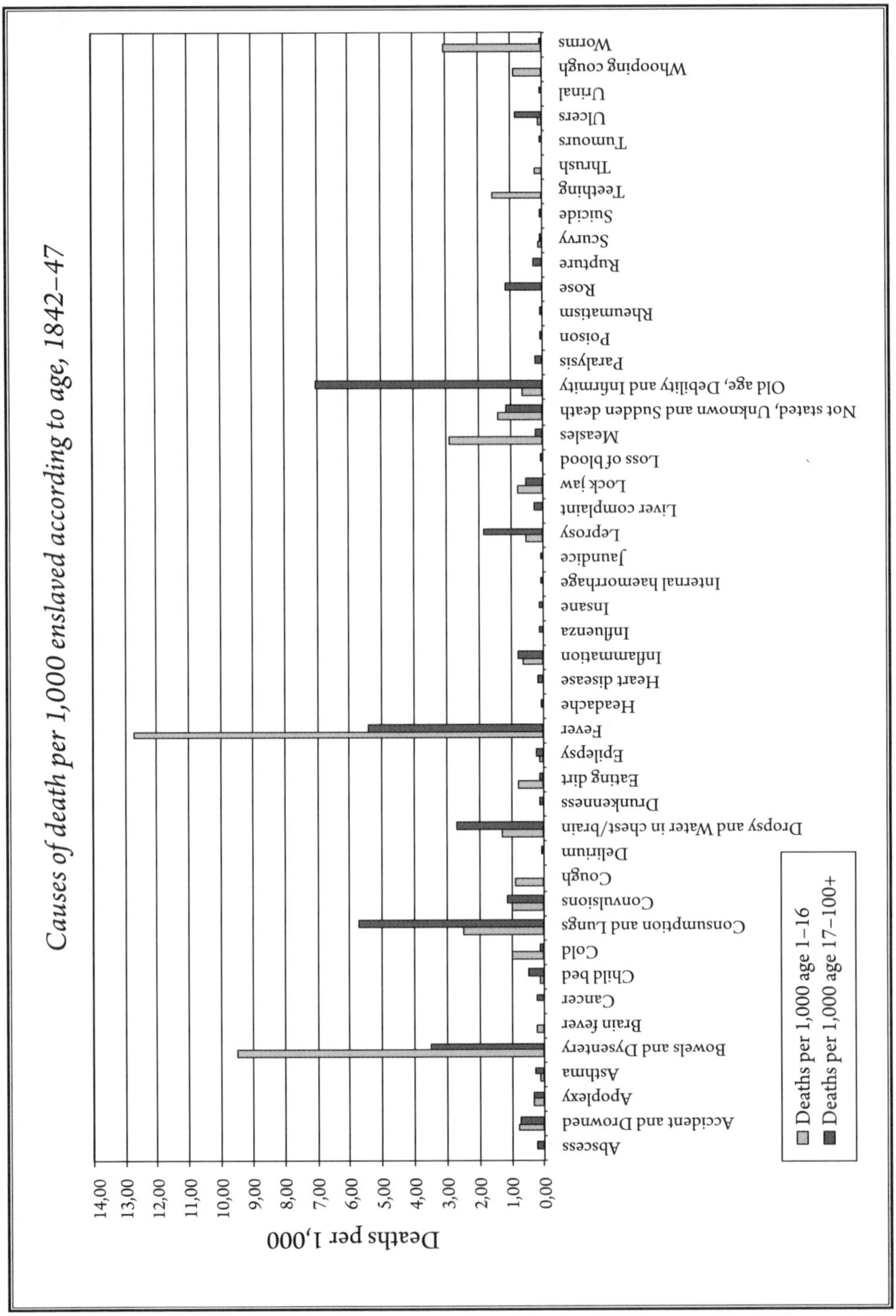

Fig. 3.13. Source: Table 3.12.

Table 3.12: Causes of death per 1,000 enslaved workers according to age, 1842–47

Age	Age 1–16	Deaths per 1,000 age 1–16	Age 17–100+	Deaths per 1,000 age 17–100+	Unknown age
Population at risk (ca. 36 % of all enslaved)	9,269.28		23,534.64		
Total number of dead	407	43.91	859	36.50	53
Abscess	0	0.00	5	0.21	0
Accident and Drowned	7	0.76	17	0.72	0
Apoplexy	3	0.32	8	0.34	0
Asthma	1	0.11	6	0.25	0
Bowels and Dysentery	88	9.49	82	3.48	4
Brain fever	2	0.22	0	0.00	0
Cancer	0	0.00	5	0.21	0
Child bed	1	0.11	11	0.47	0
Cold	9	0.97	3	0.13	0
Consumption and Lungs	23	2.48	135	5.74	2
Convulsions	9	0.97	27	1.15	0
Cough	8	0.86	0	0.00	0
Delirium	0	0.00	2	0.08	0
Dropsy and Water in chest/brain	12	1.29	63	2.68	0
Drunkenness	0	0.00	3	0.13	0
Eating dirt	7	0.76	3	0.13	0
Epilepsy	1	0.11	5	0.21	0
Fever	118	12.73	127	5.40	0
Headache	0	0.00	1	0.04	0
Heart disease	0	0.00	4	0.17	0
Inflammation	6	0.65	18	0.76	1
Influenza	0	0.00	3	0.13	0
Insane	0	0.00	3	0.13	0
Internal haemorrhage	0	0.00	1	0.04	0
Jaundice	0	0.00	1	0.04	0
Leprosy	5	0.54	43	1.83	1
Liver complaint	0	0.00	6	0.25	2
Lock jaw	7	0.76	12	0.51	0
Loss of blood	0	0.00	1	0.04	0
Measles	27	2.91	5	0.21	0
Not stated, Unknown and Sudden death	13	1.40	27	1.15	40
Old age, Debility and Infirmity	6	0.65	165	7.01	2
Paralysis	0	0.00	5	0.21	0
Poison	0	0.00	1	0.04	0
Rheumatism	0	0.00	1	0.04	0
Rose	0	0.00	27	1.15	1
Rupture	0	0.00	6	0.25	0
Scurvy	1	0.11	1	0.04	0
Suicide	0	0.00	1	0.04	0
Teething	14	1.51	0	0.00	0
Thrush	2	0.22	0	0.00	0
Tumours	0	0.00	2	0.08	0
Ulcers	1	0.11	20	0.85	0
Urinal	0	0.00	1	0.04	0
Whooping cough	8	0.86	0	0.00	0
Worms	28	3.02	2	0.08	0

Source: Church records, St Patrick, St Paul and St John, St Croix, 1842–47. Tax records, 1842–47, no. 86.69-74.

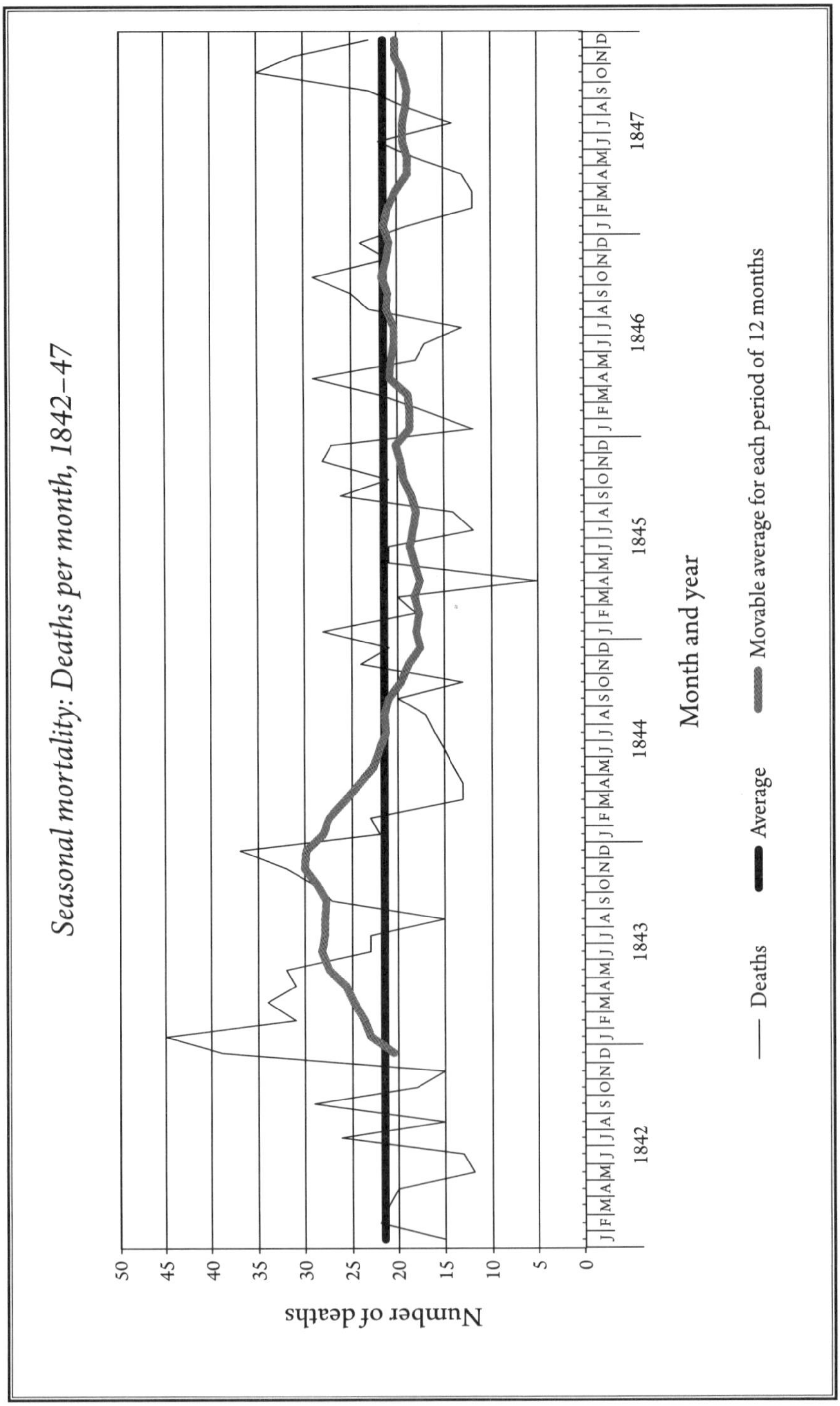

Fig. 3.14. Source: Table 3.13.

Table 3.13: Mortality per month in number of individuals and in per cent of all deaths, 1842–47

	1842	%	1843	%	1844	%	1845	%	1846	%	1847	%	Average per month	Average per month in %	Average of all years	Average of all months in %
January	15	6.12	45	12.53	22	10.43	28	11.62	12	4.80	19	7.88	16.95	9.11	21.49	8.33
February	22	8.98	31	8.64	23	10.90	18	7.47	17	6.80	12	4.98	15.07	8.10	21.49	8.33
March	21	8.57	34	9.47	13	6.16	20	8.30	22	8.80	12	4.98	14.85	7.98	21.49	8.33
April	20	8.16	31	8.64	13	6.16	5	2.07	29	11.60	13	5.39	13.42	7.21	21.49	8.33
May	12	4.90	32	8.91	14	6.64	21	8.71	18	7.20	18	7.47	13.76	7.39	21.49	8.33
June	13	5.31	23	6.41	15	7.11	21	8.71	17	6.80	22	9.13	13.21	7.10	21.49	8.33
July	26	10.61	23	6.41	16	7.58	12	4.98	13	5.20	14	5.81	12.62	6.78	21.49	8.33
August	15	6.12	15	4.18	17	8.06	14	5.81	23	9.20	19	7.88	12.40	6.66	21.49	8.33
September	29	11.84	27	7.52	20	9.48	26	10.79	25	10.00	23	9.54	18.15	9.75	21.49	8.33
October	18	7.35	29	8.08	13	6.16	21	8.71	29	11.60	35	14.52	16.99	9.13	21.49	8.33
November	15	6.12	32	8.91	24	11.37	28	11.62	21	8.40	31	12.86	17.95	9.64	21.49	8.33
December	39	15.92	37	10.31	21	9.95	27	11.20	24	9.60	23	9.54	20.73	11.14	21.49	8.33
Total	245	100.00	359	100.00	211	100.00	241	100.00	250	100.00	241	100.00	186.09	100.00	257.88	100.00

Source: Church records, St Patrick, St Paul and St John, St Croix, 1842–47.

Table 3.14: Causes of death in the British West Indies, 1817–32

	Percentage of all deaths				
	Grenada	Dominica	Tobago	Demerara-Essequibo	Berbice
Cause of death/Year	1817	1829–32	1819–21	1829–32	1819–22
Diarrhoea	25.7	19.4	20.1	18.1	16.2
Dropsy	16.0	10.7	12.1	13.9	11.4
Fever	11.3	6.0	10.6	12.3	6.2
Digestive system diseases	9.3	5.6	6.5	3.5	4.7
Nervous system diseases	8.0	7.1	5.5	11.5	11.8
Measles	6.4	—	—	—	—
Tuberculosis	4.2	12.7	8.8	11.2	9.1
Worms	3.7	9.9	4.5	3.4	3.9
Respiratory diseases	3.7	2.8	1.5	3.3	10.0
Tetanus	2.4	6.0	2.4	3.9	2.7
Leprosy	1.9	—	4.5	5.8	5.9
Accidents	1.1	7.5	3.2	6.4	3.5
Maternity	1.1	1.6	1.5	0.9	1.4
Scarlet fever	1.1	—	1.4	—	0.9
Teething	1.1	—	0.6	—	0.1
Venereal disease	0.6	—	0.9	1.5	2.3
Rheumatism	0.5	—	0.4	—	0.3
Female diseases	0.5	—	—	—	0.3
Heart diseases	0.3	—	—	—	0.1
Yaws	0.3	4.0	2.7	3.9	6.7
Neoplasms	0.2	—	0.1	0.3	0.7
Violence	0.2	—	—	—	0.3
Suicide	0.2	—	0.4	—	1.2
Diphtheria	0.2	—	—	—	0.1
Cholera	0.2	—	—	—	0.1
Whooping cough	—	—	12.1	—	0.1
Smallpox	—	6.7	—	—	—
Total	100.0	100.0	100.0	100.0	100.0
Total number of deaths	902	401	2,146	7,016	2,236
Not included above					
Unclassifiable, undefined	81	58	211	730	466
Mal d'estomac, cachexy	47	35	181	301	—
Old age, Debility	94 54	33 23	256 107	 1,342	92 176
Percentage of total	30.6	37.2	35.2	33.8	32.8

Source: Higman, *Slave Populations*, 340, table 9.8.

Table 3.15: Regrouping of causes of death following Higman

Higman's causes of death	Causes of death in the church records	Deaths	Deaths regrouped following Higman
Diarrhoea	Dysentery	41	41
Old age	Old age	74	74
Dropsy	Dropsy	69	69
Whooping cough	Whooping cough	15	15
Measles	Measles	34	34
Fever	Fever	358	
	Cold	28	
	Cough	13	399
Tuberculosis	Consumption	154	154
Digestive system diseases	Bowels	240	
	Liver complaint	8	
	Rupture	6	
	Thrush	4	
	Jaundice	2	260
Nervous system diseases	Apoplexy	11	
	Convulsions	45	
	Epilepsy	6	
	Water in the brain	4	
	Insane	3	
	Brain fever	3	
	Delirium	2	
	Paralysis	6	80
Leprosy	Leprosy	51	51
Worms	Worms	37	37
Accidents	Drowned	9	
	Accident	20	29
Yaws		0	0
Tetanus	Lockjaw	27	27
Respiratory diseases	Lungs	20	
	Asthma	7	
	Water in the chest	7	
	Influenza	6	40
Maternity	Child bed	15	15
Scarlet fever	Scarlet fever	1	1
Venereal disease		0	0
Teething	Teething	24	24
Suicide	Suicide	1	1
Rheumatism	Rheumatism	1	1
Urinary system diseases	Urinal	1	1
Neoplasms	Tumours	2	
	Cancer	5	7
Debility	Debility	79	
	Infirmity	34	
	Scurvy	3	116
Mal d'estomac	Eating dirt	10	10
Undefined	Sudden death	18	
	Unknown	19	37
Not classified	Ulcers	25	
	Inflammation	27	
	Loss of blood	2	
	Internal haemorrhage	1	
	Poison	1	
	Abscess	5	
	Drunkenness	3	
	Headache	1	
	Rose	32	97
Heart	Heart disease	4	4
Not stated	Not stated	76	76
Total			1,700

Source: Table 3.14 and the church records of St Patrick, St Paul and St John on St Croix (includes children age 0–1 years, 488 individuals in total).

Table 3.16: Causes of death from St Croix regrouped following Higman

Higman's causes of death	Church records from St Croix, number of dead	Per cent of all dead
Fever	399	30.69
Digestive system diseases	260	20.00
Tuberculosis	154	11.85
Nervous system diseases	80	6.15
Dropsy	69	5.31
Leprosy	51	3.92
Diarrhoea	41	3.15
Respiratory diseases	40	3.08
Worms	37	2.85
Measles	34	2.62
Accidents	29	2.23
Tetanus	27	2.08
Teething	24	1.85
Whooping cough	15	1.15
Maternity	15	1.15
Mal d'estomac	10	0.77
Neoplasms	7	0.54
Heart	4	0.31
Scarlet fever	1	0.08
Suicide	1	0.08
Rheumatism	1	0.08
Urinary system diseases	1	0.08
Yaws	0	0.00
Venereal disease	0	0.00
Total	1,300	100.00
Not included above		
Debility	116	8,92
Not classified	97	7,46
Not stated	76	5,85
Undefined	37	2,85
Old age	74	5,69
Total	400	30,77

Source: Table 3.15.

Table 4.1: Rations issued on the royal plantation North Star, 1832–33

	1832	1833
Total annual volume		
Corn meal, kg	10,038.70	12,445.24
Salted herring (salt fish), kg	1,811.35	2,053.68
Peas, kg	3,390.85	0.00
'Grout' (barley flour), kg	977.10	0.00
'Biscuits' (hardtack), kg	962.62	365.27
Sugar, kg	897.79	339.79
Rum, litre	500.06	875.11
Energy content in megajoules per enslaved individual per day		
Corn meal	5.87	7.27
Salted herring	0.79	0.89
Peas	1.93	0.00
Barley flour	0.56	0.00
Hardtack	0.56	0.21
Sugar	0.56	0.21
Rum	0.19	0.33
Total	10.46	8.91
Total of rations after subtraction of extra rations issued during holing	9.15	8.16
Total of rations after subtraction of extra rations and herring	8.36	7.27
Rations according to proclamation of 1817 and lease regulations of 1834 (only corn meal)		
Annual volume, kg	13,515.67	13,515.67
Energy content in megajoules per enslaved individual per day	7.91	7.91
Rations according to the customary fish ration (6 herring per enslaved per week)		
Annual volume, kg	1,080.14	1,080.14
Energy content in megajoule per enslaved individual per day	0.47	0.47
Protein content in kilograms		
Corn meal	933.60	1,157.41
Salted herring	257.03	291.42
Peas	735.81	0.00
Barley flour	102.60	0.00
Hardtack	126.10	47.85
Sugar	0.00	0.00
Rum	0.00	0.00
Total	2,155.14	1,496.67
Total of rations after subtraction of extra rations issued during holing	2,029.04	1,448.82
Amount of energy from protein in the total amount of energy issued per enslaved per day		
Excluding extra rations issued during holing, in megajoules	1.34	1.00
Including extra rations issued during holing, in megajoules	1.42	0.99
Excluding extra rations issued during holing, in per cent	14.64	12.25
Including extra rations issued during holing, in per cent	13.58	11.11

Source: Calculation 4.1 and 4.2.

Table 4.3: Rations issued on the private plantations estate Upper Bethlehem and Fredensborg, 1831

Annual volume	
Corn meal, kg	51,672.08
Salted herring, kg	7,382.50
Energy content in megajoules per enslaved individual per day	
Corn meal	8.10
Salted herring	0.86
Total	8.96
Ration according to proclamation of 1817 (only corn meal)	
Annual volume, kg	50,293.90
Energy content in megajoules per enslaved per day	7.91
Rations according to the standard fish ration (6 herring per enslaved per week)	
Annual volume, kg	4,024.80
Energy content in megajoules per enslaved per day	0.47
Protein content in kilograms	
Corn meal	4,805.50
Salted herring	1,047.58
Total	5,853.08
Amount of energy from protein in the total amount of energy per enslaved per day	
MJ	1.04
%	11.59

Source: Calculation 4.3.

Calculation 4.1

Calculation of volume and energy content in the rations issued on the royal estate North Star, 1832.

Number of enslaved individuals on North Star (1834):[19]	
Men	36
Women	24
Total adults	60
Boys	8
Girls	6
Total children	14
Total	74 (= 69.24 adult size rations)[20]

Calculation of the size of units of weight and measure:

Corn meal: 'Puncheons' (barrels):

100 enslaved people (75 on full ration and 25 on 2/3 ration) = 65 puncheons/year[21]

Standard ration of 1817 = 6 quarts/enslaved/week

6 quarts[22] × 75 enslaved × 52 weeks = 23,400 quarts/year

4 quarts × 25 enslaved[23] × 52 weeks = 5,200 quarts/year

23,400 quarts/year + 5,200 quarts/year = 28,600 quarts/year

28,600 quarts/year / 65 puncheons/year = 440 quarts/puncheon

440 quarts/puncheon = 110 imperial gallons/puncheon[24]

110 imperial gallons/puncheon × 4,546 litres/gallon[25] = 500.06 litres/puncheon

500.06 litres/puncheon × 0.550 kg corn meal/litre[26] = 275.033 kg corn meal/puncheon

19 DNA, WILA, no. 46.21.1. Inventory, North Star, 1834.

20 It is evident from a contemporary estimate made by Dr Johnson and S. Abott of the provisions needed annually on a standard plantation on St Croix that enslaved children received on average two thirds of an adult size ration. Accordingly, I have calculated the fourteen children on North Star to receive 9.24 adult rations. NARA, RG 55, Entry 82, Box 342, Some plantation inventories, Dr Johnson and S. Abott.

21 According to the contemporary estimate by Johnson and Abott.

22 1 British quart = 1,136 litres. Knut Birkeland, *Mål & Vægt* (Copenhagen: Høst and Søn Forlag, 1970), 38.

23 Twenty-five enslaved children on two thirds of adult size ration.

24 According to W. Waterston, *A Manual of Commerce* (Edinburgh: Oliver and Boyd, 1855) traditional rum puncheons contained 110–136 imperial gallons and thus we can assume that corn meal was imported in rum puncheons.

25 1 imperial gallon = 4.546 litres. Birkeland, *Mål & Vægt*, 38.

Herring: Danish herring barrels and American barrels
100 enslaved individuals = 40 Danish herring barrels or 52 American barrels a year[27]
1 Danish herring barrel = 108.205 litres[28]
40 Danish herring barrels × 108.205 litres/barrel = 4,328.2 litres herring
4,328.2 litres herring / 52 American barrels = 83.23 litres per American barrel[29]
1 Danish barrel of herring = ca. 1,200 herring (ca. 50 g/herring)[30]
40 Danish herring barrels × 1,200 herring/barrel = 48,000 herring
52 American barrels / 48,000 herring = ca. 923 herring/barrel

Total volume of rations issued:[31]
Corn meal: 36½ puncheons
36.5 puncheons × 110 imperial gallons = 4,015 imperial gallons (18,252.19 litres)
0.550 kg corn meal/litre × 18,252.19 litres = 10,038.70 kg

Herring: 39¼ barrels
1 American herring barrels = 83.23 litres
39.25 barrels × 83.23 litres = 3,266.78 litres
1 American herring barrel = 923 herring
39.25 American herring barrels × 923 herring/barrel = ca. 36,227 herring
36,227 herring × 50 g/herring = 1,811.35 kg herring

26 According to inspector Vanderbourg writing in 1798 (Tyson and Highfield, *The Kamina Folk*, 153–57) 1 gallon of corn meal weighed ca. 5 Danish pounds. 1 British gallon contains 4.546 litres and 1 Danish pound (pre 1839) weighed 0.50045 kg, which means that 5 Danish pounds equal 2.50225 kg. 2.50225 kg / 4.546 litres = 0.550 kg corn meal per litre.

27 According to the estimate of Johnson and Abott.

28 Blangstrup, *Salmonsens konversationsleksikon*, V, 619.

29 I have not been able to find any barrel size that matches 83.23 litres. In Newfoundland a barrel of herring contained 32 imperial gallons (145.47 litres), whereas an English herring barrel after 1855 contained 26 2/3 imperial gallons (121.20 litres).

30 In the eighteenth century Danish herring barrels contained somewhere between 1,040 and 1,120 herring per barrel. Bo Poulsen, *Konsekvenserne af Agger Tanges gennembrud i 1825 for fiskeriet i Limfjorden - en miljøhistorisk tolkning*. Unpublished MA thesis, University of Southern Denmark, 2002, 20.

31 DNA, WILA, no. 46.21.1. Inventory, North Star, 1834.

Peas:	34½ barrels
	1 American barrel = 115.63 litres[32]
	34.5 barrels × 115.63 litres = 3,989.24 litres
	1 litre yellow peas = ca. 850 g[33]
	3,989.235 litres × 850 g = 3,390.85 kg
'Grout':[34]	13 barrels
	1 American barrel = 115.63 litres
	13 barrels × 115.63 litres = 1,503.19 litres
	1 litre whole grain flour = ca. 650 g[35]
	1,503.19 litres × 650 g = 977.10 kg
Hardtack:	3½ puncheons[36]
	3.5 puncheons × 110 imperial gallons = 385 gallons (1,750.21 litres)
	550 g/litre[37] × 1,750.21 litres = 962.62 kg
Sugar:	¾ hogshead and 1 barrel
	1 West Indian sugar hogshead = 1,456–1,792 pounds avoirdupois[38]
	1 pound avoirdupois = 0.45359 kg[39]
	1,456–1,792 pounds avoirdupois = 660.43 kg–812.84 kg
	1 American sugar barrel = 141.58 litres = 84.95 kg[40]
	Maximum: 812.84 kg + 84.95 kg = 897.79 kg

32 I assume that this is an American 'standard dry barrel', which according to congressional resolution of 4 March 1915 (c 168 § 1, 38 Stat. 1186) contained 105 dry quarts = ca. 115.627 litres. www.sizes.com (accessed 30-05-2011).

33 'Tal og tider i køkkenet', *Ren Besked*, 6, 2001.

34 'Grout' was a coarse flour made primarily of barley but also of wheat and oats. *The Oxford English Dictionary* (2000). www.oed.com/ (accessed 30-05-2011).

35 'Tal og tider i køkkenet'.

36 I assume that these puncheons had the same size as those containing corn meal (110 imperial gallons).

37 I assume that the hardtack has the same density as corn meal.

38 Waterston.

39 Ronald Edward Zupko, *A Dictionary of Weights and Measures for the British Isles: The Middle Ages to the Twentieth Century* (Philadelphia: American Philosophical Society, 1985), xxxii.

40 Muscovado sugar weighs ca. 600 g/litre. 'Tal og tider i køkkenet'.

Rum: 1 puncheon in total
1 puncheon = 110 imperial gallons = 500.06 litres

Energy content in the above food stuffs in total and per enslaved individual:
Energy in 10,038.70 kg corn meal:

100 g corn meal = ca. 353 kcal[41]
3,530 kcal/kg corn meal × 10,038.70 kg corn meal = 35,436,626.89 kcal
1 kcal = 0.004184 MJ[42]
35,436,626.89 kcal × 0.004184 MJ/kcal = 148,266.85 MJ
148,266.85 MJ / 365 days = 406.21 MJ/day
406.21 MJ/day / 69.24 enslaved = 5.87 MJ/day/enslaved

Energy in 3,390.85 kg peas:[43]

100 g pigeon peas contain ca. 343 kcal[44]
3,390.85 kg × 3,430 kcal/kg = 11,630,615.5 kcal
11,630,615.5 kcal × 0.004184 MJ/kcal = 48,662.50 MJ
48,662.50 MJ / 365 days = 133.32 MJ/day
133.32 MJ/day / 69.24 enslaved = 1.93 MJ/day/enslaved

Energy in 977.10 kg barley flour:

100 g barley flour contain ca. 345 kcal[45]
977.10 kg × 3,450 kcal/kg = 3,370,995 kcal
3,370,995 kcal × 0.004184 MJ/kcal = 14,104.24 MJ
14,104.24 MJ / 365 days = 38.64 MJ/day
38.64 MJ/day / 69.24 enslaved = 0.56 MJ/day/enslaved

Energy in 1,811.35 kg salted herring:

100 g salted herring contain ca. 262 kcal[46]
1,811.35 kg × 2,620 kcal/kg = 4,745.737 kcal

41 Latham, appendix 3, Table A24. See: 'Maize flour, whole'.
42 *Food energy – methods of analysis and conversion factors* (Rome: FAO, 2003), chapter 3.1, www.fao.org/DOCREP/006/Y5022E/Y5022E00.HTM (accessed 30-05-2011).
43 In the West Indies and the southern USA 'peas' usually meant pigeon peas or cowpeas. *The Oxford English Dictionary* (2000). www.oed.com/ (accessed 30-05-2011). 'Tal og tider i køkkenet'.
44 Latham, appendix 3, Table A24.
45 USDA National Nutrient Database: www.nal.usda.gov/fnic/foodcomp/search/. 'Barley flour or meal' (accessed 30-05-2011).
46 USDA National Nutrient Database. 'Fish, herring, Atlantic, pickled' (accessed 30-05-2011).

4,745.737 kcal × 0.004184 MJ/kcal = 19,856.16 MJ
19,856.16 MJ / 365 days = 54.40 MJ/day
54.40 MJ/day / 69.24 enslaved = 0.79 MJ/day/enslaved

Total energy content in the issued foodstuffs:
Corn meal: 5.87 MJ/day/enslaved
Peas: 1.93 MJ/day/enslaved
Barley flour: 0.56 MJ/day/enslaved
Salted herring: 0.79 MJ/day/enslaved
Total: 9.15 MJ/day/enslaved (without herring: 8.36 MJ)

Energy in extra rations issued during holing:
Energy in 962.62 kg hardtack:
100 g hardtack contain ca. 351 kcal[47]
962.62 kg × 3,510 kcal/kg = 3,378,780.41 kcal
3,378,780.41 kcal × 0.004184 MJ/kcal = 14,140 MJ
14,140 MJ / 365 days = 38.73 MJ/day
38.73 MJ/day / 69.24 enslaved = 0.56 MJ/day/enslaved

Energy in 897.79 kg sugar:
100 g sugar contain ca. 377 kcal[48]
897.79 kg × 3,770 kcal/kg = 3,384,660.76 kcal
3,384,660.76 kcal × 0.004184 MJ/kcal = 14,161.42 MJ
14,161.42 MJ / 365 days = 38.80 MJ/day
38.80 MJ/day / 69.24 enslaved = 0.56 MJ/day/enslaved

Energy in 500.06 litres rum (= 500.06 kg)[49]
100 g rum contain ca. 231 kcal[50]
500.06 kg × 2,310 kg/kcal = 1,155,138.6 kcal
1,155,138.6 kcal × 0.004184 MJ/kcal = 4,833.10 MJ
4,833.10 MJ / 365 days = 13.24 MJ/day
13.24 MJ/day / 69.24 enslaved = 0.19 MJ/day/enslaved

47 USDA National Nutrient Database. Since hardtack is not in the database I have used whole-wheat 'Matzos', a traditional Jewish biscuit, as a reference, because it is also made only of wheat flour and water (accessed 30-05-2011).

48 USDA National Nutrient Database. 'Sugars, brown' (accessed 30-05-2011).

49 The weight of 1 litre rum is not exactly 1 kg since the density of pure alcohol is only 0.79 g/ml.

50 USDA National Nutrient Database. 'Alcoholic beverage, distilled rum, 80 proof.' (accessed 30-05-2011)

Energy in extra rations issued during holing:

Hardtack: 0.56 MJ/day/enslaved
Sugar: 0.56 MJ/day/enslaved
Rum: 0.19 MJ/day/enslaved
Total: 1.31 MJ/day/enslaved

Total energy in all rations issued on North Star (1832) per enslaved per day:

9.15 MJ + 1.31 MJ = 10.46 MJ/day/enslaved

Protein content in all foodstuffs issued as rations on North Star, 1832:

10,038.70 kg corn meal:
Protein content: 9.3 g/100 g[51]
93 g/kg × 10,038.70 kg = 933.60 kg

3,390.85 kg peas:

Protein content: 21.7 g/100 g[52]
217 g/kg × 3,390.85 kg = 735.81 kg

977.10 kg barley flour:

Protein content: 10.50 g/100 g[53]
105g/kg × 977.10 kg = 102.60 kg

1,811.35 kg salted herring:

Protein content: 14.19 g/100 g[54]
141.9 g/kg × 1,811.35 kg = 257.03 kg

962.62 kg hardtack:

Protein content: 13.10 g/100 g[55]
131 g/kg × 962.62 kg = 126.10 kg

897.788 kg sugar:

Protein content: 0 g[56]

51 Latham, appendix 3, Table A24. 'Maize flour, whole' (accessed 30-05-2011).
52 Latham, appendix 3, Table A24.
53 USDA National Nutrient Database. 'Barley flour or meal' (accessed 30-05-2011).
54 USDA National Nutrient Database. 'Fish, herring, Atlantic, pickled' (accessed 30-05-2011).
55 USDA National Nutrient Database. 'Matzos, whole-wheat' (accessed 30-05-2011).
56 USDA National Nutrient Database. 'Sugars, brown' (accessed 30-05-2011).

500.06 litres rum (500.06 kg):

Protein content: 0 g[57]

Protein content excluding extra rations:

933.60 kg + 735.81 kg + 102.60 kg + 257.03 kg = 2,029.04 kg

Energy in protein: 16.7 kJ/g = 4 kcal = 0.016672 MJ[58]

Energy in protein issued:

2,029.04 kg × 16.672 MJ/kg = 33,828.15 MJ

Energy in protein per day per enslaved:

33,828.15 MJ / 365 days = 92.68 MJ

92.68 MJ/day / 69.24 enslaved = 1.34 MJ/day/enslaved

Percentage of total energy from protein per day per enslaved:

9.15 MJ / 100 = 0.0915 MJ

1.34 MJ / 0.0915 MJ = 14.64 %

Protein content including extra rations:

126.10 kg + 2,029.04 kg = 2,155.14 kg

Energy in protein:

2,155.14 kg × 16.672 MJ/kg = 35,930.54 MJ

Energy in protein per day per enslaved:

35,930.54 MJ / 365 days = 98.44 MJ

98.44 MJ/day / 69.24 enslaved = 1.42 MJ/day/enslaved

Percentage of total energy from protein per day per enslaved:

10.46 MJ / 100 = 0.1046 MJ

1.42 MJ / 0.1046 MJ = 13.58 %

57 USDA National Nutrient Database. 'Alcoholic beverage, distilled, rum, 80 proof' (accessed 30-05-2011).

58 *Human energy requirements*, chapter 2.2 (accessed 30-05-2011).

Rations to be issued annually on North Star according to the lease regulations of 1834:[59]

Annual ration of corn meal for 60 adult enslaved workers:[60]

1 adult enslaved worker in 1 year:
6 quarts/week = 6 × 1.14 litres = 6.82 litres/week
6.82 litres/week × 52 weeks = 354.43 litres/year
354.43 litres × 550 g corn meal/litre = 194.94 kg
194.94 kg × 60 enslaved = 11,696.66 kg/year

Annual ration of corn meal for 14 enslaved children:[61]

1 enslaved child in 1 year:
4 quarts/week = 4 × 1.14 litres = 4.54 litres/week
4.54 litres/week × 52 weeks = 236.29 litres/year
236.29 litres × 550 g corn meal/litre = 129.96 kg
129.96 kg corn meal × 14 enslaved children = 1,819.42 kg/year

Amount of corn meal to be issued annually according to the lease regulations of 1834:

11,696.26 kg + 1,819.42 kg = 13,515.67 kg/year

Deficit in the amount of corn meal issued in 1832:

Amount according to regulations:	13,515.67 kg/year
Actual amount:	10,038.70 kg/year
Deficit:	3,476.97 kg/year

Energy in the ration of corn meal issued per enslaved per day compared to the energy in the rations stipulated by the lease regulations of 1834:

Lease regulations (only corn meal):
100 g corn meal = ca. 353 kcal
3,530 kcal/kg × 13,515.67 kg/year = 47,710,327.81 kcal/year

59 All enslaved individuals above the age of 15 were entitled to 6 quarts of corn meal and 'the customary quantity of herring' every week. Enslaved children between the age of 10 and 15 were entitled to 5 quarters of corn meal a week unless they worked in the so-called 'Crook gang' in which case they were entitled to the full ration. Enslaved children between the age of 6 and 10 were entitled to 3 quarts of corn meal and enslaved children under the age of 6 to 2 quarts a week.

60 I assume that the old enslaved workers continued to receive the ration they were entitled to even though they were not working as much.

61 Because the age of these children is not known, I use the same average as Johnson and Abott: 4 quarts corn meal per enslaved child per week (2/3 ration).

47,710,327.81 kcal/year × 0.004184 MJ = 199,620.01 MJ/year
199,620.01 MJ/year / 365 days = 546.90 MJ/day
546.90 MJ/day / 69.24 enslaved = 7.91 MJ/day/enslaved
The ration issued on North Star, 1832 (without herring): 8.36 MJ/day/enslaved

Energy in the customary ration of salt fish, i.e. 6 herrings a week:
Total annual volume:

Annual ration per enslaved: 6 herring/week × 52 weeks = 312 herring/year
Number of enslaved: 60 adults + 14 children = 74 individuals (69.24 full rations)
Annual total of herrings: 312 herring/year × 69.24 enslaved = 21,602.88 herrings/year
Weight per herring: 50 g
21,602.88 herring/year × 0.050 kg/herring = 1,080.14 kg herring/year

Energy in 1,080.14 kg salted herring:

100 g salted herring contain ca. 262 kcal
1,080.14 kg × 2,620 kcal/kg = 2,829,977.28 kcal
2,829,977.28 kcal × 0.004184 MJ/kcal = 11,840.62 MJ
11,840.62 MJ / 365 days = 32.44 MJ/day
32.44 MJ/day / 69.24 enslaved = 0.47 MJ/day/enslaved

Summary:
The total volume of and energy content per day per enslaved in the customary fish ration compared to the ration issued on North Star in 1832:

The customary fish ration (6 herring/week/enslaved):

Total: 1,080.14 kg herring/year
0.47 MJ/day/enslaved

The ration issued on North Star in 1832:

Total: 1,811.35 kg herring/year
0.79 MJ/day/enslaved

Calculation 4.2

Calculation of volume and energy content in the rations issued on the royal estate North Star, 1833.[62]

Total volume of rations issued:

Corn meal: 45¼ puncheons
45.25 puncheons × 110 imperial gallons = 4,977.5 imperial gallons (22,627.72 litres)
0.550 kg corn meal/litre × 22,627.72 litres = 12,445.24 kg

Herring: 44½ barrels
1 American herring barrel = 83.23 litres
44½ barrels × 83.23 litres = 3,703.74 litres
44½ American herring barrels × 923 herring/barrel = ca. 41,073.5 herring
41,073.5 herrings × 50 g/herring = 2,053.68 kg

Hardtack: 2½ barrels and ¾ puncheon
1 American barrel = 115.63 litres
2.5 barrels × 115.63 litres = 289.08 litres
0.550 kg/litre × 289.08 litres = 158.99 kg
¾ puncheon × 110 imperial gallons = 82.5 gallons (375.05 litres)
0.550 kg/litres × 375.05 litres = 206.27 kg
158.99 kg × 206.27 kg = 365.26 kg

Sugar: 4 barrels
1 American sugar barrel = 141.58 litres = 84.95 kg
84.95 kg × 4 = 339.79 kg

Rum: 1¾ puncheon
1.75 puncheon × 110 imperial gallons = 192.5 imperial gallons (875.11 litres)

62 Unless otherwise indicated the assumptions concerning barrel sizes, weights etc. are the same as in Table 4.1.

Energy content in the above foodstuffs in total and per enslaved individual:
Energy in 12,445.24 kg corn meal:

100 g corn meal = ca. 353 kcal
3,530 kcal/kg corn meal × 12,445.24 kg corn meal = 43,931,708.67 kcal
43,931,708.67 kcal × 0.004184 MJ/kcal = 183,810.27 MJ
183,810.27 MJ / 365 days = 503.59 MJ/day
503.59 MJ/day / 69.24 enslaved = 7.27 MJ/day/enslaved

Energy in 2,053.68 kg salted herring:

100 g salted herring = ca. 262 kcal
2,053.68 kg × 2,620 kcal/kg = 5,380,628.5 kcal
5,380,628.5 kcal × 0.004184 MJ/kcal = 22,512.55 MJ
22,512.55 MJ / 365 days = 61.68 MJ/day
61.68 MJ/day / 69.24 enslaved = 0.89 MJ/day/enslaved

Total energy content in the issued foodstuffs:

Corn meal: 7.27 MJ/day/enslaved
Salted herring: 0.89 MJ/day/enslaved
Total: 8.16 MJ/day/enslaved

Energy in extra rations issued during holing:
Energy in 365.266 kg hardtack:

100 g hardtack = ca. 351 kcal
365.27 kg × 3,510 kcal/kg = 1,282,083.66 kcal
1,282,083.66 kcal × 0.004184 MJ/kcal = 5,364.24 MJ
5,364.24 MJ / 365 days = 14.70 MJ/day
14.70 MJ/day / 69.24 enslaved = 0.21 MJ/day/enslaved

Energy in 339.792 kg sugar:

100 g sugar = ca. 377 kcal
339.79 kg × 3,770 kcal/kg = 1,281,015.84 kcal
1,281,015.84 kcal × 0.004184 MJ/kcal = 5,359.77 MJ
5,359.77 MJ / 365 days = 14.68 MJ/day
14.68 MJ/day / 69.24 enslaved = 0.21 MJ/day/enslaved

Energy in 875.105 litres rum (875.11 kg)

100 g rum = ca. 231 kcal

875.105 kg × 2,310 kg/kcal = 2,021,492.55 kcal

2,021,492.55 kcal × 0.004184 MJ/kcal = 8,457.92 MJ

8,457.92 MJ / 365 days = 23.17 MJ/day

23.17 MJ/day / 69.24 enslaved = 0.33 MJ/day/enslaved

Energy in extra rations issued during holing:

Hardtack: 0.21 MJ/day/enslaved

Sugar: 0.21 MJ/day/enslaved

Rum: 0.33 MJ/day/enslaved

Total: 0.75 MJ/day/enslaved

Total energy content in all rations issued on North Star (1833) per enslaved per day:

8.16 MJ + 0.75 MJ = 8.91 MJ/day/enslaved

Protein content in all foodstuffs issued as rations on North Star, 1833:

12,445.24 kg corn meal:

Protein content: 9.3 g/100 g

93 g/kg × 12,445.24 kg = 1,157.41 kg

2,053.68 kg salted herring:

Protein content: 14.19 g/100 g

141.9 g/kg × 2,053.68 kg = 291.42 kg

365.27 kg hardtack:

Protein content: 13.10 g/100 g

131 g/kg × 365.27 kg = 47.85 kg

339.79 kg sugar:

Protein content: 0 g

875.11 litres rum (= 500.06 kg):

Protein content: 0 g

Protein content excluding extra rations:

1,157.41 kg + 291.42 kg = 1,448.82 kg

Energy in protein: 16.7 kJ/g = 4 kcal = 0.016672 MJ

Energy in protein issued:

1,448.82 kg × 16.672 MJ/kg = 24,154.80 MJ

Energy in protein per day per enslaved:

24,154.80 MJ / 365 days = 66.18 MJ/day

66.18 MJ/day / 69.24 enslaved = 1.0 MJ/day/enslaved

Percentage of energy from protein per day per enslaved:

8.16 / 100 = 0.0816 MJ

1.0 MJ / 0.0816 MJ = 12.25 %

Protein content including extra rations:

1,448,82 kg + 47.85 kg = 1,496.67 kg

Energy in protein: 16.7 kJ/g = 4 kcal = 0.016672 MJ/g

Energy in protein issued:

1,496.67 kg × 16.67 MJ/kg = 24,952.55 MJ

Energy content in protein per day per enslaved:

24,952.55 MJ / 365 days = 68.36 MJ

68.36 MJ/day / 69.24 enslaved = 0.99 MJ/day/enslaved

Percentage of energy from protein per day per enslaved:

8.91 / 100 = 0.0891 MJ

0.99 MJ / 0.0891 MJ = 11.11 %

Rations to be issued annually at North Star according to the lease regulations of 1834:

13,515.67 kg corn meal/year

Deficit in the amount of corn meal issued in 1833:

Amount according to regulations:	13,515.67 kg/year
Actual amount:	12,445.24 kg/year
Deficit:	1,070.43 kg/year

Energy content in the corn meal ration issued per enslaved per day compared to the energy content in the rations stipulated by the lease regulations of 1834:

Lease regulations (only corn meal): 7.91 MJ/day/enslaved
Corn meal ration on North Star, 1833: 7.27 MJ/day/enslaved

Summary:
The total volume of and energy content per day per enslaved in the customary fish ration compared to the ration issued on North Star in 1833:
The customary fish ration (6 herring/week/enslaved):

Total: 1,080.14 kg herring/year
0.47 MJ/day/enslaved

The ration issued on North Star in 1833:

Total: 2,053.68 kg herring/year
0.89 MJ/day/enslaved

Calculation 4.3

Calculation of volume and energy content in the rations issued on estates Upper Bethlehem and Fredensborg, 1831.[63]

Number of enslaved individuals (1832):[64]

Upper Bethlehem	121
Fredensborg	161
Total	282 enslaved (= 258 adult size rations)[65]

Volume of ration-foods purchased:

Corn meal: 154 puncheons
154 puncheons × 110 imperial gallons = 16,940 imperial gallons
16,940 imperial gallons × 4.546 litres = 93,949.24 litres
93,949.24 litres × 0.550 kg/litre = 51,672.08 kg corn meal

Herring: 158 barrels of 200 pounds (90.8 kg)
1 American herring barrel = 83.23 litres (ca. 923 herring/barrel, ca. 50 g/herring)
158 barrels × 83.23 litres = 13,150.34 litres
158 barrels × 923 herring/barrel = 145,834 herring
145,834 herring × 50 g/herring = 7,291.7 kg herring
7,291.7 kg + 90.8 kg = 7,382.5 kg herring
90.8 kg herring / 0.050 kg/herring = 1,816 herring
145,834 herring + 1,816 herring = 147,650 herring

Energy content in the above foodstuffs in total and per enslaved per day:
Energy in 51,672.08 kg corn meal:

100 g corn meal = ca. 353 kcal

63 Unless otherwise indicated the assumptions concerning barrel sizes, weights etc. are the same as in Table 4.1.

64 DNA, WILA, The sheriff in Christiansted 1734–1901, Proceedings of the Sheriff's Court, no. 38.22.49. Inventories, 1832.

65 Following the estimate by Johnson and Abott mentioned above, I assume that the children make up one quarter of the enslaved and that their rations amount to two thirds of a full ration. This means that of 282 enslaved 71 (70.5) would be children who receive 47 (47.33) adult size rations. Accordingly, the number of full rations is 258.

3,530 kcal/kg corn meal × 51,672.08 kg corn meal =
182,402,449.46 kcal
182,402,449.46 kcal × 0.004184 MJ/kcal = 763,171.85 MJ
763,171.85 MJ / 365 days = 2,090.88 MJ/day
2,090.88 MJ/day / 258 enslaved = 8.10 MJ/day/enslaved

Energy in 7,382.50 kg salted herring:

100 g salted herring contains ca. 262 kcal
7,382.50 kg × 2,620 kcal/kg = 19,342,150 kcal
19,342,150 kcal × 0.004184 MJ/kcal = 80,927.56 MJ
80,927.56 MJ / 365 days = 221.72 MJ/day
221.72 MJ/day / 258 enslaved = 0.86 MJ/day/enslaved

Total energy content in the issued foodstuffs:

Corn meal: 8.10 MJ/day/enslaved
Salted herring: 0.86 MJ/day/enslaved
Total: 8.96 MJ/day/enslaved

Protein content in foodstuffs purchased for Bethlehem and Fredensborg, 1831:

51,672.08 kg corn meal:
Protein content: 9.3 g/100 g
93 g/kg × 51,672.08 kg = 4,805.50 kg

7,382.5 kg salted herring:

Protein content: 14.19 g/100 g
141.9 g/kg × 7,382.5 kg = 1,047.58 kg

Energy from protein in the foodstuffs purchased:

4,805.50 kg + 1,047.58 kg = 5,853.08 kg protein

Energy in protein: 16.7 kJ/g = 4 kcal = 0.016672 MJ/g

5,853.08 kg × 16,672 MJ/kg = 97,582.56 MJ

Energy from protein per enslaved per day:

97,582.56 MJ / 365 days = 267.35 MJ
267.35 MJ/day / 258 enslaved = 1.04 MJ/day/enslaved

Percentage of total energy from protein per enslaved per day:

8.97 MJ / 100 = 0.0897 MJ

1.04 MJ / 0.0897 MJ = 11.59 %

Annual amount of corn meal to be issued according to the proclamation of 1817:
Annual ration of corn meal for 258 adult enslaved workers:[66]

1 adult enslaved in 1 year:

6 quarts = 6 × 1.136 litres = 6.82 litres

6.82 litres × 52 weeks = 354.43 litres/year

354.43 litres/year × 0,550 kg corn meal/litre = 194.94 kg/year

194.94 kg/year × 258 enslaved = 50,293.90 kg/year

Surplus in the amount of corn meal purchased in 1831:

Amount according to the proclamation: 0,293.90 kg

Actual amount: 51,672.08 kg

Surplus: 1,378.18 kg

Energy content in the corn meal ration purchased per enslaved per day compared to the energy content in the rations stipulated by the proclamation of 1817:

The proclamation (only corn meal): 7.91 MJ/day/enslaved

The ration on Upper Bethlehem and Fredensborg, 1831:
8.10 MJ/day/enslaved

Summary:
The total volume of and energy content per day per enslaved in the customary ration of salt fish (6 herring/week) compared to the volume of fish purchased for Upper Bethlehem and Fredensborg in 1831:

The customary ration of fish:

Total: 1,080.14 kg herring/year

0.47 MJ/day/enslaved

Volume purchased in 1831:

Total: 7,382.5 kg herring/year

0.86 MJ/day/enslaved

66 I assume the enslaved children received two thirds of a full ration even though this is not specified in the proclamation.

Table 4.4: Enslaved workers vaccinated each year on St Croix (plantations and towns), 1820–48

Year	Vaccinated:
1820	702[67]
1821	0
1822	611
1823	164
1824	2,011
1825	3
1826	2
1827	675[68]
1828	2
1829	813
1830	539
1831	571
1832	542
1833	31
1834	790
1835	14
1836	974
1837	92
1838	25
1839	901[69]
1840	872
1841	242
1842	489
1843	554
1844	17
1845	805
1846	498
1847	204

Source: Unless marked by a footnote the data originate from DNA, WILA, no. 10.4.1-2, 10.5, and 10.6.1-2. I thank George Tyson for this material.

67 DNA, WILA, no. 3.81.609. Report on vaccination on St Croix in 1820.
68 DNA, BH, Med. rep., Danish West Indies. 1827.
69 DNA, BH, Med. rep., Danish West Indies. 1839.

List of figures, tables and calculations

List of Figures

List of Tables

List of Calculations

Bibliography

Archival Material

Rigsarkivet, Danish National Archive, Copenhagen, Denmark (DNA):

Danske Kancelli (Danish Chancellery), archive no. 232:

No. G125C — Fællesafdelingen, Kommission ang. en Anordning om Medicinalpolitiet 1802–1814, Indkomne Sager, Forhandlinger og Korrespondance (Common Department, Commission regarding an ordinance on medical policy 1802–1814, incoming cases, negotiations and correspondence), no. G125C, reports from St Croix, 1804

Direktionen for Statsgælden og den Synkende Fond (Directorate of the state debt and the sinking fund, DSD), archive no. 259:

No. 1113 — Sager vedr. Oxholms plantager (Cases concerning the Oxholm plantations), 1802–1830

No. 1128 — Vestindiske plantageregnskaber, St. Croix (Accounts from West Indian plantations, St Croix), 1824–1847

No. 1129 — Vestindiske plantageregnskaber, St. Croix (Accounts from West Indian plantations, St Croix), 1824–1848

Fødsels- og Plejestiftelsen (The Royal Birth and Nursing Foundation), archive no. 259:

No. 186 Kopibog, oldfrues og økonomias vilkår mv. og reglementer, samt protocol over læredøtre (Copybook of matron's instructions, regulations and a protocol on apprentices), 1806–1838

Privatarkiver (Private archives):

No. 5097 — Jens Michelsen Beck

Rentekammeret, Danske Kammer, 3. Departement (Chamber of Revenue, Danish Chamber, 3rd Department), 1771–1773:

No. 2323.2	Vestindisk Journal (West Indian Journal)
No. 2323.3	Vestindisk Journal (West Indian Journal)

Reviderede regnskaber, Vestindiske regnskaber (Audited Accounts,), arkivnr. 571:
Matrikler for St. Croix (Tax records for St Croix), 1758–1915:

No. 86.69	1842
No. 86.70	1843
No. 86.71	1844
No. 86.72	1845
No. 86.73	1846
No. 86.74	1847

Sundhedskollegiet (Royal Board of Health), archive no. 571:
Medicinalindberetninger (Medical reports), 1803–1958 (1821, 1822)
Medicinalindberetninger, Vestindien (Medical reports, Danish West Indies), 1823–1832
Medicinalindberetninger, Vestindien (Medical reports, Danish West Indies), 1833–1840
Medicinalindberetninger, Vestindien (Medical reports, Danish West Indies), 1841–1852

Vestindiske Lokalarkiver (West Indian Local Archives, WILA):
Generalguvernementet (Government-General), 1716–1882:
Plakatbøger (Proclamation books), 1733–1882:

No. 2.1.4	1733–1782
No. 2.1.5	1791–1823
No. 2.1.6	1824–1882

Korrespondance- og ordreprotokoller (Copybooks concerning orders and rules), 1815–1827:

No. 2.2.1	1815–1816
No. 2.2.2	1816–1817

Kopibøger til lokale myndigheder og personer (Copybooks concerning letters sent to local authorities and individuals), 1773–1807:
No. 2.5.3 1796–1807

Referatprotokoller for indkomne skrivelser fra myndigheder m.m. i Dansk Vestindien (Registers of letters received from authorities etc. in the Danish West Indies, journals), 1790–1854:
No. 2.16.5 1807–1815
No. 2.16.7 1816–1817
No. 2.16.8 1817
No. 2.16.9 1819

Kopibøger B (Copybooks, series B), 1829–1849:
No. 2.26.2 1829–1831

Referatprotokoller B (Registers of letters, B series), 1820–1848:
No. 2.27.6 1831
No. 2.27.12 1836
No. 2.27.14 1838

Sager for Kommissionen af 1837 ang. de ufries forhold (Records regarding the Commission of 1837 concerning the conditions of the unfree), 1832–1842:
No. 2.38.2 1832–1842

Den vestindiske Regering/Guvernementets St. Croix afdeling (West Indian Government / St Croix Department of Government), 1723–1912:
Register til ekstraktprotokoller for breve til Danske Kancelli (Index to extracts of letters received from the Danish Chancellery), 1814–1848:
No. 3.18 1814–1848

Breve fra diverse institutioner og personer (Letters received from miscellaneous institutions and individuals), 1755–1823:
No. 3.30 1755–1823

Instruktionsprotokoller (Register of instructions), 1723–1784:
No. 3.40 1723–1784

Indkomne sager til referatprotokoller for breve fra lokaladministrationen (Files relating to the registers of letters received from the local administration etc.), 1774–1801:

No. 3.42.30	1790

Indgåede skrivelser til den engelske generalguvernør (Letters received by the English Governor General), 1808–1815:

No. 3.56.2	1809–1810
No. 3.56.6	1813
No. 3.56.7	1814

Referatprotokoller B (Registers of letters received, series B, journals), 1815–1880:

No. 3.62.1	1815–1817

Gruppeordnede sager: 9. Sociale og kulturelle forhold (Subject files: 9. Social and cultural matters):

No. 3.81.592	Indgåede skrivelser vedr. Medicinalvæsenet (Letters received concerning the health service), 1780–1786
No. 3.81.599	Forhandlingsprotokol for sundheds- og karantænekommissionen i Christansted (Record of proceedings of the Health and Quarantine Commission in Christiansted), 1816–1850
No. 3.81.609	Sager vedr. vaccinationsvæsenet (Files concerning the vaccination system), 1819–1857
No. 3.81.611	Sager vedr. Ligsyn og andre af læger udstedte attester (Files concerning death certificates and other certificates issued by medical officers), 1809–1818

Gruppeordnede sager: 12. Plantagerne (Subject files: 12. Plantations):

No. 3.81.685	Sager vedr. de enkelte plantager II. (Files concerning individual plantations), 1792–1895
No. 3.81.690	Samlepakke (Miscellaneous), 1786–1899

Medicinalvæsenet på De vestindiske Øer (West Indian Medical Administration), 1753–1854:

Landfysikus' arkiv. Indkomne breve og koncepter til udgående (Archives of the Landfysikus: Letters received and drafts of letters sent), 1753–1854:

No. 10.2.1	1753–1852
No. 10.2.3	1810–1854

Landfysikus' arkiv. Vaccinationsprotokoller (Archives of the Landfysikus: Registers of vaccinations), 1820–1853

No. 10.4.1	Dr Schlegel's registers of vaccinations, 1820–1831
No. 10.4.2	Registers of vaccinations, 1848–1853
No. 10.5	Journals of vaccinations, 1829–1839

Landfysikus' arkiv. Vaccinationslister (Archives of the Landfysikus: Lists of vaccinations), 1824–1853:

No. 10.6.1	Lists of vaccinations, 1824
No. 10.6.2	Lists of vaccinations, 1827–1853

Private lægers arkiver. Dr. Søren Johannes Keutsch' Lægehovedbog (Archives of private physicians: Dr Søren Johannes Keutsch's medical ledger), 1808–1808:

No. 10.19	1808

Private lægers arkiver. Dr. Søren Johannes Keutsch' lægehovedbog (Archives of private physicians: Dr Søren Johannes Keutsch's medical ledger), 1812–1813:

No. 10.21	1812–1813

Christiansted Byfoged (Sheriff in Christiansted), 1734–1901:
Domprotokoller (Registers of sentences), 1756–1887:

No. 38.6.28	1817–1820

Politiretsprotokoller (Police Court proceedings), 1756–1841:

No. 38.9.11	1800–1803

Fogedprotokoller (Proceedings of the Sheriff's Court), 1757–1896:

No. 38.22.41	1820–1823
No. 38.22.42	1820–1823
No. 38.22.43	1822–1824
No. 38.22.48	1828–1832
No. 38.22.49	1828–1833

Sankt Croix Overformynderi (Upper Guardians' Administration on St Croix), 1755–1879:
Sager til overformynderiprotokollerne (Journal files):

No. 41.6.6	1840

Sankt Croix Borgerråd (St Croix Burgher Council), 1759–1865:
Sessionsprotokoller (Records of proceedings), 1786–1814:

No. 45.1.3	1813–1814

Den Vestindiske Gælds Likvidations Kommission på St. Croix (West Indian Debt Liquidation Commission on St Croix), 1766–1853:
Sager og rapporter vedr. de enkelte plantager på St. Croix (Files and reports concerning individual plantations on St Croix), 1787–1847:

No. 46.17.5	Boetzberg, 1805–1836
No. 46.17.6	Boetzberg, 1837–1847
No. 46.17.15	Cotton Grove, 1807–1835
No. 46.17.30	Hermon Hill, 1806–1827
No. 46.17.31	Hermon Hill, 1828–1833
No. 46.17.32	Hermon Hill, 1834–1840
No. 46.17.33	Hermon Hill, 1841–1847
No. 46.17.43	Longford with stud farm, 1830
No. 46.17.44	Longford with stud farm, 1831–1833
No. 46.17.45	Longford with stud farm, 1834–1846
No. 46.17.46	Longford with stud farm, 1829–1835
No. 46.17.53	North Star, 1831–1832
No. 46.17.54	North Star, 1833–1847
No. 46.17.55	North Star, 1830–1833
No. 46.17.72	Work and Rest, 1832–1838

Sager vedr. de kgl. plantager (Files concerning the royal plantations), 1833–1844:

No. 46.19	1833–1844

Dokumenter vedr. bortforpagtningen af de kgl. plantager (Records concerning the farming out of royal plantations), 1833–1846:

No. 46.20	1833–1846

Forpagtningskontrakter vedr. de kgl. plantager (Lease contracts concerning royal plantations), 1830–1844:
No. 46.21 1830–1844

Plantageregnskaber (Plantation accounts), 1829–1845:
No. 46.58.1 1829–1836

Provideringskommissionen for Sankt Croix af 20. marts 1823 (St Croix Provisions Commission of 20 March), 1823–1898:
No. 58.1–8 1823–1898

National Archives and Records Administration, Maryland, USA (NARA):
Record Group 55, Records of the Government of the Virgin Islands, the former Danish West Indies, 1672–1917 (RG55): http://www.virgin-islands-history.dk/nara/danmark1.pdf

Entry 56 (Box 122)	Letters received by the English Government secretary during the English occupation, including records pertaining to the transfer of the islands back to Danish administration, 1813–1815
Entry 82	General correspondence, 1848–1917:
Box 220	Midwife Matters, 1858–1917
Box 315	Doctor's Licence, P. Eggert Benzon, 1826
Box 315	Records concerning trade in medicine and poisons, 1829
Box 319	Various papers relating to free blacks
Box 342	Some plantation inventories
Entry 1089	Miscellaneous military records, 1791–1917:
Box 2407	Lists of patients in the Petersfarm Hospital, 1840–1848
Entry 1109	Correspondence relating to plantations, arranged by name of plantation, 1803–1856:
Box 2432	Estate Jolly Hill
Box 2435	Estate Jolly Hill
Box 2438	Estate Mount Victory
Box 2439	Estate Smithfield

Printed Sources

Algreen-Ussing, Tage, *Kongelige Reskripter og Resolutioner, Reglementer, Instruxer og Fundatser, samt Kollegialbreve, med flere Danmarks Lovgivning vedkommende offentlige Aktstykker* (Copenhagen, 1845).

Antonsen, Inge Mejer, 'Møbler og boligkultur i Dansk Vestindien', *Dansk Kunsthåndværk* 40, (1967–68), 187–93.

Arnold, David, 'Medicine and Colonialism', in *Companion Encyclopedia of the History of Medicine*, ed. W.F. Bynum and Roy Porter (London: Routledge, 1993), 1393–416.

Arnold, David, *Colonizing the Body: State Medicine and Epidemic Disease in Nineteenth-Century India* (London: University of California Press, 1993).

Arnold, David, ed., *Warm Climates and Western Medicine: The Emergence of Tropical Medicine, 1500–1900* (Amsterdam: Rodopi, 1996).

Asmussen, Jesper Bering, *Slavedemografi: St. Croix' Landdistrikter, 1803–1848*, unpublished MA thesis, Aarhus University, 1983.

Astrup, Arne et al., *Menneskets ernæring. Fra molekylærbiologi til sociologi* (Copenhagen: Munksgaard, 1997).

Barclay, Herman, *Bidrag til Kundskab om vestindiske Sygdomme med didhørende Bemærkninger, Samlede paa St. Thomas i Aarene 1823–1827* (Copenhagen and Schleswig, 1829 and 1830).

Barros, Juanita de, '"Setting Things Right": Medicine and Magic in British Guiana, 1803–38', *Slavery and Abolition* 25.1 (2004), 28–50.

Baumgardt, Kenneth and George F. Tyson, *A Phase 1B Archaeological Survey of Estate Coakley Bay, St. Croix, USVI*, 1987, unpublished archaeological report, copy in St Croix Landmarks Society, Research Archive and Library, Estate Whim, St. Croix, II-7, II-24 and 'artefact inventory'.

Bergsøe, Adolph Frederik, *Den danske Stats Statistik*, 4 volumes (Copenhagen, 1853).

Berlin, Ira and Philip D. Morgan, *Cultivation and Culture: Labor and the Shaping of Slave Life in the Americas* (London: University Press of Virginia, 1993).

Birkeland, Knut, *Mål & Vægt* (Copenhagen: Høst and Søn Forlag, 1970).

Blangstrup, Christian, ed., *Salmonsens Konversationsleksikon*, second edition (Copenhagen: Schultz Forlag, 1916).

Bonderup, Gerda, '"Omsorg for at afværge smitsomme sygdomme". Sundhedspolitiet ca. 1750–1900', *Årsskrift, Politihistorisk Selskab København* (1992), 5–38.

Bonderup, Gerda, *En kovending. Koppevaccinationen og dens udfordring til det danske samfund omkring 1800* (Aarhus: Aarhus University Press, 2001).

Braithwaite, Edward, *The Development of Creole Society in Jamaica 1770–1820* (Oxford: Clarendon, 1971).

Bredsdorff, Peter, et al., 'Kunstakademiets studier af byer og bygningskunst på de Dansk-Vestindieske Øer', *Arkitekten* 62 (1960), 405–13.

Bricka, Carl Frederik, *Dansk biografisk Lexikon* (Copenhagen: Gyldendalske Boghandels Forlag, 1887–1905).

Brieger, Gert, 'The Historiography of Medicine', in *Companion Encyclopedia of the History of Medicine*, ed. W.F. Bynum and Roy Porter (London: Routledge, 1993), 24–44.

Bush, Barbara, *Slave Women in Caribbean Society, 1650–1838* (London: James Curry Ltd., 1990).

Carøe, Kristian, *Den Danske Lægestand, 1479–1900* (Copenhagen: Gyldendal, Nordisk Forlag, 1977).

Carpenter, Kenneth J., *Protein and Energy: A Study of Changing Ideas in Nutrition* (Cambridge: Cambridge University Press, 1994).

Carstens, J.L., *En almindelig Beskrivelse om alle de Danske, Americanske eller West-Jndiske Ey-Lande: Dansk Vestindien for 250 år siden* (Copenhagen: Dansk Vestindisk Forlag, 1981).

Chapman, William, 'Slave Villages in the Danish West Indies', *Perspectives in Vernacular Architecture* 4 (1991), 108–120.

Collins, *Practical Rules for the Management and Medical Treatment of Negro Slaves in the Sugar Colonies* (New York: Books for Libraries Press, 1971 [Original: London, 1811]).

Collins, K.J. and D.F. Roberts, *Capacity for Work in the Tropics* (Cambridge: Cambridge University Press, 1988).

Cottias, Myriam, 'La Martinique: Babylone fertile ou terre stérile? Des discours sur la fécondité aux indicateurs démographiques et sociaux (XVIIe–XIXe siècle)', *Annales de démographie historique* (1992) 199–215.

Curtin, Philip, *Two Jamaicas: The Role of Ideas in a Tropical Colony, 1830–1865* (Cambridge, Mass.: Harvard University Press, 1955).

Curtin, Philip, *Death by Migration* (Cambridge: Cambridge University Press, 1989).

D'Alois, Lydia A., 'A Response to "Slave Mortality"', *Journal of Social History* 11.2 (1977), 292–94.

Dansk Vestindisk Regierings Avis (1802–1807, 1815–1843).

Deacon, Harriet, 'Midwives and Medical Men in the Cape Colony before 1860', *Journal of African History* 39 (1998), 271–92.

Ditlevsen, Christian, 'Om sanitære og hygiejniske Forhold i Dansk Vestindien', *Atlanten: Medlemsblad for Foreningen 'De danske Atlanterhavsøer', Særskilte Artikler og Foreningsanliggender* 4 (1917), 1–22.

Dons, P.L., 'Om den saakaldte africanske Kakexie (mal d'estomac, dirteating, jordæden)', *Journal for Medicin og Chirurgie* 9 (Copenhagen, 1833), 297–323.

Dookhan, Isaac, *A History of the Virgin Islands of the United States* (St. Thomas: Caribbean Universities Press for the College of the Virgin Islands, 1974).

Dookhan, Isaac, *A Pre-Emancipation History of the West Indies* (London: Longman, 1976).

Dorsey, Joseph C., *Slave Traffic in the Age of Abolition: Puerto Rico, West Africa, and the Non-Hispanic Caribbean, 1815–1859* (Gainesville: University Press of Florida, 2003).

Elkins, Stanley, *Slavery: A Problem in American Institutional and Intellectual Life* (Chicago: University of Chicago Press, 1959).

Elsass, Peter, *Sundhedspsykologi* (Copenhagen: Gyldendal, 1992).

Engerman, Stanley L. and B.W. Higman, 'The Demographic Structure of the Caribbean Slave Societies in the Eighteenth and Nineteenth Centuries', in *General History of the Caribbean* III, ed. Franklin W. Knight (London: UNESCO Publishing, 1997), 45–104.

Engerman, Stanley L., 'A Population History of the Caribbean', in Michael R. Haines and Richard H. Steckel, eds., *A Population History of North America* (Cambridge: Cambridge University Press, 2000).

Falbe-Hansen, V. and Dr W. Scharling, *Danmarks Statistik* V (Copenhagen, 1881), 81.

Feldbæk, Ole, 'Den lange fred, 1700–1800', in *Gyldendal og Politikens Danmarks-historie* IX, ed. Olaf Olsen (Copenhagen: Gyldendals Boghandel, Nordisk Forlag and Politikens Forlag, 1990).

Fett, Sharla M., *Working Cures: Healing, Health and Power on Southern Slave Plantations* (Chapel Hill: University of North Carolina Press, 2002).

Figueredo, A.E. and George F. Tyson, *Stage I Cultural Resources Survey of Two Structures in Plot 19, Estate Diamond, Prince's Quarter, St. Croix, US Virgin Islands*, 1986, unpublished archaeological report, copy in St Croix Landmarks Society, Research Archive and Library, Estate Whim, St Croix.

Figueredo, A.E., *Phase I Cultural Resources Survey of a 17-acre Tract in Estate Wood Cottage, East End B Quarter, Christiansted Jurisdiction*, St. Croix, US Virgin Islands, 1988, unpublished archaeological report, copy in St Croix Landmarks Society, Research Archive and Library, Estate Whim, St Croix.

Fogel, Robert W. and Stanley L. Engerman, *Time on the Cross: The Economics of American Negro Slavery* (Toronto: Little, Brown and Company, 1974).

Fogtmann, Laurids, *Kongelige Rescripter, Resolutioner og Collegialbreve for Danmark og Norge udtogsviis udgivne i chronologisk Orden* (Copenhagen, 1786–1890).

Foucault, Michel, *The Birth of the Clinic* (London: Tavistock Publications, 1979).

Geill, Torben, 'Den gule feber i Dansk Vestindien', *Dansk medicinhistorisk årbog* (1975), 140–62.

Geill, Torben, 'Spedalskheden i Dansk Vestindien', *Dansk medicinhistorisk årbog* (1977), 140–67.

Gibbs, Tyson, Kathleen Cargill, Leslie Sue Lieberman and Elizabeth Reitz, 'Nutrition in a Slave Population: An Anthropological Examination', *Medical Anthropology* 4 (1980), 175–205.

Goveia, Elsa, *Slave Society in the British Leeward Islands at the End of the Eighteenth Century* (New Haven: Yale University Press, 1965).

Grainger, James, *An Essay on the More Common West-India Diseases; and the Remedies which that Country itself Produces; to which are added, some Hints on the Management of Negroes. With practical Notes, and a Linnæan Index by William Wright, M.D.F.R.S* (Edinburgh: Mundell and Son, London: Longman and Rees, 1802 [1764]).

Green-Pedersen, Svend E., 'Slave Demography in the Danish West Indies and the Abolition of the Danish Slave Trade', in *The Abolition of the Atlantic Slave Trade: Origins and Effects in Europe, Africa, and the Americas*, ed. David Eltis and James Walvin (Madison: University of Wisconsin Press, 1981), 231–55.

Gøbel, Erik, 'Danish Trade to the West Indies and Guinea, 1671–1754', *Scandinavian Economic History Review* 31 (1983), 21–49.

Gøbel, Erik, *A Guide to Sources for the History of the Danish West Indies (US Virgin Islands), 1671–1917* (Odense: University Press of Southern Denmark, 2002). www.virgin-islands-history.dk/

Haagensen, Reimert, *Description of the Island of St. Croix in America in the West Indies* (US Virgin Islands: Virgin Islands Humanities Council, 1995).

Hall, Douglas, *Free Jamaica, 1838–1865* (New Haven: Yale University Press, 1959).

Hall, Neville A.T., *Slave Society in the Danish West Indies. St. Thomas, St. John, St. Croix*, ed. Barry W. Higman (Jamaica: The University of the West Indies Press, 1992).

Handler, Jerome S. and Robert S. Corruccini, 'Plantation Slave Life in Barbados: A Physical Anthropological Analysis', *Journal of Interdisciplinary History* 14.1 (1983), 65–90.

Handler, Jerome S., 'An Archaeological Investigation of the Domestic Life of Plantation Slaves in Barbados', *Journal of the Barbados Museum and Historical Society* 34 (1972), 64–72.

Handler, Jerome S., 'Slave Medicine and Obeah in Barbados, circa 1650 to 1834', *New West Indian Guide/Nieuwe West-Indische Gids* 74.1+2 (2000), 57–60.

Handler, Jerome S., *Africans and Creoles: Studies in Barbados Slave Life, 1627–1834*, unpublished manuscript. Personal communication with the author, January 2005.

Hannaway, Caroline, 'Environment and Miasmata', in *Companion Encyclopedia of the History of Medicine* I, ed. W.F. Bynum and Roy Porter (London: Routledge, 1993), 292–308.

Hansen, Carl Adam, 'Den "lollandske feber"', *Lolland-Falsters historiske Samfunds Aarbog* 1 (1913), 45–64.

Harrison, Mark, 'The Tender Frame of Man: Disease, Climate, and Racial Difference in India and the West Indies, 1760–1860', *Bulletin of the History of Medicine* 70.1 (1996), 68–93.

Harrison, Mark, *Climates and Constitutions: Health, Race, Environment and British Imperialism in India, 1600–1850* (Oxford: Oxford University Press, 1999).

Helman, Cecil G., *Culture, Health and Illness* (London: Hodder Arnold, 2000).

Highfield, Arnold R. and George F. Tyson, *Slavery in the Danish West Indies: A Bibliography* (US Virgin Islands: The Virgin Islands Humanities Council, 1994).

Highfield, Arnold R., ed., *Observations on the State of Negro Slavery in the Island of Santa Cruz, the Principal of the Danish West India Colonies, with Miscellaneous Remarks upon Subjects Relating to the West India Question and a Notice of Santa Cruz* (St Croix: Antilles Press, 1996 [Originally published by Simpkin and Marshall and Longman Reid and Co., London 1829]).

Highfield, Arnold R., ed., *Hans West's Accounts of St. Croix in the West Indies* (US Virgin Islands: Virgin Islands Humanities Council, 2004).

Higman, Barry W., *Slave Populations of the British Caribbean, 1807–1834* (Baltimore: Johns Hopkins University Press, 1984).

Higman, Barry. W., 'Danish West Indian Slavery in Comparative Perspective: An Appreciation of Neville Hall's Contribution to the Historiography', in *Bondmen and Freedmen in the Danish West Indies: Scholarly Perspectives,* ed. George F. Tyson (US Virgin Islands: Virgin Islands Humanities Council, 1996), 1–17.

Higman, Barry. W., 'Introduction', in *General History of the Caribbean: Methodology and Historiography of the Caribbean* VI, ed. B.W. Higman (London: UNESCO Publishing, 1999), 1–18.

Hopkins, Daniel, 'The Eighteenth-Century Invention of a Measure in the Caribbean: the Danish Acre of St. Croix', *Journal of Historical Geography* 18.2 (1992), 158–73.

Hopkins, Donald R., *Princes and Peasants: Smallpox in History* (Chicago: University of Chicago Press, 1983).

Hornby, Ove, 'Kolonierne i Vestindien', in *Danmarks historie – uden for Danmark,* ed. Svend Ellehøj and Kristof Glamann (Copenhagen: Politiken, 1980).

Hovey, Sylvester, *Letters from the West Indies: Relating Especially to the Danish Island of St. Croix and to the British Islands of Antigua, Barbados and Jamaica* (New York: Gould and Newman, 1838).

Hoxcer Jensen, Peter, et al., eds., *Dansk kolonihistorie. Indføring og studier* (Aarhus: Forlaget Historia, 1983).

Hoxcer Jensen, Peter, *From Serfdom to Fireburn and Strike: The History of Black Labour in the Danish West Indies, 1848–1916,* ed. Arnold R. Highfield (St Croix: Antilles Press, 1998).

Huss-Ashmore, Rebecca, 'The Caribbean Slave: A Biological History', *The American Anthropologist* 88 (1986), 998.

Hutson, J. Edward, ed., *On the Treatment and Management of the More Common West-Indian Diseases, 1750–1802* (Jamaica: University of the West Indies Press, 2005).

Isert, Paul Erdmann, *Reise nach Guinea und den Caribäischen Inseln in Columbien, in Briefen an seine Freunde beschrieben* (Copenhagen, 1788).

Jacobi, Keith P., Della Collins Cook, Robert S. Corruccini and Jerome S. Handler, 'Congenital Syphilis in the Past: Slaves at Newton Plantation, Barbados, West Indies', *American Journal of Physical Anthropology* 89 (1992), 145–58.

Jensen, Niklas Thode, 'En verden til forskel? Undersøgelser af lægerne og sundhedsvæsenet i Dansk Vestindien mellem 1755 og 1830', *Bibliotek for Læger* 194.4 (2002).

Jensen, Niklas Thode, *En verden til forskel? Undersøgelser af sundhedsvæsenet og lægerne i Dansk Vestindien, 1755–1830*. Unpublished MA thesis, University of Copenhagen, Department of History, 2002.

Jensen, Niklas Thode, 'Sundhed, citroner og slaver', *1066 – Tidsskrift for Historie* 33.1 (2003), 3–11.

Johansen, Hans Christian, 'Slave Demography of the Danish West Indian Islands', *The Scandinavian Economic History Review* 29 (1981), 1–20.

Johnsen, Palle, 'Snylteorme i Mennesket', *Natur og Museum* 22.4 (1983), 1–31.

Jones, Donald G., *Archaeological Survey of Estate Whim Plantation Museum, St. Croix, US Virgin Islands* (Boston: Boston University Office of Public Archaeology, 1990).

Jones, E.L., 'The Caribbean Slave: A Biological History', *The Economic History Review* 39.2 (1986), 323–24.

Jones, Trandailer, *Impressions of Nutrition Habits in the Virgin Islands* Bulletin 2 (US Virgin Islands: Virgin Islands Department of Health, Nutrition Division, 1952), 17.

Kessler, Ben, *Priceless Heritage: History and Lore of Estate St. George, Home of the St. George Village Botanical Garden of St. Croix, US Virgin Islands* (Frederiksted, 1980).

Keutsch, F., 'Medicinalbericht des constituierten Landphysicus zu St. Croix, Dr. Med. F. Keutsch, über da Westindische gelbe Fieber und andere Gegenstände des dortigen Medicinnalwesens', *Nordisches Archiv für Naturkunde, Arzneywissenschaft und Chirurgie* IV, 2.11 (Leipzig, 1805), 80–103.

Khoudabux, Mohamed Rakieb, *Effects of Life Conditions on the Health of a Negro Slave Community in Suriname*, Doctoral dissertation, University of Leiden, 1991.

Kiple, Kenneth F., *The Caribbean Slave: A Biological History* (Cambridge: Cambridge University Press, 1984).

Kiple, Kenneth F., ed., *The Cambridge World History of Human Disease* (Cambridge: Cambridge University Press, 1993).

Kleinman, Arthur, *Patients and Healers in the Context of Culture: An Exploration of the Borderland between Anthropology, Medicine and Psychiatry* (London: University of California Press, 1980).

Kuby, Ronald L., *Folk Medicine on St. Croix: An Ethnobotanical Study*, unpublished dissertation, Department of Anthropology, University of Kansas, 1979.

Lambert, M.I., E.J. Cheevers and Y. Coopoo, 'Relationship between Energy Expenditure and Productivity of Sugar Cane Cutters and Stackers', *Occupational Medicine* 44 (1994), 190–94.

Larsen, Jens, *Virgin Islands Story* (Philadelphia: Muhlenberg Press, 1950).

Larsen, Kay, *Guvernører, Residenter, Kommandanter og Chefer samt enkelte andre fremtrædende Personer i de tidligere danske Tropekolonier* (Copenhagen: Arthur Jensens Forlag, 1940).

Lawaetz, Erik J., *St. Croix 500 years: Pre-Columbus to 1990* (Copenhagen: Poul Kristensens Forlag, 1990).

Lawaetz, Eva, *A Report from Governor General P. L. Oxholm to The Royal Westindian Chamber in Copenhagen dated May 4, 1816. St. Croix*, trans. and ed. Eva Lawaetz (Christiansted, 1977).

Leti, Geneviève, *Santé et société esclavagiste à la Martinique, 1802–1848* (Paris: L'Harmatan, 1998).

Lewisohn, Florence, *St. Croix under Seven Flags* (Hollywood, FL: The Dukane Press, 1970).

Lindskog, Bengt I., *Medicinsk Ordbog* (Copenhagen: Gyldendalske Boghandel, Nordisk Forlag, 2004).

Loudon, Irvine, *Death in Childbirth: An International Study of Maternal Care and Maternal Mortality, 1800–1950* (Oxford: Clarendon Press, 1992).

Lund, Jørn, ed., *Den Store Danske Encyklopædi* (Copenhagen: Nordisk Forlag, 1998).

Løkke, Anne, 'The "Antiseptic" Transformation of Danish Midwives, 1860–1920', in *Midwives, Society and Childbirth: Debates and Controversies in the Modern Period*, ed. Hilary Marland and Anne Marie Raffery (London: Routledge, 1997), 102–33.

Løkke, Anne, *Døden i Barndommen. Spædbørnsdødelighed og moderniserings-processer i Danmark 1800 til 1920* (Copenhagen: Gyldendal, 1998).

Løkke, Anne, 'Did Midwives Matter? 1787–1845', in *Pathways of the Past: Essays in Honour of Sølvi Sogner*, ed. Hilde Sandvik, Kari Telste and Gunnar Thorvaldsen (Oslo: Novus Forlag, 2002), 59–72.

Marshall, Woodville K., 'Provision Ground and Plantation Labor in Four Windward Islands: Competition for Resources during Slavery', in *Cultivation and Culture*, ed. Ira Berlin and Phillip D. Morgan (Charlottesville: University Press of Virginia, 1993), 203–20.

McKee, Larry, 'Food Supply and Plantation Social Order: An Archaeological Perspective', in *I, Too, Am America: Archaeological Studies of African-American Life*, ed. Theresa A. Singleton (Charlottesville: University of Virginia, 1999), 218–39.

Menier, Marie-Antoinette, 'Hommes sages contre sages-femmes à la Guadeloupe (1829–1842)', *Bulletin de la Societe d'Historie de la Guadeloupe* 87–90 (1991), 3–31.

Miller, Joseph C., 'Historical Approaches to Slavery: Bibliography of Slavery', in Paul Finkelmann and Joseph C. Miller, *Macmillan Encyclopedia of World Slavery* I (New York: Macmillan Reference, 1998), 393–96.

Millspaugh, Charles Frederick, *Flora of the Islands of St. Croix* (Chicago: Field Columbian Museum, 1902).

Mintz, Sidney W. and Douglas Hall, *The Origins of the Jamaican Internal Marketing System* (New Haven: Yale University Press, 1960).

Mintz, Sidney W. and Richard Price, *The Birth of African-American Culture: An Anthropological Perspective* (Boston: Beacon Press, 1992 [1976]).

Mortensen, Theodor, *Om Fiskerierne paa vore vestindiske Øer* (Copenhagen, 1907), special edition of *Atlanten* 43–44.

Morton, Henry, *St. Croix, St. Thomas, St. John. Danish West Indian sketchbook and diary – Skitsebog og dagbog fra Dansk Vestindien, 1843–44* (Copenhagen: Dansk Vestindisk Selskab and St. Croix Landmarks Society, 1975).

Multer, H. Gray and Lee C. Gerhard, eds., *Guidebook to the Geology and Ecology of Some Marine and Terrestrial Environments, St. Croix, US Virgin Islands* (US Virgin Islands: West Indies Laboratory, Fairleigh Dickinson University, 1974), special publications no. 5.

Murphy, Patricia, *The Moravian Mission to the African Slaves of the Danish West Indies, 1732–1828* (St. Thomas: Caribbean Research Institute of the College of the Virgin Islands, 1969).

Nissen, Johan Peter, *Reminiscences of a 46 years' residence in the island of St. Thomas in the West Indies* (Nazareth, Pennsylvania: Senseman and Co. 1838).

Nutton, Vivian, 'Humoralism', in *Companion Encyclopedia of the History of Medicine* I, ed. W.F. Bynum and Roy Porter (London: Routledge, 1993), 281–91.

Nyland, Nick, *De praktiserende læger i Danmark, 1800–1910. Træk af det historiske grundlag for almen medicin* (Odense: University of Southern Denmark, 2000).

Oakes, A.J., *Poisonous and Injurious Plants of the US Virgin Islands* (Washington, D.C.: United States Department of Agriculture, Agricultural Research Service, 1962).

Oldendorp, Christian Georg Andreas, *Historie der caribischen Inseln Sanct Thomas, Sanct Crux und Sanct Jan, insbesondere der dasigen Neger und der Mission der evangelischen Brüder unter denselben* (Berlin: VWB, Verlag für Wissenschaft und Bildung, 2000 [First published Barby 1777]).

Olsen, Poul Erik, 'Danske Lov på de vestindiske øer', in *Danske og Norske Lov i 300 år*, ed. Ditlev Tamm (Copenhagen: Jurist- og Økonomforbundets Forlag, 1983), 289–321.

Olsen, Poul Erik, 'De dansk-vestindiske øer og junigrundloven', *Historie* 18.1 (1989), 1–28.

Olsen, Poul Erik, 'Fra ejendomsret til menneskeret', in *Fra slaveri til frihed. Det dansk-vestindiske slavesamfund 1672–1848*, ed. Per Nielsen (Copenhagen: Nationalmuseet, 2001), 25–52.

Olwig, Karen Fog, *Cultural Adaptation and Resistance on St. John: Three Centuries of Afro-Caribbean Life* (Gainesville: The University Presses of Florida, 1985).

Olwig, Karen Fog, 'Narrating Deglobalization: Danish Perceptions of a Lost Empire', in *Global Networks* 3.3 (2003), 207–22.

Oxholm, Peter Lotharius, *De danske Vestindiske Øers Tilstand i henseende til Population, Cultur, Finance-Forfatning i Anledning af nogle Breve fra St. Croix, indrykkede i det Politiske og Physiske Magazin for Marts og April Maaneder 1797, hvortil er føiet Beskrivelse om Sukkerets Fabrikation, med 4 Planer* (Copenhagen, 1797).

Oxholm, Peter Lotharius, *Nogle Anmærkninger over en Afhandling om Negerhandelens Ophævelse udi Maanedskriftet Minerva af Febr. 1805* (Copenhagen, 1806).

Palmié, Stephan, ed., *Slave Cultures and the Cultures of Slavery* (Knoxville: The University of Tennessee Press, 1995).

Patterson, K. David, 'The Caribbean Slave: A Biological History', *Isis* 77.2 (1986), 364–65.

Patterson, Orlando, *The Sociology of Slavery* (London: MacGibbon and Kee, 1967).

Petersen, Bernhard v., *En historisk Beretning om de dansk-vestindiske Øer, St. Croix, St. Thomas og St. Jan* (Copenhagen, 1855).

Petersen, Christian Poulsen Nørbom, *Den Danske Medicinal-Lovgivning eller Samling af de Forordninger, Placater, Kongelige Rescripter og Resolutioner, Reglementer og Instruxer, Fundatser, Collegialbreve og andre offentlige Aktstykker, som vedkomme Læger, Apothekere og Gjordemødre i Danmark* (Copenhagen, 1834).

Pluchon, Pierre, ed., *Histoire des Antilles et de la Guyane* (Toulouse: Edouard Privat, 1982).

Poulsen, Bo, *Konsekvenserne af Agger Tanges gennembrud i 1825 for fiskeriet i Limfjorden – en miljøhistorisk tolkning*, unpublished MA thesis, University of Southern Denmark, 2002.

Porter, Roy, *Ve og Vel – Medicinens historie fra oldtid til nutid* (Copenhagen: Rosinante, 2000).

Rhodes, Philip, *A Short History of Clinical Midwifery: The Development of Ideas in the Professional Management of Childbirth* (Cheshire: Books for Midwives Press, 1995).

Rigau-Perez, Jose G., 'The Introduction of Smallpox Vaccine in 1803 and the Adoption of Immunization as a Government Function in Puerto Rico', *The Hispanic American Historical Review* 69 (1989), 393–423.

Rouse-Jones, Margaret D., 'Historiography of the Leeward Islands and the Virgin Islands', in *General History of the Caribbean: Methodology and Historiography of the Caribbean* VI, ed. B.W. Higman (London: UNESCO Publishing, 1999), 531–43.

Savitt, Todd L., *Medicine and Slavery: The Diseases and Health Care of Blacks in Antebellum Virginia* (Urbana: University of Illinois Press, 1978).

Scarano, Francisco A., 'Slavery and Emancipation in Caribbean History', in *General History of the Caribbean: Methodology and Historiography of the Caribbean* VI, ed. B.W. Higman (London: UNESCO publishing, 1999), 233–82.

Schlegel, Poul, 'Beskrivelse af en Sectio Cæsarea foretaget paa negerinden Sophia paa St. Croix i Christiansstæds Bye d. 6te Febr. 1821', *Bibliothek for Læger* 3 (1823), 140–49.

Schmidt, Johan Christian, *Various Remarks Collected on and about the Island of St. Croix in America* (US Virgin Islands: The Virgin Islands Humanities Council, 1998 [First published in Copenhagen, 1788]).

Schoelcher, Victor, *Colonies Étrangères et Haiti* (Paris, 1843).

Schou, Jacob Henrie, *Chronologisk Register over de Kongelige Forordninger og Aabne Breve, samt andre trykte Anordninger, som fra Aar 1670 af ere udkomne, tilligemed et nøiagtigt Udtog af de endnu gieldende, for saavidt samme i Almindelighed angaae Undersaatterne i Danmark og Norge, forsynet med et alphabetisk Register* (Copenhagen, 1823).

Sebro, Louise, *Mellem afrikaner og kreol. Etnisk identitet og social navigation i Dansk Vestindien, 1730–1770,* University of Lund, Sweden, 2009.

Semba, Richard D. and Martin W. Bloem, *Nutrition and Health in Developing Countries* (New Jersey: Humana Press, 2001).

Sheridan, Richard, *Sugar and Slavery: An Economic History of the British West Indies, 1623–1775* (Barbados: Caribbean University Press, 1974).

Sheridan, Richard, *Doctors and Slaves: A Medical and Demographic History of Slavery in the British West Indies, 1680–1834* (Cambridge: Cambridge University Press, 1985).

Sheridan, Richard, 'The Caribbean Slave: A Biological History', *The Hispanic American Historical Review* 66.3 (1986), 584–85.

Sichler, Judith A., *Historic Period Foodways in the Danish West Indies (1718–1917): The Zooarchaeological Evidence from Cinnamon Bay and the East End, St. John, US Virgin Islands,* Ph.D. dissertation, University of Tennessee, 2003.

Simonsen, Gunvor, *En fortræffelig Constitution – om konstruktion af social orden på de Dansk Vestindiske øer i sidste halvdel af 1700-tallet,* unpublished MA thesis, Roskilde University, 2000.

Simonsen, Gunvor, 'Nye og gamle perspektiver på dansk kolonihistorie', *1066 – Tidsskrift for Historie* 33.2 (2003), 3–13.

Simonsen, Gunvor, *Slave Stories: Gender, Representation, and the Court in the Danish West Indies, 1780s–1820s,* unpublished Ph.D. dissertation, European University Institute, Department of History and Civilisation, Florence, 2007.

Smith, James, *Winter of 1840 in St. Croix with an Excursion to Tortola and St. Thomas* (New York, 1840).

Spingarn, Lawrence, 'Slavery in the Danish West Indies', *The American-Scandinavian Review* 45 (1957), 35–43.

Steensgaard, Louise, *På sporet af den 'Vestindiske Philosophie': en undersøgelse af kreoliseringen af eurocaribierne i Dansk Vestindien i det 18. Århundrede*, unpublished MA thesis, University of Copenhagen, 2002.

Stifoss-Hansen, Hans and Kjell Kallenberg, *Livssyn, sundhed og sygdom. Teoretiske og kliniske perspektiver* (Copenhagen: Hans Reitzels Forlag, 1999).

Stipriaan, Alex van, *Surinaams Contrast, Roofbouw en overleven in een Caraïbische plantagekolonie, 1750–1863* (Leiden: Koninklijk Instituut voor taal-, land- en volkenkunde, 1993).

Sveistrup, P.P., *Bidrag til de tidligere dansk-vestindiske Øers økonomiske Historie. Med særligt Henblik på Sukkerproduktion og Sukkerhandel* (Copenhagen: Institut for Historie og Samfundsøkonomi, 1942).

Svensson, Susanne Ahlmann and Signe Thylstrup, *Slaveriet i Dansk Vestindien – Ideal eller virkelighed? Den komplekse legitimering af slaveriet i Dansk Vestindien*, unpublished MA thesis, Department of History and Society, Roskilde University, 1997.

Tadman, Michael, 'The Demographic Cost of Sugar: Debate on Slave Societies and Natural Increase in the Americas', *The American Historical Review*, 105.5 (2000), 1534–75.

Taffin, Dominique, *Maladies et medicine á la Guadeloupe au XIXe siècle*, unpublished dissertation, Ecole nationale des Chartes, Paris, 1985.

'Tal og tider i køkkenet', *Ren Besked* 6 (2001).

Tannenbaum, Frank, *Slave and Citizen: The Negro in the Americas* (New York: Vintage Books, 1946).

The St. Croix Gazette, 1808–1813.

Thomas, Toni, *Traditional Medical Plants of St. Croix, St. Thomas and St. John. A Selection of 68 Plants* (St. Croix: University of the Virgin Islands Cooperative Extension Service, 1997).

Tomich, Dale W., 'Slavery in Martinique in the French Caribbean', in *Caribbean Slavery in the Atlantic World: A Student Reader*, ed. Verene Shepherd and Hilary McD. Beckles (Jamaica: Ian Randle Publishers, 2000), 413–36.

Tomich, Dale W., 'The Other Face of Slave Labour: Provision Grounds and Internal Marketing in Martinique', in *Caribbean Slavery in the Atlantic World: A Student Reader*, ed. Verene Shepherd and Hilary McD. Beckles (Jamaica: Ian Randle Publishers, 2000), 743–57.

Tuckerman, Joseph, *Letter Respecting Santa Cruz as a Winter Residence for Invalids* (Boston, 1837).

Turner, Mary, 'Slave Workers, Subsistence and Labour Bargaining: Amity Hall, Jamaica, 1805–1832', *Slavery and Abolition* 12.1 (1991), 92–106.

Tyson, George F. and Arnold R. Highfield, eds., *The Kamina Folk: Slavery and Slave Life in the Danish West Indies* (US Virgin Islands: Virgin Islands Humanities Council, 1994).

Vapereau, Gustave, *Dictionnaire universel des literatures* (Paris: Hachette, 1876).

Vibæk, Jens, 'Dansk Vestindien, 1755–1848. Vestindiens storhedstid', in *Vore gamle tropekolonier* II, ed. Johannes Brøndsted (Copenhagen: Forlaget Fremad, 1966).

Waterston, W., *A Manual of Commerce* (Edinburgh: Oliver and Boyd, 1855).

Watters, David R., 'Mortuary Patterns at the Harney Site Slave Cemetery, Montserrat, in Caribbean Perspective', *Historical Archaeology* 28.3 (1994), 56–73.

Weaver, Karol Kovalovich, *Disease in the Torrid Zone: Malady and Medicine in Eighteenth-Century Saint Domingue*, Ph.D. dissertation, Pennsylvania State University, 1999, 429–460.

Weaver, Karol Kovalovich, 'The Enslaved Healers of Eighteenth-Century Saint Domingue', *Bulletin of the History of Medicine* 76 (2002).

Weed, Thurlow, *Letters From Europe and the West Indies, 1843–1852* (Albany, 1866).

West, Hans, *Beskrivelse over St. Croix med en kort Udsigt over St. Thomas, St. Jean, Tortola, Spanishtown og Crabeneiland* (Copenhagen, 1793).

Westergaard, Waldemar, *The Danish West Indies under Company Rule* (New York, 1917).

Wetherbee, David Kenneth, *An Instant Survey of St. Croix, V.I., Natural History* (Boston, 1984).

Williamson, John, *Medical and Miscellaneous Observations Relative to the West India Islands* II (Edinburgh, 1817).

Zupko, Ronald Edward, *A Dictionary of Weights and Measures for the British Isles: The Middle Ages to the Twentieth Century* (Philadelphia: American Philosophical Society, 1985).

Online Sources

Arrowsmith, John, *Map of The Leeward Islands* (London, 1844), David Rumsey Historical Map Collection, www.davidrumsey.com (accessed 30-05-2011).

Asiedu, R., H. Mignouna, B. Odu and J.d'A. Hughes, 'Yam Breeding', in *Plant Virology in Sub-Saharan Africa: Proceedings of a Conference Organized by IITA*, ed. Jacqueline d'A Hughes and Babajide O. Odu (Ibadan: International Institute of Tropical Agriculture, 2001), 467, http://old.iita.org/cms/details/virology/pdf_files/466-475.pdf (accessed 30-05-2011).

Cappelen, John and Jens Juncher Jensen, *Jordens Klima – Guide til vejr og klima i 156 lande* (Copenhagen: Danmarks Meteorologiske Institut, 2001), www.dmi.dk/dmi/tr01-17.pdf (accessed 30-05-2011).

Davis, John R., *Soil Survey of the United States Virgin Islands* (Washington D.C: United States Department of Agriculture, Natural Resources Conservation Service in Cooperation with the Virgin Islands Department of Planning and Natural Resources, the Virgin Islands Cooperative Extension Service, and the United States Department of Interior, National Park Service. United States Dept. of Agriculture, Natural Resources Conservation Service, 2002), 12–13, www.m015.nrcs.usda.gov/technical/surveys/caribbean/VI.pdf (accessed 30-05-2011).

Hopkins, Daniel, et al., *Sketch of St. Croix showing quarters*, http://cas.umkc.edu/StCroix/ (accessed 30-05-2011).

Human energy requirements (Rome: FAO, 2004), chapter 5: Energy Requirements of Adults. The figures are taken from table 5.4, 5.5, 5.7 and 5.8, www.fao.org/docrep/007/y5686e/y5686e00.htm#Contents (accessed 30-05-2011).

Latham, Michael C., *Human nutrition in the developing world* (Rome: FAO, 1997), chapter 5, www.fao.org/DOCREP/W0073e/w0073e00.htm#TopOfPage (accessed 30-05-2011).

Lupien, J.R., et al., 'Edible Fats and Oils', *Food, Nutrition and Agriculture* 11 (1994), www.fao.org/docrep/T4660T/T4660T00.htm (accessed 30-05-2011).

Lymphatic filariasis. Fact sheet no. 102. WHO Media Centre, September 2000, www.who.int/mediacentre/factsheets/fs102/en/ (accessed 30-05-2011).

Olcott, Perry G., *Ground Water Atlas of the United States. Alaska, Hawaii, Puerto Rico and the U. S. Virgin Islands* (Virginia: U.S. Geological Survey, Cartography and Publishing Program, 1985), HA 730-N, http://capp.water.usgs.gov/gwa/ch_n/N-PR_VItext5.html (accessed 30-05-2011).

Realizing the Promise and Potential of African Agriculture (Amsterdam: InterAcademy Council, 2004), 80, www.interacademycouncil.net/CMS/Reports/AfricanAgriculture.aspx (accessed 30-05-2011).

Roots, tubers, plantains and bananas in human nutrition (Rome: FAO, 1990), table 9.2, www.fao.org/docrep/T0207E/T0207E00.htm (accessed 30-05-2011).

www.sizes.com (accessed 30-05-2011).

The Oxford English Dictionary (OED Online, Oxford University Press, 2000), www.oed.com/ (accessed 30-05-2011).

USDA *National Nutrient Database*, www.nal.usda.gov/fnic/foodcomp/search/ (accessed 30-05-2011).

Virgin Islands Social History Associates, *St Croix African Roots Project*, http://stx.visharoots.org/scarp.html (accessed 30-05-2011).

Work-Rest and Water Consumption Tables (Maryland: US Army Center for Health Promotion and Preventive Medicine, 2004), table A-3, A-5, http://safety.ucanr.org/files/2901.pdf (accessed 30-05-2011).

Index

Page numbers in italic type refer either to figures or illustrations